Immunological Aspects of
Reproduction and Fertility Control

Immunological Aspects of Reproduction and Fertility Control

EDITED BY

J. P. HEARN

Director
The Wellcome Laboratories of Comparative Physiology
The Zoological Society of London

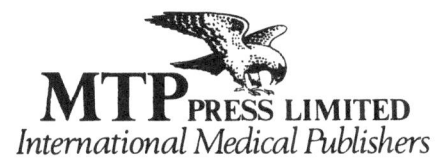

MTPPRESS LIMITED
International Medical Publishers

Published by
MTP Press Limited
Falcon House
Lancaster, England

British Library Cataloguing in Publication Data
Immunological aspects of reproduction and fer-
    tility control.
    1. Human reproduction—Immunological
    aspects
    2. Contraception, Immunological
    I. Title   II. Hearn, John P.
    612.6   QP251

ISBN 978-94-011-8041-2   ISBN 978-94-011-8039-9 (eBook)
DOI 10.1007/978-94-011-8039-9

Mather Bros (Printers) Limited, Preston

Contents

List of contributors   vii

Preface   ix

Section I
IMMUNOLOGICAL ASPECTS OF REPRODUCTION

1. Immunological relationships between mother and fetus during
   pregnancy M. Kaye   3

2. Immunological relationships between mother and conceptus
   in man D. W. Cooper   33

3. Immunological diagnosis of early pregnancy J. K. Findlay   63

4. Immunological aspects of eclampsia and pre-eclampsia
   C. W. G. Redman   83

5. Immunological factors in male and female infertility
   W. R. Jones   105

Section II
IMMUNOLOGICAL ASPECTS OF FERTILITY CONTROL

6. Inhibition of reproductive function by antibodies to
   luteinizing hormone releasing hormone H. M. Fraser   143

7. Immunization against zona pellucida antigens R. J. Aitken and
   D. W. Richardson   173

8. The current status of anti-pregnancy vaccines based on
   synthetic fractions of HCG V. C. Stevens   203

9. Vaccines based upon the Beta-subunit of HCG G. P. Talwar   217

10. The immunobiology of chorionic gonadotrophin J. P. Hearn   229

Index   245

List of Contributors

R. J. Aitken
MRC Reproductive Biology Unit,
Edinburgh EH3 9EW, UK

D. W. Cooper
School of Biological Sciences,
Macquarie University,
North Ryde,
NSW 2113, Australia

J. K. Findlay
Medical Research Centre,
Prince Henry's Hospital,
Melbourne 3004, Australia

H. M. Fraser
MRC Reproductive Biology Unit,
Edinburgh EH3 9EW, UK

J. P. Hearn
The Wellcome Laboratories of
    Comparative Physiology,
The Zoological Society of London,
London NW1 4RY, UK

W. R. Jones
Department of Obstetrics and Gynaecology,
Flinders Medical Centre,
Bedford Park 5042, South Australia

M. Kaye
Department of Obstetrics and Gynaecology,
Flinders Medical Centre,
Bedford Park 5042, South Australia

C. W. G. Redman
Nuffield Department of Obstetrics,
John Radcliffe Hospital,
Oxford OX3 9DU, UK

D. W. Richardson
MRC Reproductive Biology Unit,
Edinburgh EH3 9EW, UK

V. C. Stevens
Division of Reproductive Biology,
Department of Obstetrics and Gynecology,
Ohio State University,
Columbus, Ohio 43210, USA

G. P. Talwar
Department of Biochemistry,
All India Institute of Biomedical Research,
New Delhi-10016, India

Preface

The no-man's-land between reproductive physiology and immunology is becoming crowded. The last 10 years have seen a revolution in our understanding of many reproductive processes, brought about by the application of ever more sophisticated immunological methods. The increasing precision of these techniques has given us specific ways of assaying, enhancing or blocking hormonal mechanisms to yield more critical and interpretable information.

In this volume eleven authors have presented the current status and future prospects of some immunological aspects of reproduction and fertility control. These include the relationships between mother and fetus, the diagnosis of pregnancy, the immunological complications seen in clinical management of human reproduction and some novel approaches for immunological control of fertility.

We hope that in these chapters we have achieved an up-to-date account of a fast-moving field that calls on several disciplines. We intend the book to provide an adequate background and a current review for research workers and clinicians who wish both to understand the complex mechanisms involved and to develop improved scientific and clinical methods. We hope too that the student and newcomer will find this a useful reference book.

As editor I have tried to leave each chapter able to stand on its own, risking slight overlap in one or two places where the same topic has been approached from different angles. My thanks in full measure are due to the authors for their hard work and promptness, to Annabel Gomm and Connie Nutkins for their help with organization and to the publishers; particularly Harry Bracken, for their unfailing encouragement and support.

John Hearn
London, April 1980

Section I
Immunological Aspects of Reproduction

1
Immunological Relationships between Mother and Fetus during Pregnancy

M. KAYE

THE PHYLOGENY OF PLACENTATION

Placentation is defined as 'any intimate apposition or fusion of the fetal organs to the maternal or paternal tissues for physiological exchange'[1]. It is widespread amongst the invertebrates and vertebrates, having arisen independently in those phyla which exhibit viviparity, and has probably evolved each time from external fertilization to internal fertilization and oviparity, through ovoviviparity to viviparity.

The transition from oviparity to viviparity has involved considerably greater change in the reproductive functions of the female than the male. The trend of viviparity has been to optimize the potential of each individual egg, with a reduction in the number of eggs released. The yolk sac has been utilized for the absorption of nutrients from the uterus in vertebrates and the genital ducts have become modified to retain the embryo to an advanced stage. The synchronization of egg release with intromission and subsequent preparation of the genital tract for reception of the zygote has led to a refinement in endocrine control to synchronize mating, fertilization, pregnancy, parturition and, in the mammals, lactation. Such orchestration probably began in the specialization of a neural gland which by its proximity to the central ganglia would be in close contact with the environment through specialized sensory organs. In the phylum Chordata such a primitive pituitary gland exists in the Tunicata (sessile sea-squirts) which co-ordinates reproductive activity by

3

perceiving the sex products (pheromones) of other individuals in the water nearby[2].

In vertebrates, the reproductive functions of the maternal pituitary, ovary and corpus luteum have been extended not by the production of new hormones, but by the uses to which they are put[3]. In the mammals, 'maternal recognition' of pregnancy results in a dialogue between blastocyst and uterine epithelium, either directly or mediated via the corpus luteum. The mammalian feto-placental unit has come to intrude into the maternal endocrine environment to the point where it controls its own destiny from early in gestation so that ablation of the maternal pituitary or ovaries has no effect on gestation following implantation[4].

Invertebrate placentation

Viviparity in the invertebrates is widely distributed, having arisen many times independently. A wide range of embryonic and maternal structures have been modified to assist embryonic nutrition. Viviparity occurs in the Platy-helmynthes, Nermertea, Annelida, Onychophora, Insecta, Arachnida and Tunicata, whilst placentation is best seen in the Dermaptera, Ascidiacea, Thaliacea and the neo-tropical Onychophora. In the insects, the pseudo-placental Dermaptera, *Hemimerus talpoides* (earwigs), a few large embryos are held in the reproductive tract for long periods relative to the maternal life span. The embryo develops within the follicle surrounded by a maternally derived tunica propria. The anterior (containing the corpus luteum) and posterior pseudoplacenta develop from the follicular cells surrounding the ovum; these two maternal structures later degenerate to be replaced by two fetal placentas derived from the amnion. The embryos at birth are large and well-developed, but the function of the corpus luteum, present throughout gestation, remains unknown[5].

Within the Tunicata, a compound ascidian displays many of the adaptations seen in the mammals. The ovary of these hermaphrodite sea-squirts produces a single small egg, devoid of yolk. The extra-embryonic membranes envelop the embryo and form an avascular placenta closely applied to the lining of the brood pouch which survives some 5 months and results in the birth of a large complex tadpole. The reproductive similarities between this lowly chordate and mammals demonstrates interesting parallels in functional adaptation[6]. Some species of the tunicate salpidae also develop an embryonal placenta which is intimately applied to the maternal surface and is similar to the placental attachment in the sea-squirt[7].

The neo-tropical Onychophora of Trinidad forms a placental closely analogous to the yolk sac placenta of mammals (Figures 1.1 and 1.2). The embryo remains attached to its placenta for several months before detaching from the well-developed fetal–maternal placental zone to lie free in the oviduct where nourishment of the embryo continues from oviduct fluids prior to birth[8].

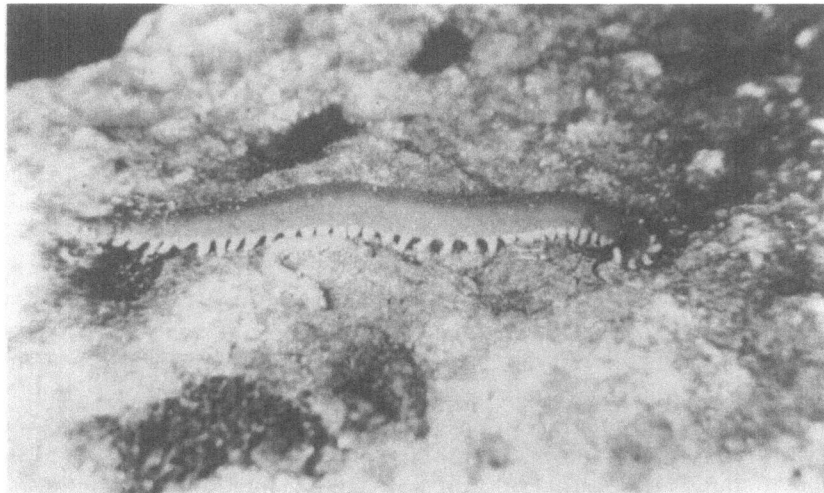

Figure 1.1 Mother and newborn *Epiperipatus* (65% of actual size). With kind permission of D. T. Anderson

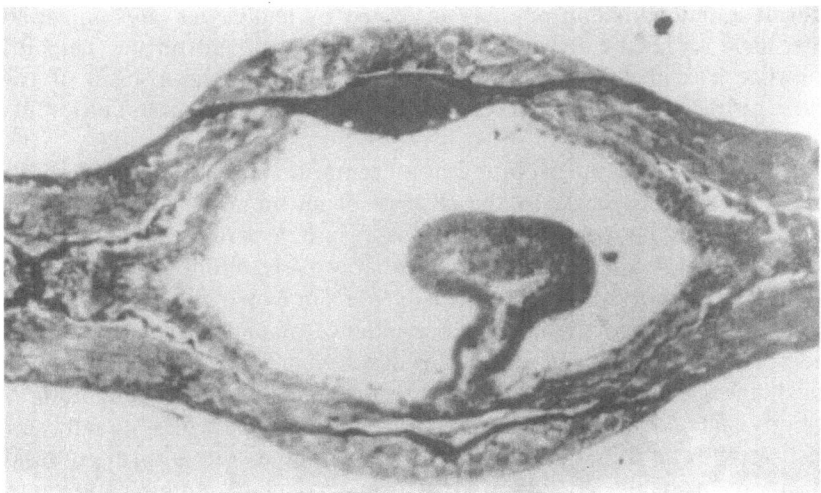

Figure 1.2 Longitudinal section through part of the oviduct of *E. trinidadensis* containing a stalked vesicle (× 130). With kind permission of D. T. Anderson

INVERTEBRATE IMMUNE RESPONSES

Although the protozoa display cell-surface macromolecules demonstrable in mating, alloincompatibility appears to be intracellular[9]. The metazoa, however, recognize differences at the cell surface and all invertebrates from

Porifera (sponges) onwards demonstrate extensive allogeneic polymorphism and discriminatory immunorecognition. The tropical sponges display an increasing rate of reaction to first-, second- and third-set grafts which is both discriminatory and displays a specific memory[10]. Among coelenterates, transplacentation reactions vary from non-fusion to acute cytotoxicity; the effector phase may be non-specific but recognition is specific. The corals display memory with first- and second-set reactions to grafting, and demonstrate extensive polymorphism of histocompatibility antigens. Transplantation reactions are mediated by leukocytes in the annelids, which show differing cell types for immunorecognition and cell-mediated cytotoxicity functions. The arthropod immunological status is somewhat ambiguous. Non-self recognition is apparent in the crustacean decapods, while insects which encapsulate xenografts may lack a subtlety in their leukocyte immunorecognition response. The hymenoptera, however, show no such lack of discrimination between isografts and allografts. Molluscan reactions are characterized by differentiation between isografts, allografts and xenografts but quantitative studies remain unknown. Memory in the form of first- and second-set reactions to allografts is apparent in the echinoderms, perhaps mediated by leukocytes. Amongst the chordates the solitary and colonial tunicates exhibit allograft reactions, again possibly mediated by leukocytes. Fusion experiments have revealed extensive histocompatibility polymorphism. Thus it is clear that a refined immunorecognition based on polymorphism of cell-surface histocompatibility markers has originated in the earliest multicellular sponges or coelenterates[11].

The importance of the evolution of placentation and immune response in the invertebrates is raised by the absence of an humoral immunoglobulin system[12, 13] which first appears in the most primitive vertebrate, the Agnatha or jawless fishes[14]. Since placentation probably evolved following the cellular immune response it follows that the change from oviparity to viviparity and placentation involved the embryo's avoidance of maternal immunorecognition. To suggest that placentation is dependent upon a specific immunological unresponsiveness of the mother mediated by an elegant humoral antibody system is irrelevant in the invertebrates, and perhaps equally so in vertebrates[15]. The ability of foreign fetal tissues and maternal tissues to reside in harmony probably depends on some form of cellular communication at the interface between the two organisms.

VERTEBRATE PLACENTATION

All the vertebrate classes exhibit placentation with the exception of aves. The placental attachment, as in invertebrates, represents an amazing diversity of adaptations of embryonal structures. The yolk sac placenta of the Chondrichthyes (cartilaginous fish) was first described by Aristotle *circa* 340 BC[16].

In the Poecilliidae of the teleosts (bony fish) placentation is the result of extensions of the hind gut or pericardial sac of the embryo to the ovarian follicle in which gestation occurs. Embryos removed from the ovarian follicle and separated from their fertilization membrane (a product of the maternally derived vitelline membrane) and transferred to the peritoneal cavity of adults were destroyed by day 14 as allografts. Embryos transplanted similarly, but within their fertilization membrane, survived, emphasizing the importance of the maternal egg membranes in protecting the 'foreign' embryo for a gestation period of 28 days[17]. In other groups of teleosts, the Jensynsii, the embryo develops in the ovarian cavity, and placentation results from a fold of ovarian tissue coming into contact with the gills of the embryo. Both maternal and fetal circulations are separated by a thin layer between ovarian and gill tissues.

The amphibians, like the fish, are mostly oviparous; however, some have adapted to terrestrial life by having the usually aquatic larval stage maintained in the maternal host. In *Salamandra atron* the embryos, having exhausted their yolk sac supply, cannibilize other embryos in the uterus and feed on the blood from uterine haemorrhages. In the Surinam toad, the externally fertilized eggs develop in skin pouches on the mother's back.

All the reproductive structures of mammals are found in the reptiles; the cleidoic egg and the extra-embryonic membranes (amnion, chorion and allantois) are present in the oviparous reptiles. The latter have been adapted to form either a vascularized yolk sac or allantoic placenta in the viviparous snakes and lizards. Perhaps an example of the advantages of placentation over oviparity in related groups of snakes and lizards is the changing ratio of oviparity to viviparity with a changing environment. From sea level to 4000 feet, oviparity is the major form of reproduction; above 4000 feet viviparity begins to predominate. Similarly, as one journeys west from the south-eastern coast of Australia to the inland plains, oviparity gives way to viviparity[18]. The role of progesterone produced by the corpus luteum of pregnancy in placental reptiles remains enigmatic[19]. For an extensive review of the evolution of placentation the reader is referred to references 4, 20 and 21.

The vertebrate egg is surrounded by a primary membrane (vitelline membrane) a product of the egg itself, and a secondary membrane (zona pellucida) secreted by the ovarian follicular cells. The tertiary membranes are products of the oviducts (mucoid coat) and uterus (shell membrane); it is well developed in monotromes but is ruptured in the last third of gestation in mammals and is absent in eutherians[22]. These egg membranes play important roles in sperm–egg recognition and may prevent recognition of the foreign zygote during its sojourn down the female genital tract.

The extra-embryonic membranes of the amniote egg, the yolk sac for nutrition and the allantois with its separate circulation for gaseous exchange and repository of embryonic excretory products, have been adapted in viviparous vertebrates to varying degrees as placental attachments. In the change from oviparity through ovoviviparity to viviparity, the yolk sac contents are reduced as the maternal–embryonic relationship becomes more intimate for the purposes of embryonic nutrition. The placental associations of the vascularized yolk sac and allantois with the non-vascular chorion (trophoblast) vary in their contribution to the definitive placenta, and their role in nutrition and gaseous exchange. In reptiles either the yolk sac or allantois takes part in nutrition and placentation[19], in marsupials the yolk sac usually forms the placenta, except in Peramelidae (bandicoots), where the allantois contributes[23].

In eutherians the yolk sac and allantois make varying contributions to the placenta. The yolk sac in the rabbit survives briefly; in the horse it survives to late gestation, and in the rat and squirrel it survives throughout gestation along with the allantoic placenta[4, 24]. The ability of some marsupials[25] and eutherian[4] chorioallantoic placenta to invade uterine tissues appears unique, while the loss of chorionic ectoderm in the allantoic placenta of viviparous lizards appears to be the result of degeneration[26]. The three forms of chorioallantoic placenta based on the differing nature of the fetal–maternal interface in reptiles[27], marsupials and eutherians has arisen independently in the three groups. The eutherian placenta may have evolved independently of the marsupial from a common oviparous ancestor some 150 million years ago[28], or from a common ancestor which was viviparous and nidiculous (young, helpless at birth and requiring extensive maternal care) with the marsupial having remained in the early state while the mammals evolved a longer gestation with a more mature embryo at birth[29].

VERTEBRATE IMMUNE RESPONSES

The evolution of the vertebrates has resulted in the continuing refinement of immune responses with the development of immunoglobulins and specialized lymphoid tissues. The thymus first appears as diffuse lymphoid tissue in the gill region of the Agnathan larval lamprey and is present in all other vertebrates. It develops early in ontogeny and provides the microenvironment for the bone-marrow lymphocytes to recognize self-antigens[30]. The secondary lymphoid organs, spleen and lymph nodes, develop later in ontogeny and unlike the thymus persist throughout adult life. The haemopoietic foci of the anterior gut of the Agnatha probably represents a primitive spleen which is present in all vertebrates. The lamina propria of the gut contain lymphocytes from the Agnatha to mammals whilst lymph nodes and lymphopoietic bone marrow emerge at the amphibian anuran level to become highly structured in the marsupials and eutherians. The source of immunoglobulin-producing B cells, which arise from the cloacal bursa of Fabricius of birds, has a possible equivalent in the fetal liver or Peyer's patches of mammals; no avian bursal equivalent has been found in other vertebrates despite the presence of B cells[31].

It is in the agnathan hagfish and lamprey that immunoglobulin-producing cells first appear with IgM synthesis; the Osteichtnyes (bony fish), amphibians and reptiles produce both IgM and IgG immunoglobulins whilst the eutherians synthesize some five classes (IgM, IgG, IgA, IgD and IgE)[13]. All vertebrates display transplantation reactions and memory, and possess lymphocytes which are the functional equivalents of thymic T cells and 'bursal' immunoglobulin-secreting B cells[31]. The process of collaboration which occurs between these cells is presaged in the annelids and results in an efficiency of immune reactions which is dependent upon shared haplotypes[32]. The perfection of this co-operation between helper and suppressor T cells, B cells and macrophages seen in the mammals may be seen to some degree in all the vertebrate classes with the exception of the Dipnoi (lungfish)[31].

The presence of IgG antigen receptors both on B cells and T cells has been described in the Chondrichthyes, teleosts, amphibians and eutherians[31]. There is, however, a difference in the manner in which mammalian T and B cells 'see' antigens. B cells 'see' the antigen with that part of the surface immunoglobulin known as the variable (V) region, whilst T cells 'see' the antigen only in association with the appropriate syngeneic major histocompatibility determinant[33].

Table 1.1 Phylogeny of the immune system

	Thymus	Spleen	Gut-associated lymploid tissue	Peripheral lymph nodes	Allograft rejection	Serum antibody class
Invertebrates	−	−	−	−	+	−
Vertebrates						
Agnatha	± (larval lamprey)	±	+	−	+	IgM
Chondrichthyes	+	+	+	−	+	IgM
Osteichthyes	+	+	+	−	+	IgM, IgG
Teleosts	+	+	+	−	+	IgM, IgG
Amphibians	+	+	+	+	+	IgM, IgG
Reptiles	+	+	+	+	+	IgM, IgG
Birds	+	+*	+	+	+	IgM, IgG, IgA
Mammals	+	+*	+	+	+	IgM, IgG, IgA, IgD, IgE

± Primitive
* Germinal centres

SPERMATOZOA AND UTERINE RESPONSES IN MAMMALS

The presence of the major histocompatibility antigens on mammalian spermatozoa[34] and the local immunological uterine responses following coitus in the rat[35] pose interesting questions for reproductive immunobiology. The ability of the rat uterus to respond to the intra-uterine inoculation of washed epididymal spermatozoa by hypertrophy of the draining para-aortic lymph nodes and transplantation immunity is in contrast to the inability of spermatozoa following coitus or pregnancy to elicit transplantation immunity despite similar hypertrophy of the para-aortic nodes. Pre-sensitization of one uterus by epididymal spermatozoa or leukocytes results in a 'local' reaction following rechallenge with the inoculum, but not when injected into the lumen of the non-sensitized contralateral uterine horn. The 'sensitized' uterus appears to gain enhanced reproductive performance over its non-sensitized homologue on an immunological basis[36].

The 'selection' of spermatozoa by the female mammalian genital tract results in only 5% of sperm reaching the oviduct. In rabbits there are two waves of sperm migration following coitus; the first is transferred within minutes to the peritoneal cavity prior to ovulation and these are non-motile. The second wave is held in the lower isthmus; these then migrate en masse to the ampulla following ovulation[37]. The probability that uterine 'selection' of spermatozoa may have an immunological basis is strengthened by the observation that sperm recovered from the uterus in the mouse and rabbit have antibodies attached, whilst those in the oviduct do not[38]. The inhospitable environment of the uterus to foreign spermatozoa may have resulted in the necessity for large numbers of sperm produced in animals. The previous suggestion that many spermatozoa are incapable of fertilization due to errors of chiasmata formation during spermatogenesis[39] has recently been refuted[40].

How spermatozoa survive long periods in the female genital tract of invertebrates or vertebrates remains unknown. The phenomenon is found in many of the vertebrates with storage occurring in any part of the genital tract from the cloaca to the ovary[41]. In the Chiroptera (bats) sperm storage may last for as long as 198 days before fertilization. The spermatozoa are occasionally found in the cells of the uterus but leukocytes have not been seen in the uterus despite the presence of the foreign spermatozoa[42].

FERTILIZATION

The evolution of species depends on reproductive isolating mechanisms to inhibit gene exchange and subsequent hybridization between populations. The prezygotic barriers are: (1) ecological or habitat isolation; (2) seasonal or temporal isolation; (3) ethological or sexual isolation; (4) mechanical isolation; and (5) gametic isolation[43]. It is (5) which, both in the past and the present, is important for the mutual recognition of male or female gametes released either into the air or the water, in those life forms exhibiting external fertilization, which prevents interspecific hybridization. This recognition at fertilization exists from seaweeds[44] to animals whose fertilization either is external or internal[45].

The unfertilized egg releases soluble products which have four varying effects on spermatozoa as they approach:

(1) Increased sperm motility.

(2) Chemotaxis, which is incompletely species-specific and is present in coelenterates, urochordates and possibly other animals[46].

(3) Sperm agglutination, which in a variety of animal species occurs in the presence of fertilizin (egg supernatant glycoprotein); it is species-specific and thought to be the initiator of the sperm acrosome reaction. The occurrence of sperm agglutination by egg supernatant has been described in molluscs, annelids, echinoderms, chordates and plants[45].

(4) The sperm acrosome reaction; beneath the plasma membrane of the sperm lies the acrosome containing hydrolytic enzymes which when released are thought to aid in sperm entry through the egg envelopes[47], together with the slicing action of the sperm head due to tail movement[48].

Recognition in sea urchins is dependent upon a glycoprotein on the egg vitelline layer (analogous to the zona pellucida of mammals) to which the sperm attaches[49]; this species-specific interaction is probably a generalized phenomenon with the receptors in the mammalian egg residing on the zona pellucida. The recognition site in mammalian spermatozoa is the inner acrosomal membrane which is uncovered following the acrosomal reaction prior to fertilization. Fusion with the microvillous areas of the egg plasma membrane occurs in the post-acrosomal region of the mammalian spermatozoa, in contrast to invertebrates where fusion of the spermatozoa and egg plasma membrane takes place at the inner acrosomal membrane. In some mammals the reaction at the zona pellucida prevents the penetration of hererologous spermatozoa; however, zona-free eggs of the hamster may be penetrated by the spermatozoa of a number of mammalian species[48].

The entry of the spermatozoa into the egg of the sea urchin results in a depolarization of the egg surface membrane within 3 s and an immediate partial block to further sperm entry. Some 30 s later the cortical granules evacuate into the perivitteline space forming the fertilization membrane which carries away from the egg surface all other unsuccessful sperm, and prevents polyspermy. The fertilizing sperm, now immotile, is engulfed by the egg cytoplasm[50].

In mammals there may also be two blocks to polyspermy. In the rabbit egg there is a cortical vesicle reaction, but no zonal reaction, the egg plasma membrane surface receptors to spermatozoa are probably lost. Other mammals have a zona reaction following the cortical reaction with perhaps loss of sperm receptors from the zona[51]. It would not be idle speculation to wonder if this loss of receptors from the zona following fertilization is responsible for the ability of transferred eggs to survive in non-related recipients prior to the development of the trophoblast.

The recognition molecules which exist for successful species-specific mating reactions from the protozoa[52] through all of the metazoa may have played an important role in speciation. It is, however, in the metazoa that the recognition molecules responsible for transplantation reactions have come to reside on the cell surface, in contrast to the protozoa where they are intracellular[9]. It would not be unreasonable to propose that the recognition molecules initially used for mating and speciation have also become responsible for transplantation reactions[53, 54].

IMPLANTATION

In mammals the egg enclosed by the cumulus oophorus is directed by the ciliated cells of the fimbria through the abdominal ostium to the ampulla, where fertilization occurs. Following a variable delay, depending on the species, the zygote moves along the isthmus through the narrow lumen of the interstitial part of the uterus[55]. Movement of the egg along the fimbria depends on ciliary action, whilst through the isthmus it depends on muscular peristalsis[56]. Once in the uterus the zygotes attach in predictable geographic areas with respect to the mesometrium and become attached at regular intervals, the result probably of uterine factors[57].

During its sojourn down the oviduct the mouse egg induces those areas through which it has passed to undergo DNA synthesis[58]. Contact of the blastocyst with the uterine wall begins the process of decidualization in which the uterine stromal cells undergo rapid DNA, RNA, protein synthesis and mitosis[59]. In the mouse the decidual cells increase their DNA content[60] as do the trophoblast cells by endoreduplication[61]. The synchronization of blastocyst, uterine and corpus luteal development for successful implantation appears to depend on the production of a signal by the blastocyst prior to uterine attachment[62].

Following compaction, the cells of the morulae recognize their position; those inside form the future inner cell mass and those on the outside the trophoblast[63]; the latter are capable of phagocytosis of uterine cells at implantation. The trophoblast differentiates into mural trophoblast (primary giant cells) and polar trophoblast (definitive placenta) cells whose continued division depends on the proximity of the inner cell mass. As both the mural and polar trophoblast cells move away from the inner cell mass they cease dividing but continue their DNA synthesis[64].

During implantation in some mammals, a curious but perhaps important event analogous to fertilization occurs; that is, cell fusion. First described in the marsupial bandicoot in 1897[65] and confirmed by light[66] and electron microscopy[23], and noted in the marsupial native cat[67], rabbit[68, 69] and hamster[70]. Although cell fusion may only occur in some animals at implantation, of equal interest is the ability of trophoblast to incorporate labelled maternal nuclear material from ectopic sites in the mouse[71] and from the uterus of rats whose uterine cells were pre-labelled by [³H]thymidine prior to blastocyst transfer[72]. Trophoblast cells incorporate exogenous DNA following parenteral injection into pregnant mice[73] and decidual cells incorporate label from the nuclei of mouse blastocysts pre-labelled with [³H]thymidine prior to their transfer to recipients[74]. Similarly of interest are the reports of reverse transcriptase present in placental and uterine tissues of mammals[75]. Although these may be viral, recent evidence has suggested that 'the distinction between an endogenous type C or type B reverse transcriptase and a cellular reverse transcriptase may ultimately prove to be semantic'[76].

These observations may have important implications in the development of a 'barrier' between the fetal and maternal tissues for the following reasons:

(1) When the cells of different species hybridize *in vitro* and nuclear mixing occurs, the resultant hybrid egg undergoes a marked alteration in its cell surface antigens[77, 78].

(2) Mammalian cells can incorporate chromosomes from other species into their genome *in vitro* and both replicate and express the new information[79].

ANTIGENIC IMMATURITY OF THE CONCEPTUS

Pre-implantation

The idea of antigenic immaturity of the conceptus was proposed in 1924[80] and although there is ample evidence that the embryo possesses transplantation antigens[81] it is possible that the fertilized egg prior to implantation also expresses immunogens on the early trophoblast precursor cells but that following implantation they disappear[82].

For a short while following fertilization the mammalian egg may be rather similar to the frog in its use of maternal messenger RNA[63]. Paternal enzymes are delayed in their production in the early embryos of hybrid sea urchins[83], frogs[84], chick-quail hybrids[85] and hybrid trout[86]. By 30 h (two-cell stage) the mouse embryonic genome is active at the transcriptional level[87], as is the paternal genome by 57 h (eight-cell stage)[88], non H-2 immunogens[89] and the H-Y (male) antigen[90]. The immunogens on the trophoblast present at pre-implantation[91] in the mouse disappear following induction of implantation[82].

It has been suggested that the major histocompatibility antigens on mouse blastocysts prior to implantation[92] may be minor immunogens[93] while others have failed to demonstrate immunogens on the trophoblast[94, 95].

If, as the evidence suggests, the blastocyst is immunogenic prior to implantation, by what means then does the blastocyst avoid 'rejection' by the maternal immune system? Several hypotheses are possible: first the decidual cell reaction may result in a 'privileged' uterine environment (discussed later).

Secondly, the maternally derived zona pellucida may protect the developing blastocyst in the uterus of the sensitized mouse[96]. Zona intact mouse blastocysts cultured *in vitro* with sensitized serum or spleen cells developed normally in host kidneys whilst zona-free blastocysts failed to develop[97] and zona-free mouse eggs died *in vitro* in the presence of a blastocyst antiserum whilst zona intact eggs developed to blastocysts[98, 99]. The role of the zona has been refuted by the suggestion that mouse eggs, presumed to be zona-free, during experimental 'delay' in the uterus of sensitized recipients develop normally following induced implantation[100]. However, rat eggs similarly maintained in 'delayed' implantation did not lose their zona pellucida[101] and the eggs in Kirby's experiments may not have been zona-free. The phenomenon of delayed implantation found in many mammals, the macropod marsupials, armadillo, roe deer, badger, seal, mouse and rats, raises the question as to how the immunogenic blastocyst can survive such long periods in the uterus. In most of these animals the blastocyst remains in the ovarian-derived zona pellucida, but in the roe deer the zona is replaced by the trophoblast[102]. Thirdly, the blastocyst which at implantation in the rat[103], man[104] and mouse induces a maternal lymphocyte response which is phagocytosed by the developing trophoblast[105], effectively removing any sensitized lymphocytes from the maternal environment. Fourthly, the surface immunogens on mouse blastocysts held in 'delayed implantation' disappear following induced implantation[82].

ANATOMICAL SEPARATION OF THE FETUS FROM THE MOTHER

Post-implantation

The ability of both the pregnant mother and fetus to reject alien tissues has led to considerable interest in the trophoblast. This specialized tissue forms a continuous layer between fetus and mother[106, 107] with the singular exception of the marsupial bandicoot where the trophoblast fuses with the uterine epithelium and disappears in the last few days of gestation[23], the anatomical separation of the maternal and fetal circulations proposed in 1953[3] remains central to the ability of two foreign immunocompetent individuals to live in harmony for the period of gestation.

The ability of the trophoblast to avoid the maternal immune response resulted in two explanations in the last decade: the 'fibrinoid barrier', whereby fibrinoid covers the immunogenic trophoblast; and the failure of the trophoblast to express immunogens.

'Fibrinoid barrier' – the presence of a non-cellular barrier lying between maternal and fetal tissues in man[108] and mouse[109], led to transplantation studies on mouse eggs and ectoplacental cones in an attempt to confirm the immunogenicity of trophoblast[110]. The inability to find a continuous layer of 'fibrinoid' at the deciduo-trophoblastic interface in the mouse[111, 112] and rat[113] led other workers to conclude from similar transplantation studies of mouse eggs and ectoplacental cones that trophoblast was not immunogenic[114]. Interpretations of these transplantation studies are difficult due to the recent observations that ectoplacental cone trophoblast requires little proliferation to survive whilst the trophoblast of the early blastocyst requires the presence of the inner cell mass to divide and proliferate[64].

Damage to the inner cell mass at transplantation might effect subsequent trophoblastic growth rather than be the result of immune responses to the host. The suggested protective effect of fibrinoid in masking the surface immunogens of trophoblast by the ability of ectoplacental cones to sensitize recipient mice to skin allografts following culture *in vitro* with neuraminidase[115] was not substantiated[116]. Mouse ectoplacental cones cultured *in vitro* were not susceptible to sensitized lymphoid cells even following pre-incubation with neuraminidase. By contrast, embryonic fibroblasts and cells from the embryonic sac were destroyed by lysis[117].

Trophoblast non-antigenicity – the absence of immunogens on the maternal surface of the mammalian (mouse) trophoblast following implantation, in contrast with pre-implantation trophoblast – is substantial[118–120]. The evidence for trophoblast immunogenicity has been partly derived from the ability of antisera raised in rabbits to placental homogenates to cause abortions following injection into pregnant mice[121] and rats[122]. This evidence suffers from two lines of investigations. First, the fetal mesenchymal elements which express the major histocompatibility complex prior to[94] and following[81] implantation may be responsible for stimulating the rabbit immune system rather than trophoblast[123]. Secondly, mouse trophoblast may be expressing tissue-specific immunogens recognized by the rabbit in a cross-species situation[91] rather than species-specific alloantigens.

In vitro culture studies on mouse trophoblast are ambiguous and difficult to interpret due to inadequate growth conditions of the culture medium which may affect expression of cell-surface antigens. Haemagglutinating antibody studies demonstrate a lack of immunogenicity of trophoblast outgrowths in contrast with other embryonic tissues[124], and both pre- and post-implantation trophoblast fail to express the Ia antigens *in vitro*[120]. Similar studies of 8-day ectoplacental cone giant cells failed to demonstrate immunogens for several days in culture whilst trophoblast from pre-implanted blastocysts and day 16 placenta were immunogenic[125, 126]. The main body of experimental evidence, however, suggests that the trophoblast following implantation fails to express alloantigens. The very circumstantial evidence that the trophoblast of *Homo sapiens* is immunogenic during pregnancy has been reviewed elsewhere[53, 127].

The presence of xenoantigens on trophoblast has been suggested by the failure of mouse ectoplacental cones[128] and mouse blastocysts[129] to survive in pre-sensitized rats, and hybrid sheep/goat embryos show a decreased survival in the uterus of goats sensitized to ram donor allografts[130].

THE UTERUS AS AN IMMUNOLOGICALLY PRIVILEGED SITE

The non-pregnant uterus is not unique for transplantation reactions; parathyroid allografts are rejected normally from the uterus in the rat[131]. This was extended by the observation that intra-uterine inoculation of lymphoid cells produced subsequent transplantation immunity and enlargement of the para-aortic lymph nodes in rats, and the uterus rejected the allografts[36].

The pregnant uterus, however, differs in its immune reactions. Repeated heterospecific pregnancies do not sensitize the female mouse to paternal antigens[132] whereas skin allografts placed in the uterus of rats do sensitize the female recipient[133]. The importance of the pregnant uterus in protecting the developing blastocyst is exemplified by the elegant demonstration that blastocysts transferred to a rabbit, previously sensitized by allografts from both the male and female donor parents, developed normally and skin allografts from the newborn were rejected by the host mother as second-set grafts[134]. Kirby's group[110] first suggested that the uterus might be a 'privileged site' from the observation that blastocysts survived in the uterus of sensitized pseudo-pregnant mice but not following transplantation to the kidney. The suggestion was confirmed by the prolonged survival of skin allografts in the pregnant uterus of rats compared with non-pregnant rats[135, 136]. Skin allografts survived longer in the uterus than on the trunk in pregnant rats, but were promptly rejected from the pregnant uterus in pre-sensitized animals or following the adoptive transfer of sensitized lymphocytes during pregnancy[133].

It would appear that the decidual response protects the immunogenic egg during the interval when the zona pellucida is lost and the non-immunogenic trophoblast develops following implantation.

The uterine response appears to affect trophoblastic development as demonstrated by the invasion of ectoplacental cone trophoblast placed in the uterus of virgin mice[137]. Kirby felt that the absence of a decidual response allowed the trophoblastic invasion to proceed through the uterine myometrium. In species such as the pig, where the trophoblast is not invasive, blastocysts transplanted into the uterine wall produce an invasive syncitial trophoblast with no evidence of a decidual reaction[138]. Perhaps such eutherian trophoblast behaviour is not surprising when one recalls that embryos of the oviparous toad fish (*Opsanus tau*) invade the abdominal organs following intraperitoneal transfer to adult toad fish[139].

SPECIFIC SUPPRESSION OF MATERNAL RESPONSES

The ability of the pregnant animal to recognize the immunogenic embryo has long been recognized in the form of rhesus incompatibility; more subtle forms of recognition may exist. When only minor incompatibilities exist between two inbred strains of mice, the paternal skin survives longer following pregnancy[132, 140] and is associated with haemagglutinating antibodies in the pregnant mouse to paternal immunogens[141].

Support for the role of 'enhancing antibodies' came from the findings *in vitro* that maternal mouse lymphocytes would inhibit the growth of hybrid embryo cells *in vitro* and that this inhibitory effect was prevented by the addition of pregnant mouse serum[142]. In rats interstrain mating decreases the haemagglutinating levels of antibody to the paternal immunogens, but prolongs survival of F_1 hybrid skin allografts on the mother; the suggested cause being the presence, in the draining para-aortic nodes of the uterus, of suppressor lymphocytes[143]. In pregnant mice the ability of the mother to react against paternal antigens on the conceptus appears to result in the interplay between sensitized cells, enhancing antibodies and suppressor cells[144]. The concept of specific suppression during pregnancy has recently been placed in confusion by the inability of Canadian workers to detect immune effector function in pregnant mice against their semi-allogeneic fetuses either by *in vitro* or *in vivo* assays[145].

Maternal lymphocyte responses

The majority of the work in this area has been in the human and has consisted of experiments designed to assess the reactivity of maternal lymphocytes in mixed lymphocyte responses to paternal and fetal lymphocytes or to mitogens in the presence of maternal plasma. The majority of workers appear to have found no decrease in maternal lymphocyte responses during pregnancy[146, 147] however the thymus, spleen and lymph nodes draining the uterus do enlarge in outbred but not inbred pregnancies in rodents[148]. For a recent review on human lymphocyte responses in pregnancy, readers are referred to references 149 and 150.

Mixed one-way lymphocyte responses of the marsupial female Tammar wallaby to her mate show altered dynamics before and after mating. As in eutherians, sensitization to male allografts or repeat pregnancies has no effect on subsequent reproductive performance[151]. Such long-awaited studies in marsupials lend little support to the suggestion that the short gestation period of marsupials is the result of the embryo's inability to survive maternal immunological rejection.

Non-specific suppression of maternal responses

The possibility of the placenta producing non-specific immunosuppressant substances has created continuing interest since its proposal in 1953[3] and the observation that skin allografts on pregnant rabbits had a prolonged survival[152]. These results have not been confirmed in pregnant animals[36, 153] except in rather special cases of closely related inbred animals discussed under

'Specific Suppression of Maternal Responses'. The observation that ortho-topic allografts do not survive longer during pregnancy raised the question that the concentrations of hormones at the materno-fetal interface would be higher at their site of production and might produce a local 'hormone barrier'[154, 155] (see also reference 156). This possibility was extended by the observation that sensitized rat lymphocyte responses were depressed in the presence of trophoblast in vitro[157] and that mouse ectoplacental cones grown in vitro with lymphocytes depressed the thymus cell dependent cytotoxicity[158]. These findings could be explained by the release of hormones by the trophoblast or perhaps by the shedding of surface antigens[159].

Several important factors are often forgotten in the proposed non-specific immunoregulation of the maternal response:

(1) The entire chorion and not just the placenta should produce the hormones.

(2) The fetal immune responses should also be depressed to prevent fetal recognition of maternal uterine tissues.

(3) The proposed placental hormones should be secreted in all placental animals.

Although steroids are found in prokaryote and eukaryote cells of plants, invertebrates and vertebrates[160] and pituitary gonadotrophins are found in the vertebrate teleosts and tetrapods[161], there is no evidence for their universal presence in all placental animals, e.g. rabbit, ferret, cat and dog placentas appear to lack gonadotrophins[62]. The pre-implantation rabbit blastocyst has recently been shown to produce a luteotrophic substance similar to human chorionic gonadotrophin[162].

Steroid hormones

The production of oestrogens and progesterones either by the corpus luteum or placenta varies during gestation. In the mammals the steroids are predominantly of ovarian (luteal) origin with increasing contributions from the placenta as gestation progresses, hence the usual abortion following ovariectomy early in pregnancy[4].

The possibility of these hormones being produced by the embryo prior to implantation has been demonstrated in the eutherian pig and rabbit blastocyst and their importance in preventing luteolysis and synchronizing implantation appears certain[62]. The ability of the marsupial placenta to produce pro-gesterone, as does the corpus luteum[163], was suggested from phylogenetic studies[53] and appears probable from in vitro steroid conversions[164].

Oestrogens given in high doses will prolong skin allograft survival in mice[165] and inhibit the rejection of corneal grafts in pre-immunized rabbits[166].

Progestational agents increased skin allograft survival when given to castrated female rabbits[167] and intact female monkeys[168]. There has been renewed interest in progesterone as a possible immunosuppressant during gestation at the feto-maternal interface with the demonstration that skin allografts transplanted with implants of progesterone under the skin of rats have a prolonged survival[169, 170]. Further support comes from the observation that the steady increase in uterine tissue leukocytes which occurs with a decreased uterine binding capacity for progesterone in late pregnancy might be due to the anti-inflammatory effect of progesterone[171].

Corticosteroids are well-known inhibitors of the inflammatory response and were shown to prolong allograft survival when administered in high doses almost 30 years ago[132, 172]. All three steroid hormones have recently been shown to depress mouse lymphocyte responses *in vitro* but have no effect on sensitized lymphocyte responses[173]. How closely these *in vitro* studies mimic those *in vivo*, however, remains unknown.

Protein hormones

The observation that human chorionic gonadotrophins might depress humoral immune responses when given to mice previously sensitized to sheep red cells[174] stimulated the work showing its depression of lymphocyte responses to phytohaemagglutinin[175, 176]. Purified human chorionic gonadotrophin does not inhibit lymphocyte blastogenic responses to mitogens or allogeneic cells[177] and the inhibitory properties could be the presence of sialoglycoproteins found in pregnancy urine rather than the presence of chorionic gonadotrophins[178]. Adult and F_1 hybrid skin allografts placed in the uterus of ovariectomized rats given human chorionic gonadotrophin were not prolonged[179, 180]. However, allografts of human skin and trophoblast treated with human chorionic gonadotrophin survived longer following transplantation into guinea-pigs than untreated controls, whilst neuraminidase treatment removed the prolonged survival of trophoblast cells[181]. Furthermore, equine endometrial cups, which are of fetal origin and produce large amounts of gonadotrophin early in pregnancy, appear to avoid the maternal lymphocyte response by this secreted layer[182].

α-Fetoprotein is a normal component of amniotic and fetal serum of several animals and was suggested as being a substance in fetal plasma responsible for the depression of adult lymphocyte responses to phytohaemagglutinin[183]. α-Fetoprotein isolated from mouse amniotic fluid suppresses the plaque-forming cells of mice *in vitro*[184]; however it remains to be determined if this effect is due to the α-fetoprotein or is artifactual[185].

The pregnancy-associated proteins include ovomucoid, fetuin, α_2-macro-globulin and β_1 glycoprotein. These proteins have been found to have varying degrees of immunosuppressive effects on various *in vitro* systems but their role in mammalian placentation awaits further elucidation. For a recent review on human studies see references 127 and 149.

TRANSFER OF IMMUNOGLOBULINS AND IMMUNO-COMPETENT CELLS DURING AND FOLLOWING GESTATION

The ability to suckle their young is one of the differentiating features of the class Mammalia. The continued exchange of antibodies and perhaps cellular components of the breast milk is a continuum of events initiated around implantation. Maternal immunoglobulins (IgG) are found in the blastocoele and trophoblast of the mouse at implantation[186]. In the rabbit, maternal cytotoxic antibodies (IgM) have been found in the blastocyst fluid but do no harm[187] and later cross via the fetal yolk sac. In ungulates, rodents, cats and dogs, the transfer of immunoglobulins is via the gut in the newborn period[188].

The passage of lymphocytes across the placenta is rather vexed: pregnant mice were found to pass T6 marker leukocytes to their hybrid offspring[189] and pregnant rodents given sensitized lymphocytes against the paternal antigens are thought to cross the placenta and cause graft-versus-host disease in the newborn[190]. However, neither of these experiments has been confirmed by other workers[191].

The passage of breast milk lymphocytes across the neonatal gut during lactation has recently created much speculation. The maternal lymphocytes (in breast milk) appear to be both viable and functional. Receipt of breast milk from allogeneic foster-mothers can alter the neonatal rodent reactivity to skin allografts, cause graft-versus-host disease and reconstitute congenitally athymic 'nude' mice[192]. However, others have failed to demonstrate the passage of breast milk lymphocytes in neonatal rats and mice[193, 194].

DEVELOPMENT OF IMMUNOCOMPETENCE BY THE CONCEPTUS

The ontogeny of the immune system was much neglected with the resultant belief that the developing conceptus was immunologically incompetent despite the reported ability of a fetal goat to produce antibodies to heterologous blood injected *in utero* in 1904[195]. Similarly forgotten was the report in 1953 by experiments in Australia showing that a fetal lamb could reject skin allografts *in utero*[196].

Immune competence arises early in fetal development (despite the small numbers of immunocompetent cells raising the possibility of multipotential cells) in a controlled manner with humoral responses to certain antigens developing in a stepwise fashion. The maturation of immune competence occurs prior to maturation of lymph nodes, spleen- or gut-associated nodes, presumably arising in the lymphoid cells of the fetal liver, the mammalian equivalent of the avian bursa of Fabricius[197]. In both the fetal monkey and lamb, orthotopic skin allografts are rejected as efficiently as the adult and immunoglobulins are made in the same sequence (ovine, IgM, IgG_1 and IgG_2)

nd titres, using similar proportions of its lymphocyte population as does the dult[198].

The ontogeny of the thymus, so important in the generation of cellular nmunity, varies depending on the species; its removal at birth in mice results l loss of cell-mediated immunity[199]. Intra-uterine thymectomy of the fetal imb early in gestation has no effect on general immunologic competence or /ith the maturation of functions related to thymic-derived (T) cells[198] whilst in rimates the thymus matures prior to parturition[200]. It is within the micronvironment of the thymus that precursor 'thymic cells' learn to recognize s 'self' the histocompatibility antigens expressed on the thymic epithelium[30]. `he debate as to whether pregnancy restores immunocompetence in female odents previously thymectomized at birth[201] continues with a recent report hat immunocompetence is not restored by pregnancy[202].

EFFECTS OF ANTIGENIC DISPARITY ON FETAL–MATERNAL NTERACTION

Placental mass has been used as an expression of immunological differences)etween mother and conceptus. Hybrid mouse placentas were found to be arger in matings between histoincompatible strains than in syngeneic[203, 204]. Previous sensitization of the mother to paternal antigens produced even larger)lacentas, and tolerance in female mice prior to mating produced small)lacentas[205]. These studies have been confirmed in rats, mice and hamsters with the added observation that removal of the para-aortic lymph nodes or spleen of the mother prior to mating reduces the mass of the feto-placental unit[206].

A review, however, of the hypothesis[207] that antigenic disparity between mother and conceptus is beneficial and contributes to the maintenance of histocompatibility polymorphisms suggests that it is no longer tenable. Further, the increase in weight of the feto-placental unit appears to be the result of heterosis rather than antigenic disparity[208] and maternal sensitization to paternal antigens has not been found to increase feto-placental weight or litter size in mice[209].

CONCLUSIONS

It will be apparent to the reader that much of the evidence for each of the hypotheses concerning the success of placentation is far from conclusive. By approaching placentation from the broadest possible aspects of comparative placentation and immune responses from 'Monas to Man', the writer has endeavoured to ascertain key events at placentation which probably exist in all placental animals and thereby enable the fetal allograft to avoid maternal cellular recognition.

Several criteria may be necessary for the placental allograft to succeed.

(1) A 'barrier' must be established between fetal and maternal tissues which prevents mutual recognition of each other's foreign cell surface antigens.

(2) Bidirectional cellular traffic of immune effector cells must be kept to a minimum across this 'barrier' if recognition and rejection are not to occur in either of the maternal or fetal compartments.

(3) Placentation had first to deal with cellular rejection in its evolution; the recent appearance of immunoglobulins in the vertebrates may have required further placental evolution to avoid recognition.

(4) The absence of immunogens on the maternal aspect of the trophoblast does not account for the failure of the fetal immunocompetent cells to recognize foreign maternal uterine cells.

If the 'barrier' between the maternal and fetal tissues in non-immunogenic both to the mother and fetus then all of the hypotheses other than an 'anatomical barrier' are redundant. At the moment, it would appear that the embryo prior to implantation, at least in the eutherians, is immunogenic and that these immunogens are no longer expressed following implantation. Thus the events around the time of implantation are perhaps critical to successful placentation. The 'anatomical barrier' may result from a group of cells which, having exchanged informative molecules such as DNA, are able to express varying maternal or fetal surface immunogens, thereby presenting to the maternal and fetal immune systems 'self' antigens. This possibility is being investigated in the writer's laboratory.

References

1. Mossman, A. W. (1937). Comparative morphogenesis of the fetal membrane and accessory uterine structures. *Contrib. Embryol. Carneg. Inst. Wash.*, **26**, 129
2. Barrington, E. J. W. (1964). *Hormones and Evolution*, p. 34 (London: English and Universities Press)
3. Medawar, P. B. (1953). Some immunological and endocrinological problems raised by the evolution of viviparity in vertebrates. *Symp. Soc. Exp. Biol.*, **7**, 320
4. Kaye, M. D. (1971). The evolution of placentation. *Aust. N.Z. J. Obstet. Gynaecol.*, **11**, 197
5. Hagan, H. R. (1951). *Embryology of the Viviparous Insects*, p. 261 (New York: Ronald Press Co.)
6. Brewin, B. I. (1956). The growth and development of a viviparous compound ascidian *Hypsistozoa fasmeriana. Q. J. Microsc. Sci.*, **97**, 435
7. Sutton, M. F. (1960). The sexual development of the *Salpa fusiformis. J. Embryol. Exp. Morphol.*, **8**, 268
8. Anderson, D. T. and Manton, S. M. (1972). Studies on the onychophora. VIII. The relationship between the embryos and the oviduct in the viviparous onychopherans,

Epiperipatus trinidadensis and *Macroperipatus torquatus* from Trinidad. *Philos. Trans. R. Soc. Lond. B. (Biol. Sci.)*, **264**, 161

9. Tartar, V. (1970). Transplantation in protozoa. *Transplant. Proc.*, **2**, 183

10. Hildemann, W. H., Johnson, I. S. and Jokiol, P. L. (1979). Immunocompetence in the lowest metazoan Phylum: transplantation immunity in sponges. *Science*, **204**, 420

11. Hildemann, W. H. (1979). Immunocompetence and allogeneic polymorphism among invertebrates. *Transplantation*, **27**, 1

12. Jenkin, C. R. (1976). In Marchalonis, J. J. (ed.), *Comparative Immunology*, p. 80. (Oxford: Blackwell Scientific Publications)

13. Marchalonis, J. J. (1977). *Immunity in Evolution*, p. 43. (Massachusetts: Harvard University Press)

14. Hildemann, W. H. (1970). Transplantation immunity in fishes Agnatha, Chondrichthyes and Osteichthyes. *Transplant. Proc.*, **2**, 53

15. Kaye, M. D., Jones, W. R. and Anderson, D. T. (1972). Immunology and placentation in viviparous invertebrates. *J. Reprod. Fertil.*, **31**, 335

16. Aristotle. In Peck, A. L. (ed.) (1970). *Historia Animalium HA565B*. The Loeb Classical library. (London: Heinemann)

17. Hogarth, P. J. (1968). Immunological aspects of feto-maternal relations in lower vertebrates. *J. Reprod. Fertil.* (Suppl. 3), 15

18. Weekes, H. C. (1933). On the distribution, habitat and reproductive habits of certain European and Australian snakes and lizards with particular regard to their adaptation to viviparity. *Proc. Linn. Soc. NSW*, **58**, 271

19. Yaron, Z. (1977). In Calaby, J. H. and Tyndale-Biscoe, C. H. (eds.) *Reproduction and Evolution*, p. 271. (Australian Academy of Sciences)

20. Amoroso, E. C. (1964). In Parkes, A. S. (ed.) *Marshall's Physiology of Reproduction*, Vol. 2, p. 127. (London: Longmans)

21. Amoroso, E. C. (1968). The evolution of viviparity. *Proc. R. Soc. Med.*, **61**, 1188

22. Hughes, R. L. (1977). In Calaby, J. H. and Tyndale-Biscoe, C. H. (eds.) *Reproduction and Evolution*, p. 281. (Australian Academy of Sciences)

23. Padykula, H. A. and Taylor, J. M. (1977). In Calaby, J. H. and Tyndale-Biscoe, C. H. (eds.) *Reproduction and Evolution*, p. 303. (Australian Academy of Sciences)

24. Steven, D. (1975). *Comparative Placentation*, p. 58. (London: Academic Press)

25. Hughes, R. L. (1974). Morphological studies on implantation in marsupials. *J. Reprod. Fertil.*, **39**, 173

26. Weekes, H. C. (1927). Placentation and other phenomena in the scincid lizard *Lygosoma quoyi*. *Proc. Linn. Soc. NSW*, **55**, 499

27. Weekes, H. C. (1935). A review of placentation among reptiles with particular regard to the function and evolution of the placenta. *Proc. Zool. Soc. Lond.*, 625

28. Sharman, G. B. (1970). Reproductive physiology of marsupials. *Science*, **167**, 1221

29. Lillegraven, J. A. (1975). Biological considerations of the marsupial–placental dichotomy. *Evolution*, **29**, 707

30. Zinkernagel, R. M., Callahan, G. N., Klein, J. and Dennert, G. (1978). Cytotoxic T cells learn specificity for self H-2 during differentiation in the thymus. *Nature (London)*, **271**, 251

31. Borysenko, M. (1979). Evolution of lymphocytes and vertebrate alloimmune reactivity. *Transplant. Proc.*, **11**, 1123

32. Toivanen, A. (1979). Interactions of leucocytes in phylogenetic perspective. *Transplant. Proc.*, **11**, 1131

33. Robertson, M. (1979). Recognition, restriction and immunity. *Nature (London)*, **280**, 192

34. Erickson, R. P. (1977). In Edidin, M. and Johnson, M. H. (eds.) *Immunobiology of Gametes*, p. 85. (Cambridge University Press)

35. Marcus, G. J. and Shelesnyak, M. C. (1968). Studies on the mechanism of nidation. *Acta Endocrinol.*, **57** (Suppl. 123), 136

36. Beer, A. E. and Billingham, R. E. (1974). Host responses to intrauterine tissue, cellular and fetal allografts. *J. Reprod. Fertil.* (Suppl. 21), 59
37. Overstreet, J. W. and Cooper, G. W. (1979). Effect of ovulation and sperm motility on the migration of rabbit spermatozoa to the site of fertilization. *J. Reprod. Fertil.*, **55**, 53
38. Cohen, J. and Werrett, D. J. (1975). Antibodies and sperm survival in the female genital tract of the mouse and rabbit. *J. Reprod. Fertil.*, **42**, 301
39. Cohen, J. and McNaughton, D. C. (1974). The probable selection of a small population by the genital tract of the female rabbit. *J. Reprod. Fertil.*, **39**, 297
40. Overstreet, J. W. and Katz, D. F. (1977). In Johnson, M. H. (ed.) *Development of Mammals*, Vol. 2, p. 31. (Amsterdam: North Holland Publ. Co.)
41. Thibault, C. (1973). Sperm transport and storage in vertebrates. *J. Reprod. Fertil.*, (Suppl. 18), 39
42. Racey, P. A. (1975). In Duckett, J. G. and Racey, P. A. (eds.) Biology of the male Gamete. *Biol. J. Linn. Soc.*, **7** (Suppl. 1), 385
43. Dobzhansky, T. (1977). In Dobzhansky, T., Ayala, F. J., Stebbins, G. L. and Valentine, J. W. (eds.) *Evolution*, p. 171. (San Francisco: W. H. Freeman)
44. Bolwell, G. P., Callow, J. A., Callow, M. E. and Evans, L. V. (1977). Cross fertilization in fucoid seaweeds. *Nature (London)*, **268**, 626
45. Metz, C. B. (1978). Sperm and egg receptors involved in fertilization. *Curr. Top. Devel. Biol.*, **12**, 107
46. Miller, R. L. (1977). In Adiyodi, K. G. and Adiyodi, P. G. (eds.) *Advances in Invertebrate Reproduction*, **1**, 99. (India: Peralam-Kenoth Kariueller)
47. Franklin, L. E. (1970). Fertilization and the role of the acrosomal region in non-mammals. *Biol. Reprod.* (Suppl. 2), 159
48. Yanagimachi, R. (1978). Sperm–egg associations in mammals. *Curr. Top. Devel. Biol.*, **12**, 83
49. Vacquier, V. D. and Moy, G. W. (1977). Isolation of bindin: the protein responsible for adhesion of sperm to sea urchin eggs. *Proc. Natl. Acad. Sci.*, **74**, 2456
50. Epel, D. (1978). Mechanisms of activation of sperm and eggs during fertilization of sea urchin gametes. *Curr. Top. Devel. Biol.*, **12**, 185
51. Austin, C. R. (1978). Patterns in metozoan fertilization. *Curr. Top. Devel. Biol.*, **12**, 1
52. Miyake, A. (1978). Cell communication, cell union and initiation of meiosis in ciliate conjugation. *Curr. Top. Devel. Biol.*, **12**, 37
53. Kaye, M. D. (1973). Immunological studies in mammalian placentation. *PhD Thesis*, Sydney University
54. Monroy, A. and Rosati, F. (1979). The evolution of the cell–cell recognition system. *Nature (London)*, **278**, 165
55. Halbert, S. A., Tam, P. Y. and Blandau, R. J. (1976). Egg transport in the rabbit oviduct: the roles of cilia and muscle. *Science*, **191**, 1052
56. Eddy, C. A., Flores, J. J., Archer, D. R. and Paverstein, C. J. (1979). The role of cilia in fertility: an evaluation by selective microsurgical modification of the rabbit oviduct. *Am. J. Obstet. Gynecol.*, **132**, 814
57. Finn, C. A. (1977). In Wynn, R. M. (ed.) *Biology of the Uterus*, p. 245. (New York: Plenum Press)
58. Freese, V. E., Ormans, S. and Pavlos, G. (1973). An autoradiographic investigation of epithelium egg interaction in the mouse oviduct. *Am. J. Obstet. Gynecol.*, **117**, 364
59. Ledford, B. E., Rankin, J. C., Froble, F. L., Serra, M. J., Markwald, R. R. and Baggett, B. (1978). The decidual cell reaction in the mouse uterus: DNA synthesis and autoradiographic analysis of responsive cells. *Biol. Reprod.*, **18**, 506
60. Ansell, J. D., Barlow, P. W. and McLaren, A. (1974). Binucleate and polyploid cells in the decidua of the mouse. *J. Embryol. Exp. Morphol.*, **31**, 223
61. Chapman, V. M., Ansell, J. D. and McLaren, A. (1972). Trophoblast giant cell

differentiation in the mouse: expression of glucose phosphate isomerase variants in transferred chimeric embryos. *Develop. Biol.*, **29**, 48

62. Heap, R. B., Flint, A. P. F., Gadsby, J. E. and Rice, C. (1979). Hormones, the early embryo and the uterine environment. *J. Reprod. Fertil.*, **55**, 267

63. Johnson, M. H. (1979). Intrinsic and extrinsic factors in pre-implantation development. *J. Reprod. Fertil.*, **55**, 255

64. Gardner, R. (1975). In Edwards, R. G., Howe, C. W. S. and Johnson, M. H. (eds.) *Immunobiology of Trophoblast*, p. 43. (Cambridge University Press)

65. Hill, J. P. (1897). The placentation of perameles. *Q. J. Microsc. Sci.*, **40**, 385 and **43**, 1

66. Flynn, T. (1923). Placentation of parameles. *Q. J. Microsc. Sci.*, **67**, 123

67. Hill, J. P. (1900). On the fetal membranes, placentation and parturition of the native cat. *Anat. Anz.*, **18**, 364

68. Larsen, J. F. (1961). Electron microscopy of the implantation site in the rabbit. *Am. J. Anat.*, **109**, 319

69. Schlafke, S. and Enders, A. C. (1975). Cellular basis of interaction between trophoblast and uterus at implantation. *Biol. Reprod.*, **12**, 41

70. McLennan, J. G. (1974). Ultrastructural studies of early nidation in pregnancy and pseudopregnancy. *Am. J. Obstet. Gynecol.*, **120**, 319

71. Avery, G. B. and Hunt, C. V. (1969). The differentiation of trophoblast giant cells in the mouse studied in kidney capsule grafts. *Transplant. Proc.*, **1**, 61

72. Galassi, L. (1967). Reutilization of maternal nuclear material by embryonic and trophoblastic cells in the rat for the synthesis of DNA. *J. Histochem. Cytochem.*, **15**, 573

73. Ledoux, L. and Charles, P. (1967). Uptake of exogenous DNA by mouse embryos. *Exp. Cell. Res.*, **45**, 498

74. Kaye, M. D. (1977). An autoradiographic study of the implantation of transferred mouse blastocysts. *Aust. J. Biol. Sci.*, **30**, 577

75. Daniel, J. C. and Chilton, B. S. (1978). In Johnson, M. H. (ed.) *Development in Mammals*, Vol. 3, p. 131. (Amsterdam: North Holland Publ. Co.)

76. Kantor, J. A., Lee, Y. H., Chirikjian, J. G. and Fellow, W. F. (1979). DNA polymerase with characteristics of reverse transcriptase purified from human milk. *Science*, **204**, 511

77. Harris, H., Sidebottom, E., Grace, D. M. and Bramwell, M. E. (1969). The expression of genetic information: a study with hybrid animal cells. *J. Cell. Sci.*, **4**, 499

78. Croce, C. M. and Koprowski, H. (1978). The genetics of human cancer. *Sci. Am.*, **238**, 117

79. Marx, J. L. (1977). Gene transfer in mammalian cells mediated by chromosomes. *Science*, **197**, 146

80. Little, C. C. (1924). The genetics of tissue transplantation in mammals. *J. Cancer Res.*, **8**, 75

81. Edidin, M. (1976). Embryogenesis in mammals. *CIBA Foundation Symp.*, **40** (new series), p. 177

82. Hakansson, S., Heyner, S., Sundquist, K. and Bergstrom, S. (1975). The presence of paternal H-2 antigens on hybrid mouse blastocysts during experimental delay of implantation and the disappearance of the antigens after onset of implantation. *Int. J. Fertil.*, **20**, 137

83. Barrett, D. and Angelo, G. M. (1969). Maternal characteristics of hatching enzymes in hybrid sea urchin embryos. *Exp. Cell. Res.*, **57**, 159

84. Wright, D. A. and Subtelny, S. (1969). The expression of genes controlling enzymes in the diploid and androgenetic haploid hybrid frog embryos. *J. Cell. Biol.*, **43**, 160a

85. Castro-Sierra, E. and Ohno, S. (1968). Allelic inhibition of the autosomally inherited gene locus for liver alcohol dehydrogenase in chicken-quail hybrids. *Biochem. Genet.*, **1**, 323

86. Hitzeroth, H., Klose, J., Ohno, S. and Wolf, V. (1968). Asynchronous activation of parental alleles at the tissue specific gene loci observed on hybrid trout during early development. *Biochem. Genet.*, **1**, 287

87. Chapman, V. M., Adler, D., Labarca, C. and Wudl, L. (1976). *Embryogenesis in Mammals.* Ciba Foundation Symp., **40** (new series), p. 115
88. Wudl, L. and Chapman, V. M. (1976). The expression of β glucuronidase during pre-implantation development of mouse embryos. *Dev. Biol.* **48**, 104
89. Muggleton-Harris, A. L. and Johnson, M. H. (1976). The nature and distribution of serologically detectable alloantigens on the pre-implantation mouse embryo. *J. Embryol. Exp. Morphol.*, **35**, 59
90. Krco, C. J. and Goldberg, E. H. (1976). H-Y antigen: detection on eight cell mouse embryos. *Science*, **193**, 1134
91. Searle, R. F. and Jenkinson, E. J. (1978). Localization of trophoblast defined surface antigens during early mouse embryogenesis. *J. Embryol. Exp. Morphol.*, **43**, 147
92. Carter, J. (1976). Expression of maternal and paternal antigens on trophoblast. *Nature (London)*, **262**, 292
93. Sellens, M. H. (1977). Antigen expression on early mouse trophoblast. *Nature (London)*, **269**, 60
94. Webb, C. B., Gall, W. E. and Edelman, G. M. (1977). Synthesis and distribution of H-2 antigens in pre-implantation mouse embryos. *J. Exp. Med.*, **146**, 923
95. Parr, E. L. and Moore, H. A. (1977). In Calaby, J. H. and Tyndale-Biscoe, C. H. (eds.) *Reproduction and Evolution*, p. 363. (Australian Academy of Sciences)
96. Simmons, R. L. and Russell, P. S. (1966). The histocompatibility antigens of fertilized mouse eggs and trophoblast. *Ann. N.Y. Acad. Sci.*, **129**, 35
97. James, D. A. (1960). Antigenicity of the blastocyst masked by the zona pellucida. *Transplantation*, **8**, 846
98. Heyner, S., Brinster, R. L. and Palm, J. (1969). Effect of isoantibody on pre-implantation mouse embryos. *Nature (London)*, **222**, 783
99. Moskalewski, S. and Koprowski, H. (1972). Presence of egg antigen in immature oocytes and pre-implantation embryos. *Nature (London)*, **237**, 167
100. Kirby, D. R. S. (1969). On the immunological function of the zona pellucida. *Fertil. Steril.*, **20**, 933
101. Dickmann, Z. and De Feo, V. J. (1967). The rat blastocyst during normal pregnancy and during delayed implantation, including an observation on the shedding of the zona pellucida. *J. Reprod. Fertil.*, **13**, 3
102. Short, R. V. and Hay, M. F. (1966). Comparative reproduction in mammals. Delayed implantation in the roe deer *Capreolus capreolus*. *Symp. Zool. Soc. Lond.*, **15**, 173
103. Lobel, B. L., Levy, E. and Shelesnyak, M. C. (1967). Studies on the mechanism of nidation. *Acta Endocrinol.* (Suppl. 123), 7
104. Hamilton, W. J. (1970). In Hubinont, P. O., Le Roy, F., Robyn, C. and Leleux, P. (eds.) *Ovoimplantation, Human Gonadotropins and Prolactin*, p. 149. (New York: S. Karger)
105. Mulnard, J. G. (1970). In Hubinont, P. O., Le Roy, F., Robyn, C. and Leleux, P. (eds.) *Ovoimplantation, Human Gonadotropins and Prolactin*, p. 9. (New York: S. Karger)
106. Grosser, O. (1927). *Fruheutwicklumg eihautbildung und placentation des menschen und der saugestierre.* (Munchen: J. F. Bergmann, VIII U454S)
107. Enders, A. C. (1965). A comparative study of the fine structure of the trophoblast in several hemochorial placentae. *Am. J. Anat.*, **116**, 29
108. Bardawil, W. A. and Toy, B. L. (1959). The natural history of choriocarcinoma. Problems of immunity and spontaneous regression. *Ann. N.Y. Acad. Sci.*, **80**, 197
109. Kirby, D. R. S., Billington, W. D., Bradbury, S. and Goldstein, D. J. (1964). Antigen barrier of the mouse placenta. *Nature (London)*, **204**, 548
110. Kirby, D. R. S., Billington, W. D. and James, D. A. (1966). Transplantation of eggs to the kidney and uterus of immunised mice. *Transplantation*, **4**, 713
111. Simmons, R. L., Cruse, V. and McKay, D. G. (1967). The immunologic problem of

pregnancy. II. Ultrastructure of isogenic and allogenic transplants. *Am. J. Obstet. Gynecol.*, **97**, 218

112. Wynn, R. M. (1967). Comparative electron microscopy of the placental junctional zone. *Obstet. Gynecol.*, **29**, 644

113. Martinek, J. J. (1970). Fibrinoid and the fetal maternal interface of the rat placenta. *Anat. Rec.*, **166**, 587

114. Simmons, R. L. and Russell, P. S. (1966). The histocompatibility antigens of fertilized mouse eggs and trophoblast. *Ann. N.Y. Acad. Sci.*, **129**, 35

115. Currie, G. A., Van Doorninck, W. and Bagshawe, K. D. (1968). The effect of neuraminidase on the immunogenicity of early mouse trophoblast. *Nature (London)*, **219**, 191

116. Simmons, R. L., Lipschultz, M. L., Rios, A. and Ray, P. K. (1971). Failure of neuraminidase to unmask histocompatibility antigens on trophoblast. *Nature (London)*, **231**, 111

117. Jenkinson, E. J. and Billington, W. D. (1974). Differential susceptibility· of mouse trophoblast and embryonic tissue to immune cell lysis. *Transplantation*, **18**, 286

118. Edidin, M. (1972). In Kahan, B. D. and Reisfeld, R. A. (eds.) *Transplantation Antigens*, p. 75. (New York: Academic Press)

119. Bagshawe, K. and Lawler, S. (1975). In Edwards, R. G., Howe, C. W. S. and Johnson, M. H. (eds.) *Immunobiology of Trophoblast*, p. 171. (Cambridge University Press)

120. Jenkinson, E. J. and Searle, R. F. (1979). Ia-antigen expression on the developing mouse embryo and placenta. *J. Reprod. Immunol.*, **1**, 3

121. Koren, Z., Abrams, G. and Behrman, S. J. (1968). Antigenicity of mouse placental tissue. *Am. J. Obstet. Gynecol.*, **102**, 340

122. Beer, A. E., Billingham, R. E. and Yang, S. L. (1972). Further evidence concerning the auto-antigenic status of the trophoblast. *J. Exp. Med.*, **135**, 1177

123. Kirby, D. R. S. (1969). Antigenicity of mouse placental tissue. *Am. J. Obstet. Gynecol.*, **105**, 289

124. Schlesinger, M. (1964). Serologic studies of embryonic and trophoblastic tissues of the mouse. *J. Immunol.*, **93**, 255

125. Carter, J. (1978). The expression of surface antigens on three trophoblastic tissues in the mouse. *J. Reprod. Fertil.*, **54**, 433

126. Sellens, M. H., Jenkinson, E. J. and Billington, W. D. (1978). Major histocompatibility complex and non-major histocompatibility complex antigens on mouse ectoplacental cone and placental trophoblastic cells. *Transplantation*, **25**, 173

127. Loke, Y. W. (1978). *Immunology and Immunopathology of the Human Fetal and Maternal Interaction.* (Amsterdam: Elsevier/North Holland Biomedical Press)

128. Simmons, R. L. and Russell, P. S. (1967). Xenoantigens in mouse trophoblast. *Transplantation*, **5**, 85

129. Dehem, A., Sobis, H. and Vandeputte, M. (1971). Effect of immunosuppression on the development of xenogenic trophoblast under the kidney capsule. *Transplantation*, **11**, 578

130. Dent, J., McGovern, P. T. and Hancock, J. L. (1971). Immunological implications of ultrastructural studies of goat sheep hybrid placentae. *Nature (London)*, **231**, 116

131. Poppa, G., Simmons, R. L., David, D. S. and Russell, P. S. (1964). The uterus as a recipient site for parathyroid homotransplantation. *Transplantation*, **2**, 496

132. Medawar, P. B. and Sparrow, E. M. (1956). The effects of adreno cortical hormones, adreno corticotrophic hormone and pregnancy on skin transplantation immunity in mice. *J. Endocrinol.*, **14**, 240

133. Beer, A. E., Billingham, R. E. and Hoerr, R. A. (1971). Elicitation and expression of transplantation in the uterus. *Transplant. Proc.*, **3**, 609

134. Lanman, J. T., Herod, L. and Fekrig, S. (1964). Homograft immunity in pregnancy: Survival rates in rabbits born of ova transplanted into sensitised mothers. *J. Exp. Med.*, **119**, 781

135. Watnick, A. S. and Russo, R. A. (1968). Survival of skin homografts in uteri of pregnant and progesterone and estrogen treated rats. *Proc. Soc. Exp. Biol. Med.*, **128**, 1

136. Kaye, M. D., Jones, W. R. and Ing, R. M. Y. (1974). An investigation of privilege in the pregnant rat uterus. *J. Reprod. Fertil.*, **36**, 467

137. Kirby, D. R. S. (1969). *Adv. Biosc.*, **4**, 255

138. Samuel, C. A. and Perry, J. S. (1972). The ultrastructure of pig trophoblast transplanted to an ectopic site in the uterine wall. *J. Anat.*, **113**, 139

139. Galtsoff, P. S. and Galtsoff, E. (1953). Destruction, survival and disorganised growth of embryonic organs and tissues of *Opsanus tau* after homoplastic transplantation of whole embryos in the adult toad fish. *Anat. Rec.*, **117**, 601

140. Breyere, E. J. and Barrett, M. K. (1960). Prolonged survival of skin homografts in parous female mice. *J. Natl. Cancer Inst.*, **25**, 1405

141. Goodlin, R. C. and Herzenberg, L. A. (1964). Pregnancy induced haemagglutinins to paternal H-2 antigens in multiparous mice. *Transplantation*, **2**, 357

142. Hellstrom, K. E., Hellstrom, I. and Brown, J. (1969). Abrogation of cellular immunity to antigenically foreign mouse embryonic cells by a serum factor. *Nature (London)*, **224**, 914

143. Beer, A. E., Head, J. R., Smith, W. G. and Billingham, R. E. (1976). Some immunoregulatory aspects of pregnancy in rats. *Transplant. Proc.*, **8**, 267

144. Chaouat, G., Voisin, G. A., Escalier, D. and Robert, P. (1979). Facilitation reaction (enhancing antibodies and suppressor cells) and rejection reaction (sensitised cells) from the mother to the paternal antigens of the conceptus. *Clin. Exp. Immunol.*, **35**, 13

145. Wegmann, T. G., Waters, C. A., Drell, D. W. and Carlson, G. A. (1979). Pregnant mice are not primed but can be primed to fetal alloantigens. *Proc. Natl. Acad. Sci.*, **76**, 2410

146. Kaye, M. D. (1973). Human lymphocyte responses during pregnancy. *J. Reprod. Fertil.*, **32**, 333

147. Hawes, C. S., Kemp, A. S., Jones, W. R. and Need, J. A. Personal communication

148. Forster, P. M., McLean, J. M. and Gibbs, A. C. C. (1979). Lymphoid response to pregnancy and pseudopregnancy in the rat. *J. Anat.*, **128**, 837

149. Gusdon, J. P. (1976). In Scott, J. S. and Jones, W. R. (eds.) *Immunology of Human Reproduction*, p. 103. (London: Academic Press)

150. Rocklin, R. E., Kitzmiller, J. L. and Kaye, M. D. (1979). Immunobiology of the maternal fetal relationship. *Ann. Rev. Med.*, **30**, 375

151. Walker, K. Z. and Tyndale-Biscoe, C. H. (1978). Immunological aspects of gestation in the Tammar wallaby *Macropus eugenii. Aust. J. Biol. Sci.*, **31**, 173

152. Heslop, R. W., Kohn, P. L. and Sparrow, E. M. (1954). The effect of pregnancy on the survival of skin allografts in rabbits. *J. Endocrinol.*, **10**, 325

153. Billingham, R. E. (1971). Transplantation biology of mammalian gestation. *Am. J. Obstet. Gynecol.*, **111**, 469

154. Zipper, J., Ferrando, G., Saez, G. and Tehernitchin, A. (1966). Intra uterine grafting in rats of autologous and homologous adult rat skin. *Am. J. Obstet. Gynecol.*, **94**, 1056

155. Nelson, J. H., Hall, J. E., Manuel-Limson, G., Friedberg, H. and O'Brien, F. J. (1967). Effect of pregnancy on the thymolymphatic system. I. Changes in the intact rat after exogenous HCG, estrogen and progesterone administration. *Am. J. Obstet. Gynecol.*, **98**, 895

156. Amoroso, E. C. and Perry, J. S. (1975). The existence during gestation of an immunological buffer zone at the interface between fetal and maternal tissues. *Phil. Trans. R. Soc. Lond. Ser. B.*, **271**, 343

157. Kaye, M. D. and Jones, W. R. (1973). *In vitro* activity of sensitised maternal lymphocytes to paternal and embryonic tissues in the rat. *IRCS* (73–12), 3.10.37

158. Berg, M., Burton, R. C., Smith, J. A., Luckenbach, G. A., Decker, J. and Mitchell, G. F. (1978). Effects of placental tissue on immunological responses. *Clin. Exp. Immunol.*, **34**, 441

59. Alexander, P. (1974). Escape from immuno destruction by the host through shedding of surface antigens. Is this a characteristic shared by malignant and embryonic cells? *Cancer Res.*, **34**, 2077

60. Sander, T., Sonea, S. and Mead, A. Z. (1975). The possible role of steroids in evolution. *Am. Zool.*, **15** (Suppl. 1), 227

61. Licht, P., Papkoff, H., Farmer, S. W., Muller, C. H., Tsuitt, W. and Crews, D. (1977). Evolution of gonadotropins, structure and function. *Recent Prog. Horm. Res.*, **33**, 169

62. Channing, C. P., Stone, S. L., Sakai, C. N., Haour, F. and Saxena, B. B. (1978). A stimulatory effect of the fluid from the pre-implantation rabbit blastocysts upon luteinization of monkey granulosa cell cultures. *J. Reprod. Fertil.*, **54**, 215

163. Tyndale-Biscoe, C. H., Hearn, J. P. and Renfree, M. B. (1974). Control of reproduction in Macropodid marsupials. *J. Endocrinol.*, **63**, 589

164. Renfree, M. B. (1977). In Calaby, J. H. and Tyndale-Biscoe, C. H. (eds.) *Reproduction and Evolution*, p. 325. (Australian Academy of Sciences)

165. Simmons, R. L., Price, A. L. and Oserkis, A. J. (1968). The immunologic problems of pregnancy. V. The effect of estrogen and progesterone on allograft survival. *Am. J. Obstet. Gynecol.*, **100**, 908

166. Waltman, S. R., Burde, R. M. and Barrios, J. (1971). Prevention of corneal homograft rejection by estrogens. *Transplantation*, **11**, 194

167. Hulka, J. F., Mohr, K. and Liberman, M. W. (1965). Effect of synthetic progestational agents on allograft rejection and circulating antibody production. *Endocrinology*, **77**, 897

168. Munroe, J. S. (1971). Progesteroids as immunosuppressive agents. *J. Reticuloendoth. Soc.*, **9**, 361

169. Siiteri, P. K., Febres, F., Clemens, L. E., Chang, R. J., Gondos, B. and Stites, D. (1977). Progesterone and maintenance of pregnancy. Is progesterone Nature's immunosuppressant. *Ann. N.Y. Acad. Sci.*, **286**, 384

170. Beer, A. E. and Billingham, R. E. (1979). *Maternal Recognition of Pregnancy*. Ciba Foundation Symp., **64** (new series), p. 293

171. Padykula, H. A. and Tansey, T. R. (1979). The occurrence of uterine stromal and intra epithelial monocytes and heterophils during normal late pregnancy in the rat. *Anat. Rec.*, **193**, 329

172. Billingham, R. E., Krohn, P. L. and Medawar, P. B. (1951). Effect of locally applied cortisone acetate on survival of skin allografts in rabbits. *Br. Med. J.*, **2**, 1049

173. Pavia, C., Siiteri, P. K., Perlman, J. D. and Stites, D. P. (1979). Suppression of immune allogeneic cell interactions by sex hormones. *J. Reprod. Immunol.*, **1**, 33

174. Younger, J. B., St. Pierre, R. L. and Zmijewski, C. M. (1969). Effect of human chorionic gonadotrophin on antibody production. *Am. J. Obstet. Gynecol.*, **105**, 9

175. Kaye, M. D. and Jones, W. R. (1971). Effect of human chorionic gonadotrophin on *in vitro* lymphocyte transformation. *Am. J. Obstet. Gynecol.*, **109**, 1029

176. Contractor, S. F. and Davies, H. (1973). Effect of human chorionic somatomammotrophin and hCG on phytohemagglutinin induced lymphocyte transformation. *Nature (London)*, **243**, 284

177. Caldwell, J. L., Stites, D. P. and Fudenberg, H. H. (1975). Human chorionic gonadotrophin. Effects of crude and purified preparations on lymphocyte responses to phytohaemagglutinin and allogeneic stimulation. *J. Immunol.*, **115**, 1249

178. Morse, J. H., Stearn, C., Arden, J., Agosto, G. M. and Canfield, R. E. (1976). The effects of crude and purified human gonadotropin on *in vitro* stimulated human lymphocyte cultures. *Cell. Immunol.*, **25**, 178

179. Kaye, M. D., Jones, W. R., Ing, R. M. Y. and Markham, R. (1971). Effect of human chorionic gonadotrophin on intrauterine skin allograft survival in rats. *Am. J. Obstet. Gynecol.*, **110**, 640

180. Kaye, M. D., Jones, W. R. and Ing, R. M. Y. (1973). Effect of human chorionic gonadotrophin on intrauterine skin graft survival in F-1 hybrid rats. *Am. J. Obstet. Gynecol.*, **116**, 39

181. Borland, R., Loke, Y. W. and Wilson, D. (1975). In Edwards, R. G., Howe, C. W. S. and Johnson, M. H. (eds.) *Immunobiology of Trophoblast*, p. 157. (Cambridge University Press)

182. Allen, W. R. (1975). In Edwards, R. G., Howe, C. W. S. and Johnson, M. H. (eds.) *Immunobiology of Trophoblast*, p. 217. (Cambridge University Press)

183. Ayoub, J. and Kasakura, S. (1971). *In vitro* response of fetal lymphocytes to PHA and a plasma factor which suppresses the PHA response of adult lymphocytes. *Clin. Exp. Immunol.*, **8**, 427

184. Murgita, R. A. and Tomasi, T. B. (1975). Suppression of the immune response by alpha feto protein. I. Primary and secondary response. *J. Exp. Med.*, **141**, 269

185. Littman, B. H., Alpert, E. and Rocklin, R. E. (1977). Effect of purified alpha feto protein on *in vitro* assays of cell mediated immunity. *Cell. Immunol.*, **30**, 35

186. Bernard, O., Ripoche, M. A. and Bennett, D. (1977). Distribution of maternal immunoglobulins in the mouse uterus and embryo in the days after implantation. *J. Exp. Med.*, **145**, 58

187. Lanman, J. T. and Herod, L. (1965). Homograft immunity in pregnancy: The placental transfer of cytotoxic antibodies in rabbits. *J. Exp. Med.*, **122**, 579

188. Brambell, F. W. R. (1970). *The Transmission of Passive Immunity from Mother to Young.* (Amsterdam: North Holland Publ. Co.)

189. Barnes, R. D. and Tuffrey, M. (1971). Maternal cells in the newborn. *Adv. Biosc.*, **6**, 457

190. Beer, A. E. and Billingham, R. E. (1973). Maternally acquired runt disease. *Science*, **179**, 240

191. Billington, W. R. (1976). In Scott, J. S. and Jones, W. R. (eds.) *Immunology of Human Reproduction*, p. 93. (London: Academic Press)

192. Head, J. R., Beer, A. E. and Billingham, R. E. (1977). Significance of the cellular component of the maternal immunologic endowment in milk. *Transplant. Proc.*, **9**, 1465

193. Silvers, W. K. and Poole, T. W. (1975). The influence of foster nursing on the survival and immunologic competence of mice and rats. *J. Immunol.*, **115**, 1117

194. Trentin, J. J., Gallagher, M. T. and Priest, E. L. (1977). Failure of functional transfer of maternal lymphocytes to F_1 hybrid mice. *Transplant. Proc.*, **9**, 1473

195. Kreidl, A. and Mandl, L. (1904). Uber den mebergang der immonhamolysine non der frucht auf die muher. *Wein Klin Weschscht.*, **17**, 611

196. Schinkel, P. G. and Ferguson, K. A. (1953). Skin transplantation in the fetal lamb. *Aust. J. Biol. Sci.*, **6**, 533

197. Owen, J. J., Cooper, M. D. and Ralt, M. C. (1974). *In vitro* generation of B lymphocytes in mouse fetal liver, a mammalian bursa equivalent. *Nature (London)*, **249**, 361

198. Silverstein, A. M. (1977). In Cooper, M. C. and Dayton, D. (eds.) *Development of Host Defences*, p. 1. (New York: Rowen Press)

199. Miller, J. F. A. P. (1961). Immunological function of the thymus. *Lancet*, **2**, 748

200. Solomon, J. B. (1971). *Fetal and Neonatal Immunology*, p. 234. (Amsterdam: North Holland Publ. Co.)

201. Osoba, D. (1965). Immune reactivity in mice thymectomised soon after birth: normal response after pregnancy. *Science*, **147**, 298

202. Clancy, J. (1978). Failure of pregnancy to restore immune competence in neonatally thymectomised rats. *Transplantation*, **26**, 454

203. Billington, W. D. (1964). Influence of immunological dissimilarity of mother and fetus on size of placenta in mice. *Nature (London)*, **202**, 317

204. McLaren, A. (1965). Genetic and environmental effects on fetal and placental growth in mice. *J. Reprod. Fertil.*, **9**, 79

205. James, D. A. (1967). Some effects of immunological factors on gestation in mice. *J. Reprod. Fertil.*, **14**, 265

206. Beer, A. E. and Billingham, R. E. (1977). Histocompatibility gene polymorphisms and maternal fetal interaction. *Transplant. Proc.*, **9**, 1393

207. Clarke, B. C. and Kirby, D. R. S. (1966). Maintenance of histocompatibility polymorphisms. *Nature (London)*, **211**, 999

208. McLaren, A. (1975). In Edwards, R. G., Howe, C. W. E. and Johnson, M. H. (eds.) *Immunobiology of Trophoblast*, p. 255. (Cambridge University Press)

209. Hetherington, C. M. (1978). Absence of effect of maternal immunization to paternal antigens on placental weight, fetal weight and litter size in the mouse. *J. Reprod. Fertil.*, **53**, 81

2
Immunological Relationships between Mother and Conceptus In Man

D. W. COOPER

INTRODUCTION

The evolution of viviparity in placental mammals has involved numerous modifications to the anatomy and physiology of the mother and her conceptus. Many of these changes have been described and the reasons for them understood; but despite much experimental work in the last three decades, one basic question at least remains unanswered. How is the conceptus retained for such a long period in the womb in the face of the mother's immunological system? The conceptus with its foreign paternally derived antigens is seen as violating the basic immunogenetic rules for the acceptance or rejection of transplanted tissue. Medawar[1] first posed the immunological problem in these terms and since then many writers have referred to the conceptus as being analogous to an allograft within the womb. The extent to which this analogy is valid has now become debateable[2]. Nonetheless the comparison of the conceptus with an allograft is a convenient starting point for a consideration of the conceptus–maternal relationship; their similarities and their differences are both instructive.

The allograft comparison has dominated the field to the virtual exclusion of other possible approaches. This is a natural result of the high level of understanding of transplantation phenomena which has been attained over the last 20 years. The fact that a solution to the problem still seems elusive, however, suggests that these other approaches should now be explored.

Burnet has shown that immunological problems may be illuminated by first considering them in basic Darwinian terms. This review is accordingly also an attempt to examine the problem from the standpoint of evolutionary biology and genetics. Attention will be confined largely to man although many of the general points are applicable to other organisms (see Kaye, Chapter 1). Other recent treatments of the data and ideas of the subject as they pertain to man may be found in Loke[3] and in articles by several authors in volumes edited by Scott and Jones[4] and Boettcher[5].

IN WHAT SENSE IS THE CONCEPTUS ANALOGOUS TO AN ALLOGRAFT?

An allograft is a piece of tissue transplanted from one individual to another genetically different individual of the same species. If the donor possesses antigens not possessed by the recipient, the recipient will usually reject the transplanted tissue. Antigens provoking such rejection responses are termed transplantation or histocompatibility antigens. This rejection is usually mediated by T lymphocytes rather than by antibodies. The antigens of the transplanted tissue exist on the surface of cells which are directly exposed to the cells of the recipient's circulatory system. The attack upon the transplanted tissue is a direct one: no physical barrier exists between it and the recipient's immune system.

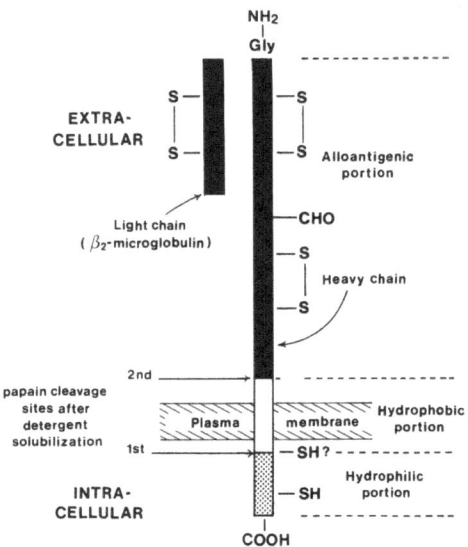

Figure 2.1(a)   Proposed structure of HLA-A and HLA-B antigens (after Strominger *et al.*[121] with kind permission) β_2-microglobulin seems to be an indispensable part of the A, B and C antigens

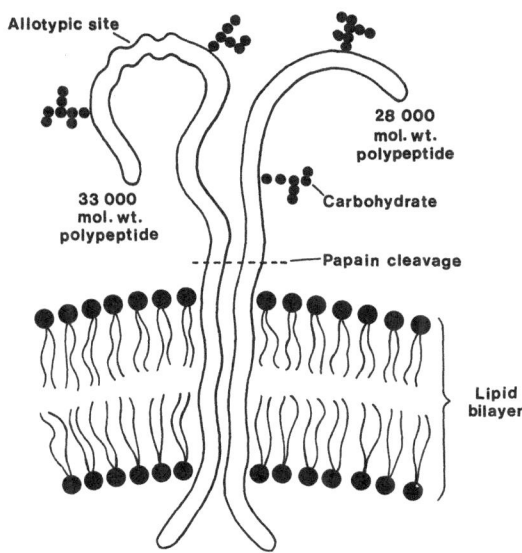

Figure 2.1(b) Proposed structure of HLA-DR$_w$ antigens (after Snary *et al.*[122] with kind permission)

Reactions against some transplantation antigens lead to much faster removal than reactions against others. For reasons which are still obscure, the antigens which provoke the fastest removal of tissue are always under the control of one particular group of closely linked loci, the major histocompatibility loci. This is true of all species so far investigated. In man the major histocompatibility (MHC) loci are the HLA loci of which four (A, B, C and D) have so far been identified. Skin transplant survival time is strongly influenced by all four of these loci[6]. The suggested chemical structure of these antigens is shown in Figure 2.1, and present information on the linkage map of the chromosomal region which controls them is shown in Figure 2.2. As in other organisms, these loci have many alleles. It is therefore very likely that a particular individual will be heterozygous, i.e. will possess two different antigens at any locus, and very unlikely that any two individuals selected at

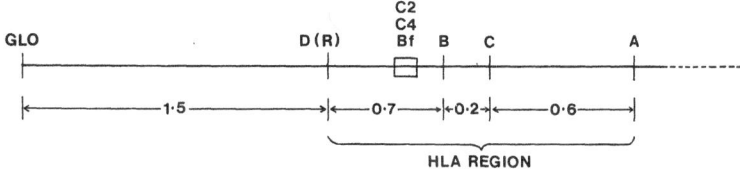

Figure 2.2 The linkage map of the HLA region on chromosome 6. A, B, C, and D represent the HLA loci, C2, C4 and Bf are loci which control the structure of complement proteins, and GLO is the locus for the enzyme glyoxalase

random will possess the same two antigens. It is also unlikely that mother and fetus will have the same HLA types.

The antigens which provoke weaker responses are controlled by gene loci collectively referred to as minor histocompatibility (MIH) loci. In man skin grafts which are ABO compatible (O → O, O → A, etc.) survive longer than ABO-incompatible grafts (A → O, B → O, etc.)[7]. Compatibility at the P-locus may possibly also increase skin graft survival time, but other human blood group systems examined (MN and RhD antigen) do not have any detectable effect. Thus the ABO and possibly the P loci are human MIH loci. No other human MIH loci appear to have been identified[8]. However, by analogy with the mouse many would be expected to exist. In this species there are at least 35 MIH loci. Grafts of mouse skin across an MHC barrier are always rejected within 3 weeks, whereas MHC-compatible grafts across an MIH barrier take at least 3 weeks and some are never rejected at all. Murine grafts of tissues like tumours, ovaries and teeth are not rejected if the only difference is an MIH one. A comprehensive account of the biology of mouse transplantation phenomena may be found in reference 9, while studies on both man and mouse are fully reviewed in reference 10. The fact that kidney transplants in man may be maintained with immunosuppressive agents which leave other parts of the immunological system functional, or in a few cases without immunosuppression (see reference 11 for an example of the latter) suggests that the effects of human MIH loci could also be fairly easily overridden.

While DR_w antigens of the D locus are restricted to B lymphocytes and monocytes[69], the HLA A, B and C antigens in man are found on most but not all tissues[12]. It is therefore clearly of fundamental importance in the present context to establish whether the placenta, and in particular its outermost layer, the syncytiotrophoblast, possesses HLA antigens. A summary of some investigations of this question is shown in Table 2.1.

Superficially the results are conflicting, since some investigations suggest that the HLA antigens are on the trophoblast and others do not. Tumours of trophoblastic origin stimulate the production of HLA antibodies in about 50% of women and five normal pregnancies do so in about 30% of women[10]. HLA antibodies can be eluted from the full-term placenta[2, 13]. However, the inhibition of MLC reactions caused by these placental eluates is non-specific, and cannot be attributed to the specific HLA antibodies they contain[14, 15]. Cells cultured from explants of placental tissue also have HLA antigens[16]. The relation of these cells to the trophoblast *in vivo* is unclear. Since cells which grow readily in culture are usually the most undifferentiated components of the explanted tissue, it is likely that in this case they come from the villous stroma and not from the trophoblast layer itself.

Several other types of data indicate that while HLA antigens are present in the villous stroma, they are absent from, or in much reduced level on, the trophoblast. This was first suggested by the data of Seigler and Metzgar[17], who used goat anti-human immunoglobulin in an attempt to adhere human

Table 2.1 HLA antigens on human trophoblast

References	Technique	Age of trophoblast (No. studied)	Other tissues examined	Antigen present	Evidence and comments
Seigler and Metzgar[17]	mixed agglutination and antibody absorption	weeks to full term (not stated, at least 7)	brain, lung, thymus, spleen stomach, gut, adrenals, kidney, skin, testis, sperm, cells cultured from various organs	no	both techniques showed antigens on all tissues except sperm and syncytiotrophoblast
Loke et al.[16]	cytotoxic tests on cultured trophoblast cells	full term (4)	fetal skin	yes	antisera with HLA specificity killed cultured cells from placenta; relation of these cells to placenta in vivo not known
Faulk et al.[14]	MLC tests in presence of eluates from placenta	full term (20)	thyroid, kidney and lung basal membranes	no	IgG from placenta inhibits MLC reactions non-specifically, i.e. inhibiting factors are not HLA antibodies; IgG was specific for trophoblast basal membrane
Lawler et al.[123]; Lawler[124]	HLA of women with trophoblastic tumours and their husbands	trophoblast tumours of indeterminate age (227)	—	yes	HLA antibodies persist in women bearing these tumours, but seldom in normal women after the end of their pregnancy
Goodfellow et al.[18]	HLA A and B, Ia and β_2 microglobulin levels in plasma membrane assayed by inhibition of fluorochromatic cytotoxicity	full term (6)	spleen lymphocytes, and one lymphoblastoid cell line	small amounts	low levels of antigen (5% that of lymphocytes) found in purified placental plasma membrane
Doughty and Gelsthorpe[13]	antibody specificity of placental eluates	full term (40)	none	yes	HLA antibodies in maternal serum were also usually found in the placental eluates
Faulk and Temple[20]; Faulk et al.[125]	immunohistological tests on cryostat sections of placenta using antisera to β_2 microglobulin, HLA antigens, and Ia antigens; also immunoperoxidase tests	week one (1); 13 weeks (1), and full term (40)	trophoblast, trophoblast basal membrane, cells of villous stroma, and endothelial cells of placental vessels	no	no immunofluorescence for HLA, Ia, or β_2M on trophoblast or trophoblast basal membrane. However HLA and β_2M are found on cells of villous stroma including the vascular endothelium; Ia antigens only seen on occasional monocytes (presumably fetal B cells)
Sundquist* et al.[126]	immunofluorescence	6–13 weeks	—	no	no HLA on trophoblast

* Not seen: information from reference 3

erythrocytes coated with chimpanzee anti-human erythrocyte to trophoblast treated with HLA antibodies. If both red cells and trophoblast were coated with human Ig, mixed agglutination of red cells and trophoblast should have occurred. It did not, although the same technique showed HLA antibodies capable of reacting with many other tissues (Table 2.1). Goodfellow et al.[18] isolated plasma membrane from placenta and measured the level of HLA A and B, Ia and β_2 microglobulin (β_2M). The β_2M protein is found associated with HLA A, B and C antigens and appears to be an indispensable part of their structure[19]. Its level is thus a direct measure of the level of HLA and its absence from any tissue shows that HLA A, B and C are also absent. Goodfellow et al.[18], concluded that HLA A and B were present in a very small amount; 5% or less of the level in most other tissues. Contamination was thought to be an unlikely explanation for the small amounts found, i.e. the HLA antigens are genuinely present. Faulk and his colleagues[2, 20] used a fluorescein-labelled antiserum to β_2M and a similarly labelled antiserum with specificity against HLA-A2 and A28 (one, the other or both of which occur in the European population in about 35% of individuals). They found that syncytiotrophoblast, cytotrophoblast, and basement membrane did not stain, but strong fluorescence was seen over the villous stroma.

In summary, these investigations show that components of the placenta, or tumour tissue derived from it, can stimulate the production of HLA antibodies or interact with them. But when attempts are made to demonstrate HLA antigens on the trophoblast itself, the results are largely negative. Billington[21] has reviewed studies on the mouse H-2 antigens and concluded that 'although . . . the placenta possesses transplantation antigens, there is as yet no unequivocal evidence to implicate the trophoblastic elements'.

A diagram of the probable distribution of HLA antigens in a trophoblast villus is shown in Figure 2.3.

The same rule probably applies to the ABO antigens. Gross[22] claimed to have demonstrated A antigen on the trophoblast, but the results are not convincing. Most workers agree that A, B, and H antigens are either absent[23-26] or sparse[27]. The techniques used have been the immunofluorescent and electron microscope immunoferritin methods of detection of antigens. Goto et al.[26] ruled out the possibility that the antigens were masked by some overlying substance, such as the sialomucin suggested by Currie and Bagshaw[28] for the mouse. They incubated their trophoblast preparations with neuraminidase, chondroitinase, hyaluronidase, trypsin, pepsin, and pronase. None of these digestions revealed any masked antigen. Goto et al.[26] examined material from 10 to 40 weeks of gestation and Szulman from 5 weeks to full term. Thus although immunologically mediated selection appears to operate at the ABO locus[29], it presumably does so by affecting fetal tissues other than the trophoblast, the most likely possibility being haemolytic disease. Caucasian women with trophoblastic tumours have the same distribution of ABO antigens as the control population[30].

While it is desirable to have further data on the actual level of expression of HLA and ABO on the trophoblast, as well as data for other so far unexamined HLA antigens, it seems likely that both HLA and ABO antigens are either absent or sparse in this tissue. If so, the conclusion is straightforward: *the conceptus is not analogous to allografts made across either the MHC barrier or across one at least of the MIH barriers.* It may be that other presently undiscovered alloantigenic systems are expressed on the trophoblast surface.

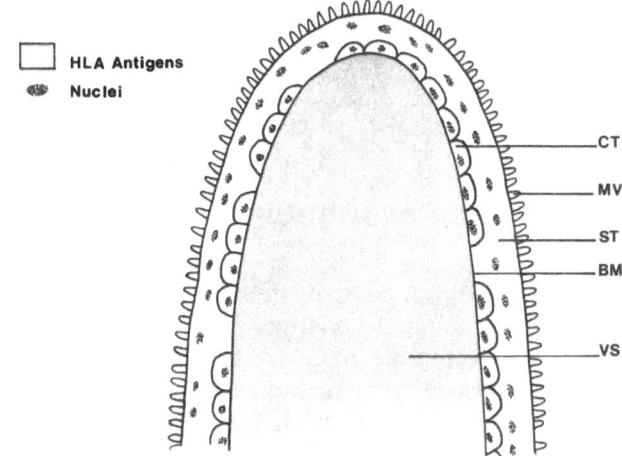

Figure 2.3 Diagram of a human chorionic villus showing the probable distribution of HLA antigens. They are either not present or very sparse on the syncytiotrophoblast (ST), cyto-trophoblast (CT) and basal membrane of the syncytiotrophoblast (BM), but are present on the cells of the villous (= mesenchymal) stroma (VS). The villous stroma contains placental capillaries lined with endothelial cells, fibroblasts, macrophages (Hofbauer cells), and occasional monocytes. Note that the cytotrophoblast or Langhans cells do not form a continuous layer, especially in the mature placenta. The syncytiotrophoblast has the endoplasmic reticulum and Golgi bodies characteristic of a tissue which manufactures and secretes protein. Microvilli (MV) occur on the surface of the trophoblast. The total thickness of the trophoblast varies from 0.025 to 0.002 mm. Data on the distribution of HLA from references given in the text. Data on general structure and properties of the villus from references 117 and 122a

This possibility has been raised by Faulk *et al.*[2] when discussing the maternal immunoglobulin which is found attached to the trophoblast basement membrane. As Faulk *et al.*[2] imply, the identification of the antigens against which the antibody activity of this immunoglobulin is directed is one of the next steps which should be taken in order to understand how the conceptus evades maternal immune rejection. In the meantime, judgment upon the validity of allograft analogy should be reserved.

Specific xenoantigens, i.e. antigens defined by antisera produced in another species such as a rabbit, are found on the membrane of the trophoblast[31, 32] or are produced by trophoblast, e.g. SPI[33]. Faulk *et al.*[32] have defined two classes of antigen: the TA1 group is shared by trophoblast and human cultured cell lines and TA2 by placental blood vessel endothelium, periphereal monocytes, and leukocytes. They suggest that normal human pregnancy involves maternal immune recognition of TA2 antigens and non-recognition of TA1. Failure to recognize TA2 may lead to recognition of TA1, with likely abnormal pregnancy or termination of pregnancy. Implicit in this hypothesis is the notion that the TA2 group has some alloantigenic variation, although direct evidence for this is lacking. Many xenoantigens are of course monotypic within a species. Xenoantigens are useful in order to recognize trophoblast components, but they are not of direct relevance to the immunological problem posed by pregnancy. Alloantigens and their distribution in the placenta are the essence of this problem.

DOES NON-SPECIFIC IMMUNOSUPPRESSION OCCUR IN PREGNANCY?

Allograft survival can be prolonged if the recipient is given immunosuppressive treatment. Does this mean that the survival of the conceptus is also due to immunosuppression in the mother? This implication of the allograft analogy has led to a series of investigations designed to discover pregnancy-specific substances with immunosuppressive properties.

Most of this work has been pursued without taking account of the reservations outlined above concerning the allograft nature of the conceptus. If it is not clear that the trophoblast presents alloantigens for the mother to attack, is it not premature to search for substances in the mother which would prevent this attack?

Notwithstanding this, there are many claims of immunosuppressive substances in pregnancy, and so it is necessary to examine the evidence upon which these are based. The questionable nature of much of the evidence immediately becomes apparent when the several uses of the terms immunosuppression and immunosuppressive agents are spelled out. There are at least three broad classes of biological entities which have been referred to as having immunosuppressive properties.

(1) The original or 'classical' immunosuppressive agents are purine analogues, cortisone and related oxycorticosteroids, high-energy radiation, and anti-lymphocyte serum. These act mainly by preventing division of cells essential for an active immune response or by destroying these cells. All of them used at a sufficient level or intensity will prolong the life of an allograft of skin or other tissue. In other words, they are agents which are immunosuppressive *in vivo*. The general effects of most agents in this class on an organism, apart from their particular ones on its immunological system, are severe and even destructive.

(2) As suggested by Gershon[34], there is a class of T lymphocytes which will prevent or prematurely terminate certain immune responses. They are called suppressor T cells. Two biological functions have been attributed to them[35]. Some suppressor T lymphocytes appear to be involved in the mechanism for switching off an immune response once it has reached a certain level. Others may hold in check clones of cells which would otherwise attack self-antigens. Both antigen-specific suppressor T cells and suppressor T cells with more generalized suppressive effects have been described[36]. There is no doubt that these cells act as immuno-suppressive agents *in vivo*. Unlike the original agents described in (1) there is no evidence that they drastically effect the cells involved in the active immune response. Their presence and activities are assumed to be normal and indeed essential components of a properly functioning immune system.

(3) The term has been extended to a heterogeneous collection of agents which will modify one or more of several immunological tests, such as the mixed lymphocyte reaction (MLR), the mitogen-induced division of lymphocytes, or the rosette inhibition test (Table 2.2). With the exception of steroids such as cortisone, there is little if any direct evidence that these agents do in fact have an immunosuppressive effect *in vivo*. That is, they are immunosuppressive only in the restricted sense that they can modify or inhibit an immunological test *in vitro*. When the term is used in reproductive biology, and particularly when the relationship between mother and conceptus is under discussion, it is usually in this sense.

Table 2.2 Some postulated agents of 'pregnancy immunosuppression'

(a) *Proteins*
  Alpha-fetoprotein (AFP)
  Chorionic gonadotrophin (HCG)
  Pregnancy-associated α_2-glycoprotein (α_2 PAG)
  Early pregnancy factor (EPF)
  Pregnancy-specific β_1-glycoprotein (SP1)[a]
  Somatomammotrophin = placental lactogen[b]
  Placental transcortin[c]

(b) *Steroids*
  Cortisol
  Progesterone and other sex steroids

(c) *Fluids with several or many components*
  Pregnancy serum (blocking factors)[d]
  Placental eluates (contain maternal and fetal immunoglobulins)[e]

[a] Not dealt with in text: see Horne *et al.*[33].
[b] Not dealt with in text: see Contractor and Davies[126a].
[c] Not dealt with in text: see Werthamen *et al.*[127].
[d] Not dealt with in text: see Bernard[128].
[e] Not dealt with in text: see Revillard *et al.*[129]; and Faulk *et al.*[14].

It is obvious that the three usages of the term are very different, and that there is some danger that, for example, the attributes of the agents in (1) may, without justification, be ascribed to the agents in (3). In what follows, the term 'pregnancy immunosuppression' will be used to refer collectively to the effects of the agents in (3). The inverted commas are meant to convey scepticism concerning the reality of the phenomenon. Pregnancy undoubtedly has many observable effects upon the immune system, but whether these amount to suppression in a proper biological sense is doubtful.

The data advanced in support of the hypothesis of 'pregnancy immuno-suppression' are necessarily circumstantial for each of the agents in Table 2.2. Moreover there is a great deal of disagreement. It is not possible here to review all the literature on the agents in Table 2.2; the discussion below is to illustrate the general nature of the evidence. A more detailed summary may be found in reference 3.

Alpha-fetoprotein (AFP)

Most of the general problems in assessing the biological reality of effects of proteins upon the immune system in pregnancy may conveniently be delineated using AFP as an example. The bulk of the evidence upon the immunosuppressive properties of this protein comes from studies on labora-tory rodents (see reference 37 for a recent review). Its effects are mainly on T cells. Apart from its suggested immunosuppressive role, the function of this protein is not known. In humans and other mammals it exists in high concentrations in fetal plasma but is in ng/ml quantities in adults. The maternal plasma level rises progressively during pregnancy. Increased levels in amniotic fluid indicate a neural tube defect[38].

Because several previous studies had indicated an immunosuppressive role for human AFP, Murgita et al.[39] examined its effect upon human lymphocyte cultures stimulated with a B-cell mitogen (protein A released by a particular Staphylococcus aureus strain), upon a T-cell mitogen (PHA), and upon the one-way MLR test, in which the response of one of the two allogeneic cells is prevented by prior irradiation. PHA responses were inhibited in the range 18–300 µg/ml in a dose-dependent manner. However, AFP preparations varied in their potency and one was inactive. Yachnin and Lester[40] have also found that hepatoma-derived AFP was less inhibitory in the PHA test than fetal-derived AFP. Figueredo et al.[41] were unable to find a consistent cor-relation between AFP levels and PHA-stimulated cell growth for cultured lymphocytes from pregnant women. Murgita et al.[39] found that MLR responses were inhibited by 300–600 µg/ml levels, a result also obtained by Muchmore and Blaese[42]. Charpentier et al.[43], however, observed augmen-tation of MLR responses by AFP.

The levels found in the plasma of pregnant women are in the range 18–550 ng/ml[44] while for newborn infants the range is 100–600 µg/ml, with the upper values being for premature infants[45]. Thus the observed inhibition of T-cell reactivity may perhaps take place in fetal blood, but not in the mothers'.

Murgita *et al.*[39] found that the response to protein A was unaffected by AFP level, in keeping with the mouse data showing no effect upon B-cell responses.

The inconsistency of the results from preparation to preparation suggests that contaminants may play a part in the observed inhibition, as has now been found for different HCG preparations (see below). Moreover it is not clear how the *in vitro* inhibition relates to the biological *in vivo* function of the protein. Certainly some genuine immunosuppressive agents inhibit MLR or PHA tests; but it does not follow that all agents which affect these tests are necessarily immunosuppressive. They may simply exert a rather non-specific effect upon cell growth in general, an effect made possible only because the cells are growing in the sub-optimal conditions provided by the standard methods of culture in which cell density, control of pH, and ionic, nutrient, and metabolite concentrations are very far from those within the organism. Cell growth in culture is notoriously sensitive to a number of factors, such as batch of serum or medium, and others which are less well-defined. Some understanding of the specificity of the inhibitory effects of the agents in Table 2.2 would be obtained by a study of their effect upon the growth of a broader range of cell type than is customary.

Chorionic gonadotrophin (HCG)

This protein is dealt with elsewhere in this volume. Here it is sufficient to note that immunosuppressive properties have often been attributed to it (see references 3 and 46 for reviews). The validity of these suggestions has been called in question by the demonstration by Muchmore and Blaese[42] that the inhibitors of PHA responses, one-way MLR responses, and responses to streptolysin-O can be dialysed away from commercial preparations of HCG usually used to investigate the question. They suggest that this contaminant, which was not characterized, had ideal immunosuppressive properties, since it was non-toxic, and had reversible activity at low concentrations which operated over a broad range of cellular immune functions.

Pregnancy associated α_2-glycoprotein (α_2PAG) $\equiv$ pregnancy zone protein (PZP) and several other synonyms

This protein occurs in the serum of pregnant women and women taking oestrogen-containing oral contraceptives. The range varies from 0.5 to $2\,\mu g/ml$. Its increased production in pregnancy appears to be induced by oestrogen; in non-pregnant individuals it occurs in much lower concentrations ($10–20\,ng/ml$). Work on it has been comprehensively reviewed by Horne *et al.*[47]. Like AFP and HCG, its presence inhibits the response of lymphocytes to PHA[48–50]. Stimson[50] also found it inhibited responses to other

T-cell mitogens (concanavalin A, allogeneic cells and tuberculin), but was less effective in inhibiting the response to lipopolysaccharide and goat anti-human $F(ab')_2$ serum, both B-cell stimulators. It thus resembles AFP and EPF (see below) in seeming to affect cell-mediated immunity rather than the humoural component.

Early pregnancy factor (EPF) ≡ inhibitor of E-rosette formation

If sheep red blood cells (SRBC) are mixed with human lymphocytes, some of the lymphocytes bind the SRBC. This creates a flower-like structure, called a rosette. In the absence of any other agent, SRBC bind specifically to T cells, creating what are called E rosettes. Antilymphocyte serum (ALS) will block the formation of these rosettes at quite high titres. Morton et al.[51] have observed that lymphocytes from pregnant women fail to form rosettes at even higher titres of ALS than do lymphocytes from other people. The factor responsible for this behaviour is found in the serum, since incubation in pregnancy serum causes lymphocytes from non-pregnant individuals to behave in the same way as pregnancy lymphocytes. Morton et al.[51] have attributed immunosuppressive properties to this serum factor and proposed that it is necessary for continued viability of the early embryo. Its level declines in the third trimester.

A similar factor or possibly factors is found in pregnant mice[52, 53] and in pregnant sheep[54]. Indirect evidence for its immunosuppressive nature has been obtained for mice[55].

While ALS is undoubtedly immunosuppressive in a biological sense it is not necessarily true that an agent which enhances its capacity to block rosette formation is also biologically immunosuppressive. It also appears that only a minority of ALS preparations interact with EPF. Cooper and Aitken[56] tested 12 different antisera and did not find any difference between pregnancy sera and other sera in their capacity to enhance the inhibition of rosette formation.

The protein nature of mouse EPF is suggested because of its heat lability at 72 °C[52].

Cortisone

Corticosteroids can have inhibitory effects on lymphocytes *in vivo* and *in vitro*[57, 58]. They are used routinely to promote acceptance of kidney grafts. Since the level of cortisol increases markedly in pregnancy, it is natural to ask whether this leads to 'pregnancy immunosuppression'. Kasakura[59] measured cortisol levels in pregnancy plasma and the degree to which these plasmas inhibited the MLC reaction. He found no correlation. Human peripheral lymphocytes are not easily killed by high cortisol levels, unlike mouse lymphocytes[57]. Mendolsohn et al.[58] found that *in vitro* suppression of responses of human lymphocytes to PHA and concanavalin A, caused by high levels of cortisol, could be reversed by removing the hormone from the medium. These results make it unlikely that cortisol has an *in vivo* suppressive effect in human pregnancy.

Progesterone and other sex steroids

This steroid reaches levels in the plasma of 50 ng/ml in the 20th–30th week of pregnancy and 120 ng/ml at 36 weeks. These values understate the production of hormone by the placenta, since 90% of blood progesterone is removed by the liver within 25 min of entry[60]. It is sometimes suggested that progesterone is immunosuppressive[61]. Attempts to test this hypothesis have produced conflicting results. Early investigations produced no evidence of prolonged skin graft survival in mice and rabbits[62, 63] while later investigations found the reverse[64–66]. A very recent investigation has found no evidence of prolonged survival of skin grafts in rabbits using doses up to 200 mg three times weekly[67].

Studies of the effect of progesterone and other steroids on responses to PHA and other mitogens do not support the hypothesis. Schiff *et al.*[68] and Mendolsohn *et al.*[58] did not find any consistent effects upon cell division by oestrogen, oestradiol, progesterone and testerone below levels of 10 μm (approximately 3 μg/ml–3000 ng/ml), far higher than the levels which occur in pregnancy. However, as Mendolsohn *et al.*[58] point out, there is so far no information upon possible synergistic effects of steroid hormones on the immune system in pregnancy.

That steroid hormones at physiological concentrations do affect the immune system in a significant manner is suggested by the results of Mathur *et al.*[70]. They studied the effects of progesterone and oestradiol titres of antibodies to *Candida albicans* in normal females, females with gonadal dysgenesis, females using oral contraceptives, and normal males. Normal females were studied in the luteal and follicular phases of the menstrual cycle. Their results suggested that production of antibodies was positively correlated with progesterone and oestradiol levels at low concentrations. However, higher concentrations of oestradiol were correlated with reduced antibody titre. The antibodies studied were predominantly IgA, i.e. secretory antibodies.

Other evidence

The large number of agents which have been invoked as possible 'pregnancy immunosuppressants' is confusing. Clearly not all of them can really have such an effect. If they did, one would wonder how a pregnant woman had any immune capacity at all! The ability of the various *in vitro* tests used to detect *specific* effects upon the immune system, rather than more general effects upon cells *in vitro*, is called in question. Alternative ways of testing the hypothesis of 'pregnancy immunosuppression' are necessary. Comparative data upon the ability of pregnant and non-pregnant women to respond to infectious agents and other antigenic material offer a more direct way of assessing the biological reality of 'pregnancy immunosuppression'. There seem to be at least four main sources of these data.

(1) Llewellyn-Jones[71] states that pregnant women are not more susceptible to infectious disease than non-pregnant women. There is however a suggestion that some viral diseases may be more common in pregnant women[72]. Some of the evidence for this appears to depend upon acceptance of the questionable assertion that pregnancy depresses cell-mediated immunity. The epidemiological evidence concerns polio-myelitis which in epidemic years between 1940 and 1950 affected pregnant women more frequently than would be expected on a chance basis[73–75]. Buck and Hasenclever[76] have shown that *Candida albicans* chronic infection may be more common in pregnancy.

(2) The abilities of pregnant and non-pregnant women to make humoral responses to alloantigens can be compared in a crude way. Table 2.3 summarizes some data on the immunological responsiveness of pregnant women compared to other people for the three classes of alloantigens: HLA, Rhesus, and Gm immunoglobulins. The pregnant women have been immunized solely by their conceptuses, whereas the others have been immunized by deliberate injection or transfusion. The latter are probably more efficient routes for provoking immune responses; indeed it is unclear how many of the pregnant women are challenged by these antigens in pregnancy. Allowing for this, there seems to be little suggestion that the proportions of women responding to HLA or Rhesus are diminished by pregnancy. Far fewer pregnant women develop Gm antibodies than do individuals transfused more than once, but this difference is plausibly ascribed to the differences in the amount and frequency of antigen administration.

Besides the three classes of antigen referred to in Table 3, some pregnant women also respond to non-HLA antigen on the white cells of their fetuses[77, 78].

(3) The transplacental transfer of maternal immunoglobulin to the neonate is another indication that the humoral arm of the immune response is largely intact in late pregnancy at least, given that this transfer confers such efficacious passive protection.

(4) Cell-mediated immunity (CMI) in pregnant women has been the subject of fewer investigations. Maternal CMI against fetal antigens in humans can be demonstrated. The macrophage migration-inhibition test indicates CMI against placental antigens[79] and paternal lymphocytes[80] during the course of pregnancy. Timonen and Saksela[81] have shown CMI cytotoxicity against fetal lung cells in pregnancies from 15

Table 2.3 Immunization of women by conceptuses or trophoblastic tumours compared with immunization of non-pregnant individuals

Nature of immunogen and route of injection	No. of challenges	Percentage of challenged individuals responding	Effect on fetus	Reference
Rhesus				
Red cells from Rh-positive fetus which is ABO-compatible with mother: transplacental passage	2 pregnancies	17% of Rh-negative women respond	haemolytic disease	Woodrow[130]
Red cells from Rh-positive fetus: transplacental passage	6 pregnancies	33% of Rh-negative women respond	haemolytic disease	Clemens and Walsh[131]
Deliberate injection of Rh-positive cells into Rh-negative male volunteers	7–9 intravenous injections[a]	37% 'high' responders 26% 'low' responders 37% 'non' responders	n.a.	Tovey (cited by Tovey and Maroni[88])
HLA				
Presumably trophoblast liberated into maternal circulation	5 pregnancies	30% develop cytotoxic HLA antibodies	none	Vives (cited by Snell *et al.*[10], Figure 9.1)
Trophoblast liberated from tropho-blastic tumours	indeterminate: age of tumour usually unknown	50% develop lymphocytotoxins	no apparent effect on tumour	Lawler[124]
Blood transfusion	5 transfusions	13% develop lymphocytotoxins	n.a.	Opelz *et al.*[132]
Blood transfusion	26–30 transfusions	46% develop lymphocytotoxins	n.a.	Opelz *et al.*[132]
Immunoglobulin antigens				
Blood transfusions with Gm antigens	3–40 transfusions	71% develop Gm antibodies	n.a.	Allen and Kunkel[133]
Gm antigens: transplacental	not stated; data on 1763 white, Puerto Rican and black women	1.6% develop Gm antibodies	none	Nathenson *et al.*[134]

[a] Estimated from indirect information in the reference
n.a. = not applicable

to 23 weeks. Oddly enough they could not demonstrate CMI against cultured amnion cells when the effector cells of mothers at full term were used. No explanation for this finding was obvious and the interval from 23 weeks to full term was not examined, presumably for the lack of experimental material. While no comparison with non-pregnant individuals is possible, the results obtained in these investigations show at the very least that there is no gross impairment of CMI in pregnancy.

Andresen and Monroe[82] carried out reciprocal skin transplants between two pregnant women and two non-pregnant individuals. One of these pregnant women was challenged with a second transplant in a later pregnancy. The results obtained suggested that rejection of skin grafts may be slower in pregnancy, but the small number of subjects involved makes firm assessment difficult.

It is not surprising that maternal humoral and cellular responses should be made against the conceptus because both trophoblast[83, 84]; and fetal lymphocytes[85–87]; enter the circulation of at least some mothers.

In simple Darwinian terms, immunosuppression which affects the immune system of a pregnant mammal in any general way is an unlikely idea. Mammals are a highly successful group with good defences against viral and bacterial disease. Any female mammal which chose the time of reproduction to lower these defences would be at a strong selective disadvantage compared to another of the same species which employed a different method of protecting her conceptus. Likewise any male which contributed genes to the conceptus which caused it to produce immunosuppressive substances affecting the mother would also be at a strong selective disadvantage. Prevention of attack against alloantigens only, i.e. antigen-specific immunosuppression, is a much more plausible hypothesis.

The seriousness with which the possibility of generalized 'pregnancy immunosuppression' has been taken is a tribute to the extent to which the allograft analogy has dominated thinking on the subject. That it has not been possible to test the idea fully is a consequence of a basic difference between an allograft and a pregnancy as experimental systems. The former is far more manipulable. An allograft usually fails, but this failure can be prevented. A pregnancy usually succeeds, and it cannot be terminated in a way which gives insight into the immunological problem. It is possible to demonstrate the immunosuppressive properties of various agents by showing that their administration to the recipient of the graft prevents rejection. It is not possible to remove any of the agents listed in Table 2 from an otherwise normally pregnant female in order to see whether or not this leads to the immune rejection of the conceptus. By correlating the behaviour of a transplant and an *in vitro* immunological test, it is possible to assess the usefulness of the latter for predicting the fate of the former. Inability to terminate a pregnancy immunologically in the same way as is possible for an allograft prevents evaluation of the relevance of these tests for assessing the biological integrity of the immune system in pregnancy, or of the ability of various agents to impair this integrity. This inability to manipulate a pregnancy as easily as an allograft is the largest single barrier to further understanding of the immunology of pregnancy. It has also helped to conceal the fact that they are two rather different phenomena.

IS PRE-ECLAMPSIA A GENETICALLY DETERMINED FAILURE OF PREGNANCY IMMUNOSUPPRESSION?

Some understanding of the processes which lead to normal development can often be obtained by examining inherited abnormalities of development. It is therefore worthwhile to ask whether there are any inherited conditions in which the mother's immunological system attacks the conceptus. The blood group incompatibilities are well-known examples. They usually involve the passive transfer of IgG at or near term with subsequent effects upon the neonate. Until the widespread use of prophylactic doses of anti-D, Rhesus incompatibility was particularly frequent and severe because (1) the D antigen is highly immunogenic; (2) the antibodies produced against it are often high-titre IgG which will cross the placenta; and (3) the D antigen is entirely confined to the red cell[88]. These three factors combined lead to massive red-cell breakdown. The existence of the D/d polymorphism in human populations in the face of the strong selection against it has never been satisfactorily explained. It is a clear example of the selective cost which mammalian viviparity imposes; presumably the losses from maternal–fetal blood group incompatibility are outweighed in the long term by the immunological protection which the passive transfer of maternal immunoglobulin confers upon the neonate.

But while the blood group incompatibilities show that mammalian viviparity does sometimes lead to an immunologically based selective disadvantage for some alloantigens, they do not help a great deal in understanding how other tissues of the conceptus, particularly the placenta, evade the mother's immune system. In this respect, a potentially more informative condition is severe pre-eclampsia, also known as pregnancy-induced hypertension, pregnancy toxaemia, or gestosis. Clinically the most obvious manifestations are high blood pressure, oedema, and proteinuria, all occurring in the last trimester. A minority of cases may proceed to eclamptic fitting, hence the name pre-eclampsia. Fortunately, modern obstetric management makes this a very rare event. Many theories have been put forward to explain this condition[89]. The family data suggest that susceptibility is largely if not wholly inherited, with environmental influences being minor[90]. These data are compatible with a recessive mode of inheritance, although whether the genes act through the mother herself, through her fetus, or in both together, is not entirely clear. Further family data collected by Sutherland (personal communication) implicates the maternal genotype more strongly than the fetal. In the remainder of this discussion, I shall assume the correctness of the hypothesis that the condition is the result of a homozygosity for a recessive gene acting in the mother.

Recessive inheritance usually implies defective or absent gene product, in this case in some part of the immunological system. The evidence which suggests an immunological basis has been reviewed several times recently (see references 91, 92 and see Chapter 4 [Redman] in this volume). In brief, immunofluorescent studies of placental bed vessels suggest that they may have suffered immune attack[93]. The kidney lesions typical of pre-eclampsia could be due either to disseminated intravascular coagulation precipitated by an immunological reaction against placental antigens[94,95] or to a direct auto-immune reaction against the kidney[96,97] which shares antigens with the placenta[98]. Pathological states resembling pre-eclampsia may be induced in experimental animals by the passive administration of anti-placental serum[99].

Table 2.4 Incidence of pre-eclampsia in a series of 2872 women in their first and second pregnancies (data of Macgillivray[102])

Grade	First pregnancy		Second pregnancy	
	No.	*Percentage*	*No.*	*Percentage*
Severe	161	5.8	11	0.4
Mild	476	18.4	218	7.6
No pre-eclampsia	2235	75.7	2643	92.0

Jenkins *et al.*[100] have shown increased HLA antigen sharing and Redman *et al.*[101] have shown that homozygosity at the HLA B locus is more frequent in affected women and their spouses. The interpretation of these findings is difficult. One possibility suggested by Redman *et al.*[101] is that maternal immune response (*Ir*) genes are involved. Such genes have been found linked to the murine MHC locus, H-2. Given the apparent homology between mouse H-2 and human HLA, it may be assumed that Ir genes are also linked to HLA, but direct proof of this is lacking. Ir genes control the ability to respond, or failure to respond, to particular immunogens, with ability to respond being dominant.

If there is a maternal immune attack against the placenta and the maternal kidney, it is a seeming paradox that the condition should occur so much more frequently in first pregnancy, as opposed to later pregnancies. The dramatic nature of this drop in frequency of occurrence is shown in Table 2.4. Macgillivray[102] spoke of 'immunization' against pre-eclampsia through experience of first pregnancy. Recent work in mice suggests that his suggestion may indeed resolve the paradox[103]. In these experiments mice injected with rat red cells developed an autoimmune haemolytic anaemia which in normal strains eventually disappeared[104]. A secondary challenge resulted in an accelerated disappearance of autoantibody, even while heteroantibody to rat-specific antigens continued to rise in titre. Thus repeated immunization resulted in the suppression rather than the enhancement of the autoimmune response. Transfer of suppressor T cells from the spleen of immunized mice to syngeneic mice caused significant suppression of autoantibody production after the first challenge, but did not affect production of heteroantibody. Suppression could not be effectively induced in NZB × BALB/C mice which have a genetically determined tendency to develop autoimmune anaemia. The repressive response in this system is analogous to a classical rejection response. Both have memory and specificity for particular antigens, and there are genetically determined differences in the capacity to respond (rejection or repression of rejection). The results obtained also support the hypothesis that one function of suppressor cells is to hold in check 'forbidden clones' of lymphocytes capable of responding against self-antigens.

This mouse autoimmune anaemia parallels pre-eclampsia in being less severe with each exposure to the antigen which elicits the disease, and it offers a framework in which to consider possible immunogenetic bases for pre-eclampsia. Two are outlined here:

(1) The primary lesion in pre-eclampsia may lie in altered suppressor T cells which, because of a defective component, are unable to respond quickly enough to a first challenge of placental antigen, although they function effectively in most later pregnancies. The antigens involved are presumed to be very common in the population, and some at least not confined to the placenta within the individual. Reaction against them normally does not occur because of the T suppressor cells rather than because the appropriate clone of lymphocytes is absent. The defective suppressor cells are unable to cope with the extra antigen in pregnancy and so an immune attack on the placenta may occur. The kidney lesion may also be the result of an autoimmune attack, or the result of the deposition of immune complexes, or even both. Severity of pre-eclampsia would depend upon the number and nature of the antigens to which the mother is responding. The occasional observation of severe pre-eclampsia in a second pregnancy when the first has been by a different father may be because a strongly immunogenic antigen was encountered for the first time in the second pregnancy.

(2) The second possibility is that individuals with the putative genotype are unable to make enough blocking antibody in their first pregnancy to prevent attack upon the placenta by other components of the immunological system[105] (see Figure 2.4). Their secondary response in later pregnancies would usually be adequate. This hypothesis also accounts

for the decline in incidence after the first pregnancy. Faulk *et al.*[32] have put forward a more complicated version of this hypothesis. Billington[21] has suggested that low levels of antigen expression may favour the production of blocking antibody.

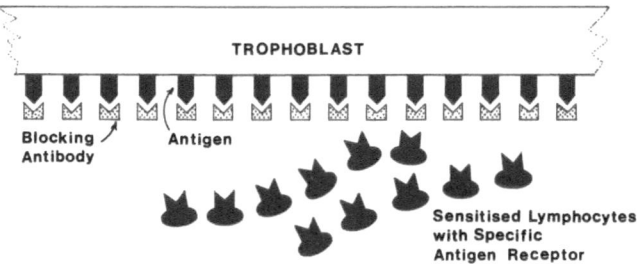

Figure 2.4   Illustration of the mechanism by which blocking antibodies prevent the attack of sensitized lymphocytes (immunological enhancement)

Clearly, investigations designed to examine T-suppressor cell activity and other agents such as blocking antibody in pre-eclampsia may be fruitful not only in understanding the cause of the disease itself, but also in understanding how the conceptus evades the maternal immunological system in the latter part of normal pregnancy.

HOW DOES THE CONCEPTUS SURVIVE ATTACK BY PASSIVELY TRANSFERRED ANTIBODIES?

At least 30% of multiparous mothers develop HLA antibodies (summarized in reference 10; see also reference 106). About 20% of the offspring of immunized mothers have HLA antibodies in their cord sera[107]. Nonetheless the fetus appears to be unaffected; no deleterious effects have been ascribed to HLA antibodies, despite much searching[108, 109]. Doughty and Gelsthorpe[13, 106] have studied the maternal and neonatal HLA types and the HLA antibodies in maternal sera, neonatal sera, and placental eluates in a large series of mother–offspring combinations. They conclude that:

'Where a foetus possesses an antigen to a maternal lymphocytotoxic antibody, antibody can be detected in the placental eluate, but not in the neonatal serum, and conversely where the foetus lacks an antigen to maternal antibodies, antibody is not found in the eluate, but in the neonatal serum'[106].

Similar results have been obtained by Tongio *et al.*[110]. Together these results constitute an elegant demonstration of the validity of the hypothesis that the placenta acts as an immunoadsorbent, filtering out at least some of the HLA ntibodies which might otherwise attack other components of the fetus. The nouse placenta appears to act in the same way[111]. How the placenta itself, or nore particularly the cells of the villous stroma, are able to combine with these ntibodies and yet continue to survive and proliferate, has not been decided. There are, however, some possibilities.

Doughty and Gelsthorpe[106] suggest that 'antibody/antigen complexes are removed from the placental surface once combination has taken place'. They nvoke the hypothesis of 'escape from sensitization' put forward by Miyajima *t al.*[112]. These authors observed that human lymphocytes sensitized with HLA antibodies could not be killed if addition of complement was delayed, .e. did not place until 1 h or more after addition of the HLA antisera. They suggested that active release or pinocytosis of HLA antigens with attached antibody was responsible. The evidence for this is the inability of the cells treated with antibiotics which inhibit protein synthesis to escape from sensitization. Cells which have escaped from sensitization can be readily resensitized with antibody and killed by immediate addition of complement.

The results of Tiilikainen *et al.*[113] are of interest here. They found that fetal lymphocytes from cord blood expressed the maternally derived HLA antigen normally, but that the paternally derived antigen was often difficult to demonstrate. Overnight incubation in tissue culture medium restored the paternally derived antigen to normal levels. Moreover antibodies to paternal antigens were not cytotoxic unless the cord cells had been incubated. Fetal plasma possesses all complement components from the 18th week of pregnancy (reviewed in reference 114). Hence 'escape from sensitization' is presumably not the mechanism by which fetal lymphocytes reduce their level of paternally derived antigen, unless fetal white cells are able to release an anticomplement factor. Since blood cells would be the first fetal component to encounter HLA antibodies which escaped the filtering action of the placenta, it may be that the reduced expression of the paternally derived antigen on white cells, however accomplished, is a secondary defence mechanism.

A somewhat different suggestion has been made by Wild[115] who has discussed the way in which immunoglobulin is transferred into and across the placenta. This is an active and selective process, which may involve attachment of the Fc portion of the immunoglobulin to structures called coated vesicles, which are seen in electron micrographs. These vesicles are abundant at the surface of human syncytiotrophoblast[116, 117]. Attachment of Fc portion to the coated vesicle would prevent or hinder binding of the Fab portion to its target cell[118]. If Fc binding were greater than Fab binding within the placenta, potentially injurious antibody would be kept to a minimum. This proposed mechanism would affect all immunoglobulin and would not by itself account for selective filtering of HLA antibodies demonstrated by Doughty and Gelsthorpe[13, 106] or Tongio *et al.*[110].

In addition to the well-known blood group incompatibilities, non-HLA antibodies to white cells are the cause of some infrequent deleterious conditions. Neonatal purpura has been attributed to rare antibodies against platelet antigens of the P1^A and P1^E systems[119]. Neutropenia is caused by rare anti-neutrophil antibodies in the NA and NB system[120]. These platelet and neutrophil antigens presumably resemble the Rhesus antigens in being confined to a particular cell type. The transfer of a small amount of antibody directed against them therefore interferes with a specific fetal function. Given the virtual ubiquity of the HLA antigens and the filtering action of the placenta, a much higher titre of HLA would have to be present in the maternal plasma to cause significant effects in the fetus.

SUMMARY AND FURTHER WORK

In man, the placenta is not an allograft in the same sense as a piece of skin or kidney transplanted to another allogeneic individual. The rejection of these tissues occurs largely because of their major histocompatibility antigens, which are either sparse or not present on the trophoblastic surface of the placenta. The almost ritual repetition of the formula 'the fetus is an allograft', which usually begins discussion of maternal–fetal immunological relationships, is now becoming a barrier rather than an aid to understanding.

Much effort has been expended upon searching for substances which inhibit the immune system in a pregnant woman in order to allow her to accept her 'allograft'. Since alloantigens have not been demonstrated on the human trophoblast surface, this search is premature. It has produced a list of substances which will interfere with various *in vitro* tests commonly used in immunology. These substances have been called immunosuppressant. This extension of the use of a term which was originally applied to other agents which unquestionably act as immunosuppressants *in vivo* has still to be justified. Pregnancy undoubtedly modifies the maternal immune system; however, the notion implied in much of this work is that it suppressed in a generalized way and this is unappealing from a basic Darwinian point of view.

The principal question now to be answered is whether there are any immunogenic alloantigens expressed on the surface of the trophoblast. If there are, it will be necessary to show how they evade maternal attack. If there are not, a part of the immunological puzzle posed by pregnancy will be answered by the hypothesis of antigenic neutrality. It is certainly a tall order to investigate the genetic control of antigens of a tissue like the trophoblast, because family data can only be accumulated very slowly. If it could be shown that the putative trophoblast alloantigenic system were expressed on another tissue, this difficulty would be overcome. A promising inherited condition with which to begin is pregnancy toxaemia, which seems to have an immunological basis.

Although the trophoblast may act as a barrier which cannot be attacked immunologically, antibodies can cross it. The HLA antibodies which are

:ommonly produced in pregnancy enter the placenta. If the placenta has the :orresponding antigen, these antibodies are trapped and go no further. How he cells of the trophoblastic villous stroma which bear the antigens evade mmunological damage in this circumstance is not clear. Further work is 1eeded to understand the mechanism involved.

References

1. Medawar, P. B. (1953). Some immunological and endocrinological problems raised by the evolution of viviparity in vertebrates, *Symp. Soc. Exp. Biol.*, **7**, 320
2. Faulk, W. P., Sanderson, A. R. and Temple, A. (1977). Distribution of MHC antigens in human placental chorionic villi. *Transplant. Proc.* **9**, 1379
3. Loke, Y. W. (1978). *Immunology and Immunopathology of the Human Foetal–Maternal Interaction.* (Amsterdam, New York and Oxford: Elsevier/North Holland Biomedical Press)
4. Scott, J. S. and Jones, W. R. (eds.) (1976). *Immunology of Human Reproduction.* (London: Academic Press)
5. Boettcher, B. (ed.) (1978). *Immunological Influence on Human Fertility.* (Sydney, Australia: Academic Press)
6. Dausset, J., Contu, L., Legrand, L., Marcelli-Barge, A., Meo, T. and Rapaport, F. L. (1979). Role of Ia-like products of the main histocompatibility complex in conditioning skin allograft survival in man. *J. Clin. Invest.*, **63**, 893
7. Cepellini, R., Curtoni, E. S., Mattiuz, P. L., Leigheb, G., Viselti, M. and Colombi, A. (1966). Survival of test skin grafts in man: effect of genetic relationship and of blood group incompatibility. *Ann. N.Y. Acad. Sci.*, **129**, 421
8. Kissmeyer-Nielsen, F. and Thorsby, E. (1969). Human transplantation antigens. *Transplant Rev.*, **4**, 11
9. Klein, J. (1975). *Biology of the Mouse Histocompatibility-2 Complex.* (Berlin, Heidelberg and New York: Springer-Verlag.)
10. Snell, G. D., Dausset, J. and Nathenson, S. (1976). *Histocompatibility.* (New York: Academic Press)
11. Naik, R. B., Abdeen, H., English, J., Chabrakorty, J., Slapak, M. and Lee, H. A. (1979). Prednisolone withdrawal after 2 years in renal transplant patients receiving only this form of immunosuppression. *Transplant. Proc.*, **11**, 39
12. Berah, M., Hors, J. and Dausset, J. (1970). A study of HL-A antigens in human organs. *Transplantation*, **9**, 185
13. Doughty, R. W. and Gelsthorpe, K. (1976). Some parameters of lymphocyte antibody activity through pregnancy and further eluates of placental material. *Tissue Antigens*, **8**, 43
14. Faulk, W. P., Jeannet, M., Creighton, W. D. and Carbonara, A. (1974). Immunological studies of the human placenta: characterization of immunoglobulins on trophoblastic basement membrane. *J. Clin. Invest.*, **54**, 1011
15. Jeannet, M., Werner, Ch., Ramirez, E., Vassalli, P. and Faulk, W. P. (1977). Anti-HLA, anti-human 'Ia-like' and MLC blocking activity of human placental IgG. *Transplant. Proc.*, **9**, 1417
16. Loke, Y. W., Joysey, V. C. and Borland, R. (1971). HL-A antigens on human trophoblast cells. *Nature (London)*, **232**, 403
17. Seigler, H. F. and Metzgar, R. S. (1970). Embryonic development of human transplantation antigens. *Transplantation*, **9**, 478
18. Goodfellow, P. N., Barnstaple, C. J., Bodmer, W. F., Snary, D. and Crumpton, M. J. (1976). Expression of HLA system antigens on placenta. *Transplantation*, **22**, 595

19. Nilsson, K., Evrin, P. E. and Welsh, K. I. (1974). Production of β_2-microglobulin by normal and malignant human cell lines and peripheral lymphocytes. *Transplant. Rev.*, **21**, 53

20. Faulk, W. P. and Temple, A. (1976). Distribution of β_2-microglobulin and HLA in chorionic villi of human placentae. *Nature (London)*, **262**, 799

21. Billington, W. D. (1976). The immunobiology of trophoblast. In Scott, J. S. and Jones, W. R. (eds.) *Immunology of Human Reproduction*. (London: Academic Press; New York: Grune & Stratton)

22. Gross, S. J. (1966). Human blood group A substance in human endometrium and trophoblast localised by chromatographed rabbit antiserum. *Am. J. Obstet. Gynecol.*, **95**, 1149

23. Witebsky, E. and Reich, H. (1932). Zur gruppenspezifischen differenzierung der placenta-organe. *Klin. Wochenschr.*, **11**, 1960

24. Thiede, H. A., Choate, J. W., Gardner, H. H. and Santay, H. (1965). Immunofluorescent examination of the human chorionic villus for blood group A and B substance. *J. Exp. Med.*, **121**, 1039

25. Szulman, A. E. (1972). The A, B, and H blood group antigens in human placenta. *N. Engl. J. Med.*, **286**, 1028

26. Goto, S., Hoshino, M., Tomoda, Y. and Ishizuka, N. (1976). Immunoelectron microscopy of the human chorionic villus in search of blood group A and B antigens. *Lab. Invest.*, **35**, 530

27. Loke, Y. W. and Ballard, A. (1973). Blood group A antigens on human trophoblast cells. *Nature (London)*, **245**, 329

28. Currie, G. A. and Bagshawe, K. D. (1967). The masking of antigens on trophoblast and cancer cells. *Lancet*, **1**, 708

29. Cohen, B. H. (1970). ABO and Rh incompatibility. 1. Fetal and neonatal mortality with ABO and Rh incompatibility. *Am. J. Hum. Genet.*, **22**, 412

30. Mittal, K. K., Kachru, R. B. and Brewer, J. I. (1975). The HL-A and ABO antigens in trophoblastic diseases. *Tissue Antigens*, **6**, 57

31. Whyte, A. and Loke, Y. W. (1979). Antigens of the human trophoblast plasma membrane. *Clin. Exp. Immunol.*, **37**, 359

32. Faulk, W. P., Temple, A., Lovins, R. E. and Smith, N. (1978). Antigens of human trophoblasts: a working hypothesis for their role in normal and abnormal pregnancies. *Proc. Natl. Acad. Sci.*, **75**, 1947

33. Horne, C. H. W., Bohn, H. and Towler, C. M. (1976a). Pregnancy associated α_2-glucoprotein. In A. Klopper (ed.) *Plasma Hormone Assays in Evaluation of Fetal Wellbeing*. (Edinburgh: Churchill-Livingstone)

34. Gershon, R. K. (1973). T cell control of antibody production. *Contemp. Topics Immunobiol.*, **3**, 1

35. Basten, A., Loblay, R., Chia, E., Collard, R. and Pritchard-Briscoe, H. (1977). Suppressor T cells in tolerance to non-self and self antigens. *Cold Spring Harbor Symp. Quant. Biol.*, **41**, 93

36. Waksman, B. H. (1977). Tolerance, the thymus, and suppressor cells. *Clin. Exp. Immunol.*, **28**, 63

37. Peck, A. B., Murgita, R. A. and Wigzell, H. (1978). Cellular and genetic restrictions in the immunoregulatory activity of alpha-fetoprotein. I. Selective inhibition of anti-Ia associated proliferative reactions. *J. Exp. Med.*, **147**, 667

38. Brock, D. J. H. (1976). Prenatal diagnosis – chemical methods. *Br. Med. Bull.*, **32**, 16

39. Murgita, R. A., Anderson, I. C., Sherman, M. S., Bennich, H. and Wigzell, H. (1978). Effects of human alpha-foetoprotein on human B and T lymphocyte proliferation *in vitro*. *Clin. Exp. Immunol.*, **33**, 347

40. Yachnin, S. and Lester, E. (1976). Inhibition of human lymphocyte transformation by human alpha-foetoprotein (HAFB): comparison of foetal and hepatoma HAFP and kinetic studies of *in vitro* immunosuppression. *Clin. Exp. Immunol.*, **26**, 484

41. Figueredo, M. A., Palomino, P. and Ortiz, F. (1979). Lymphocyte response to phyto-haemagglutinin in the presence of serum from pregnant women: correlation with serum levels of alpha-foetoprotein. *Clin. Exp. Immunol.*, **37**, 140

42. Muchmore, A. V. and Blaese, R. M. (1977). Immuno-regulatory properties of fractions from human pregnancy urine: evidence that human chorionic gonadotrophin is not responsible. *J. Immunol.*, **118**, 881

43. Charpentier, B., Guttmann, R. D., Shuster, J. and Gold, P. (1977). Augmentation of proliferation of human mixed lymphocyte culture by human α fetoprotein. *J. Immunol.*, **119**, 897

44. Seppälä, M. and Ruoslahti, E. (1972). α-fetoprotein in normal and pregnancy sera. *Lancet*, **1**, 375

45. Nörgaard-Pedersen, B. (1973). α_1-foetoprotein. *Scand. J. Immunol.*, **2** (Suppl. 1), 107

46. Amoroso, E. C. and Perry, J. S. (1975). The existence during gestation of an immunological buffer zone at the interface between maternal and foetal tissues. *Proc. R. Soc. Ser. B.*, **271**, 343

47. Horne, C. H. W., Towler, C. M., Pugh-Humphreys, R. G. P., Thomson, A. W. and Bohn, H. (1976b). Pregnancy specific β_1-glycoprotein – a product of the syncytiotrophoblast. *Experientia*, **32**, 1147

48. Von Schoultz, B. (1974). *Studies on PZ.* Umea University Medical Dissertations, No. 2

49. Than, G. N., Csaba, I. F., Karg, N. J., Szabo, D. G. and Novak, P. F. (1975). Pregnancy-associated α_2 globulin antigen in pathological pregnancies. *ICRS Med. Sci.*, **3**, 94

50. Stimson, W. H. (1976). Studies on the immunosuppressive properties of a pregnancy associated α-macroglobulin. *Clin. Exp. Immunol.*, **25**, 199

51. Morton, H., Rolfe, B., Clunie, G. J. A., Anderson, M. J. and Morrison, J. (1977). An early pregnancy factor detected in human serum by the rosette inhibition test. *Lancet*, **1**, 394

52. Morton, H., Hegh, V. and Clunie, G. J. A. (1976). Studies on the rosette inhibition test in pregnant mice: evidence of immunosuppression. *Proc. R. Soc. Ser. B*, **193**, 413

53. Clarke, F. M., Morton, H. and Clunie, G. J. A. (1978). Detection and separation of two serum factors responsible for depression of lymphocyte activity in pregnancy. *Clin. Exp. Immunol.*, **32**, 318

54. Morton, H., Nancarrow, C. D., Scaramuzzi, R. J., Evison, B. M. and Clunie, G. J. A. (1979). Detection of early pregnancy in sheep by the rosette inhibition test. *J. Reprod. Fertil.*, **56** (In press)

55. Noonan, F. P., Halliday, W. J., Morton, H. and Clunie, G. J. A. (1979). Early pregnancy factor is immunosuppressive. *Nature (London)*, **278**, 649

56. Cooper, D. W. and Aitken, R. J. (1980). Failure to detect changed E-rosette inhibition titre in human pregnancy (submitted)

57. Claman, H. N. (1972). Corticosteroids and lymphoid cells. *N. Engl. J. Med.*, **287**, 388

58. Mendolsohn, J., Multer, M. M. and Bernheim, J. L. (1977). Inhibition of human lympho-cyte stimulation by steroid hormones: cytokinetic mechanisms. *Clin. Exp. Immunol.*, **27**, 127

59. Kasakura, S. (1973). Is cortisol responsible for inhibition of MLC reactions by pregnancy plasma? *Nature (London)*, **246**, 496

60. MacDonald, R. R. (1978). Clinical pharmacology of progestogens. In MacDonald, R. R. (ed.) *Scientific Basis of Obstetrics and Gynaecology*, 2nd Edn. (Edinburgh, London and New York: Churchill-Livingstone)

61. Siiteri, P. K., Febres, F., Clemens, L. E., Chang, R. J., Gondos, B. and Stites, D. (1977). Progesterone and maintenance of pregnancy: is progesterone nature's immunosuppressant? *Ann. N.Y. Acad. Sci.*, **286**, 384

62. Krohn, P. L. (1954). Effect of ACTH on reaction to skin homografts in rabbits. *J. Endocrinol.*, **11**, 71

63. Medawar, P. B. and Sparrow, E. M. (1956). Effects of adrenocortical hormones, adreno-corticotropic hormone, and pregnancy on skin transplantation in mice. *Endocrinology*, **14**, 240

64. Hulka, J. F., Mohr, K. and Lieberman, M. W. (1965). Effect of synthetic progestational agents on allograft reaction and circulating antibody production. *Endocrinology*, **84**, 897

65. Pelner, M. V. and Rhoades, M. G. (1965). Host–tumor antagonism. 34. The use of progestational agents to retard homograft rejection in rabbits: a pilot study. *J. Am. Geriatr. Soc.*, **13**, 765

66. Turcotte, J. G., Hains, R. F., Brody, G. L., Meyer, T. J. and Schwartz, S. A. (1968). Immunosuppression with medroxyprogesterone acetate. *Transplantation*, **6**, 248

67. Kountz, S. L. and Wechter, W. J. (1977). Immunosuppression with melengestrol. *Transplant. Proc.*, **9**, 1447

68. Schiff, R. I., Mercier, D. and Buckley, R. C. (1975). Inability of gestational hormones to account for the inhibitory effects of pregnancy plasma on lymphocyte responses *in vitro*. *Cell. Immunol.*, **20**, 69

69. Barnstaple, C. J., Jones, E. A., Bodmer, W. F., Bodmer, J. C., Acre-Gomez, B., Snary, D. and Crumpton, M. J. (1977). Genetics and virology of HL-A-linked human Ia antigens. *Cold Spring Harbor Symp. Quant. Biol.*, **41**, 443

70. Mathur, S., Mathur, R. S., Dowda, H., Williamson, H. O., Faulk, W. P. and Fudenberg, H. H. (1978). Sex steroid hormones and antibodies to *Candida albicans*. *Clin. Exp. Immunol.*, **33**, 70

71. Llewellyn-Jones, D. (1969). Infectious diseases in pregnancy. In *Fundamentals of Obstetrics and Gynaecology*, p. 245. (London: Faber & Faber)

72. Menser, M. A. (1976). Immunological aspects of maternal infection. In Scott, J. S. and Jones, W. R. (eds.) *Immunology of Human Reproduction*. (London: Academic Press)

73. Aycock, W. L. (1941). The frequency of poliomyeletis in pregnancy. *N. Engl. J. Med.*, **225**, 405

74. Weinstein, L., Aycock, W. L. and Feemster, R. F. (1951). The relation of sex, pregnancy, and menstruation to susceptibility to poliomyelitis. *N. Engl. J. Med.*, **245**, 54

75. Priddle, M. D., Lenz, W. R., Young, D. C. and Stevenson, C. S. (1952). Poliomyelitis in pregnancy and puerperium: experience in Detroit epidemics of 1949 and 1950. *Am. J. Obstet. Gynecol.*, **63**, 408

76. Buck, A. A. and Hasenclever, H. F. (1963). Epidemiological studies of skin reactions and serum agglutinins to *Candida albicans* in pregnant women. *Am. J. Hyg.*, **78**, 232

77. Ferrone, S., Mickey, M. R., Terasaki, P. I., Reisfeld, R. A. and Pellegrina, M. A. (1976). Humoral sensitisation in parous women: cytotoxic antibodies to non-HLA antigens. *Transplantation*, **22**, 61

78. Winchester, R. J., Fu, S. M., Wernet, P., Kunkel, H. G., Dupont, B. and Jersild, C. (1975). Recognition by pregnancy serums of non-HLA alloantigens selectively expressed on B lymphocytes. *J. Exp. Med.*, **141**, 924

79. Yontananukam, V., Matangkosombut, P. and Osathapondh, V. (1974). Onset of human maternal cell-mediated immune reaction to placental antigens during the first pregnancy. *Clin. Exp. Immunol.*, **16**, 593

80. Pence, H., Petty, W. H. and Rocklin, R. E. (1975). Suppression of maternal responsiveness to paternal antigens by maternal plasma. *J. Immunol.*, **114**, 525

81. Timonen, T. and Saksela, E. (1976). Cell-mediated anti-embryo cytotoxicity in human pregnancy. *Clin. Exp. Immunol.*, **23**, 462

82. Andresen, R. H. and Monroe, C. W. (1962). Experimental study of the behaviour of adult human skin homografts during pregnancy. *Am. J. Obstet. Gynecol.*, **84**, 1096

83. Thomas, L., Douglas, G. W. and Carr, M. C. (1959). The continual migration of syncytial trophoblast from the foetal placenta into the maternal circulation. *Trans. Assoc. Am. Physicians*, **72**, 140

84. Attwood, H. D. and Park, W. W. (1961). Embolism to the lungs by trophoblast. *J. Obstet. Gynaecol. Br. Commonw.*, **68**, 611

85. Walkanowska, J., Conte, F. A. and Grumbach, M. M. (1969). Practical and theoretical implications of fetal–maternal lymphocyte transfer. *Lancet*, **1**, 1119
86. Schröder, J. and De La Chappelle, A. (1972). Fetal lymphocytes in the maternal blood. *Blood*, **39**, 153
87. Schröder, J. (1974). Passage of leucocytes from mother to foetus. *Scand. J. Immunol.*, **4**, 279
88. Tovey, L. A. D. and Moroni, E. S. (1976). Rhesus isoimmunisation. In Scott, J. S. and Jones, W. R. (eds.) *Immunology of Human Reproduction*. (London: Academic Press)
89. Chesley, L. C. (1978). *Hypertensive Disorders in Pregnancy*. (New York: Appleton-Century Crofts)
90. Cooper, D. W. and Liston, W. A. (1979). Genetic control of severe pre-eclampsia. *J. Med. Genet.* **16**, 409
91. Scott, J. S. and Jenkins, D. M. (1976). Immunogenetic factors in aetiology of pre-eclampsia/eclampsia (gestosis). *J. Med. Genet.*, **13**, 200
92. Beer, A. E. (1978). Possible immunologic bases of pre-eclampsia/eclampsia. *Semin. Perinatol.*, **2**, 39
93. Kitzmiller, J. L. and Benirschke, K. (1973). Immunofluorescent study of placental bed vesseles in pre-eclampsia of pregnancy. *Am. J. Obstet. Gynecol.*, **115**, 248
94. Thompson, D., Paterson, W. G., Smart, G. E., MacDonald, H. K. and Robsin, J. S. (1972). The renal lesions of toxaemia and abruptis placentae studied by light and electron microscopy. *J. Obstet. Gynaecol. Br. Commonw.*, **79**, 311
95. Howie, P. W. (1977). The haemostatic mechanisms in pre-eclampsia. *Clin. Obstet. Gynecol.*, **4**, 685
96. Irino, T., Okuda, T. and Grollman, A. (1967). Changes induced in the glomeruli of the kidney of rats by placental extracts as observed with the electron microscope. *Am. J. Pathol.*, **50**, 421
97. Petrucco, O. M., Thomson, N. M., Lawrence, J. R. and Weldon, W. M. (1974). Immunofluorescent studies in renal biopsies in pre-eclampsia. *Br. Med. J.*, **1**, 473
98. Boss, J. H. (1965). Antigenic relationships between placenta and kidney in humans. *Am. J. Obstet. Gynecol.*, **93**, 574
99. Koren, Z., Abrams, G. and Behrman, S. J. (1968). Antigenicity of mouse placental tissue. *Am. J. Obstet. Gynecol.*, **102**, 340
100. Jenkins, D. M., Need, J. A., Scott, J. S., Morris, H. and Pepper, M. (1978). Human leucocyte antigens and mixed lymphocyte reaction in severe pre-eclampsia. *Br. Med. J.*, **1**, 542
101. Redman, C. W. G., Bodmer, J. G., Bodmer, W. F., Beilin, L. J. and Bonnar, J. (1978). HLA antigens in severe pre-eclampsia. *Lancet*, **2**, 397
102. Macgillivray, I. (1958). Some observations on the incidence of pre-eclampsia. *J. Obstet. Gynaecol. Br. Emp.*, **65**, 536
103. Cooke, A., Hutchings, P. R. and Playfair, J. H. L. (1978). Suppressor T cells in experimental autoimmune haemolytic anaemia. *Nature (London)*, **273**, 154
104. Playfair, J. H. L. and Marshall-Clarke, S. (1973). Induction of red cell autoantibodies in normal mice. *Nature New Biol.*, **243**, 213
105. Jones, W. R. (1978). Immunological aspects of pregnancy. In Macdonald, R. R. (ed.) *Basis of Obstetrics and Gynecology*. (Edinburgh, London and New York: Churchill-Livingstone)
106. Doughty, R. W. and Gelsthorpe, K. (1974). An initial investigation of lymphocyte antibody activity through pregnancy and in eluates prepared from placental material. *Tissue Antigens*, **4**, 291
107. Payne, R. (1964). Neonatal neutropenia and leukoagglutinins. *Pediatrics*, **33**, 193
108. Ahrons, S. (1971). HL-A antibodies: influence on the human foetus. *Tissue Antigens*, **1**, 121
109. Nymand, G. (1974). Complement-fixing and lymphocytotoxic antibodies in serum of pregnant women at delivery. *Vox. Sang.*, **27**, 322
110. Tongio, M. M., Mayer, S. and Lebec, A. (1975). Transfer of HLA antibodies from the mother to the child. *Transplantation*, **20**, 163

111. Wegmann, T. G., Singh, B. and Carlson, G. A. (1979). Allogeneic placenta is a paternal strain antigen immunoabsorbent. *J. Immunol.*, **122**, 270

112. Miyajima, T., Hirata, A. A. and Terasaki, P. I. (1972). Escape from sensitisation by HLA antibodies. *Tissue Antigens*, **2**, 64

113. Tiilikainen, A., Schröder, J. and De La Chapelle, A. (1974). Fetal leukocytes in the maternal circulation after delivery. *Transplantation*, **17**, 355

114. Jones, W. R. (1976). Fetal and neonatal immunology. In Scott, J. S. and Jones, W. R. (eds.) *Immunology of Human Reproduction*. (London: Academic Press; New York: Grune & Stratton)

115. Wild, A. E. (1979). Cellular mechanisms effecting antibody transport and immunological protection in the placenta. In Beaconfield, P. and Villee, C. A. (eds.) *Placenta – A Neglected Experimental Animal.* (Oxford: Pergamon Press)

116. Ockleford, C. D. (1976). A three dimensional reconstruction of the polygonal pattern on the placental-coated vesicle membranes. *J. Cell. Sci.*. **21**. 83

117. Ockleford, C. D. and Whyte, A. (1977). Differentiated regions of human placental cell surface associated with exchange of materials between maternal and foetal blood coated vesicles. *J. Cell Sci.*, **25**, 293

118. Ockleford, C. D. (1977). Antibody clearance by micropinocytosis: a possible role in foetal immunoprotection. *Lancet*, **1**, 310

119. Shulman, N. R., Marder, J. V., Hiller, M. C. and Collier, E. M. (1964). Platelet and leucocyte isoantigens and their antibodies: serologic, physiologic and clinical studies. *Progr. Haematol.*, **4**, 222

120. Lalezair, P. and Radel, F. (1974). Neutrophil specific antigens: immunology and clinical significance. *Semin. Haematol.*, **11**, 281

121. Strominger, J. L., Mann, D. L., Parham, P., Robb, R., Springer, T. and Teshorst, C. (1977). Structure of HL-A A and B antigens isolated from cultured human lymphocytes. *Cold Spring Harbor Symp. Quant. Biol.*, **41**, 323

122. Snary, D., Barnstable, C. J., Bodmer, W. F. and Crumpton, M. J. (1975). Human Ia antigens – purification and molecular structure. *Cold Spring Harbor Symp. Quant. Biol.*, **41**, 379

122a. Wynn, R. M. (1968). Morphology of the placenta. In Assali, N. S. (ed.) *Biology of Gestation.* (New York: Academic Press)

123. Lawler, S. D., Klouda, P. T. and Bagshawe, K. D. (1974). Immunogenicity of molar pregnancies in the HLA system. *Am. J. Obstet. Gynecol.*, **120**, 857

124. Lawler, S. D. (1978). HLA and trophoblastic tumours. *Br. Med. Bull.*, **34**, 305

125. Faulk, W. P. and Johnston, P. M. (1977). Immunological studies of human placentae: identification and distribution of proteins in mature chorionic villi. *Clin. Exp. Immunol.*, **27**, 365

126. Sundquist, K., Bergstrom, S. and Håkansson, S. (1977). Surface antigens of human trophoblasts. *Devel. Comp. Immunol.*, **1**, 241

126a. Contractor, S. F. and Davies, H. (1973). Effect of human chorionic somatomammotrophin and human chorionic gonadotrophin on phytohaemagglutinin-induced lymphocyte transformation. *Nature New Biol.*, **243**, 284

127. Werthamen, S., Govindaraj, S. and Amoral, C. (1976). Placental transcortin and localised immune response. *J. Clin. Invest.*, **57**, 1000

128. Bernard, O. (1977). Possible protecting role of maternal immunoglobulins on embryonic development in mammals. *Immunogenetics*, **5**, 1

129. Revillard, J. P., Brochier, J., Robert, M., Bonneau, M. and Traeger, J. (1976). Immunologic properties of placental eluates. *Transplant. Proc.*, **8**, 275

130. Woodrow, J. C. (1970). Rh immunisation and its prevention. *Ser Haemat.*, **3**, 1

131. Clemens, K. and Walsh, R. J. (1954). The frequency of immunisation of Rh negative women by Rh antigen. *Med. J. Aust.*, **2**, 707

32. Opelz, G., Mickey, M. R. and Terasaki, P. I. (1973). Blood transfusions and unresponsive-r.ess to HLA. *Transplantation*, **16**, 649

33. Allen, J. C. and Kunkel, H. G. (1963). Antibodies to genetic types of gamma globulin after multiple transfusions. *Science*, **139**, 418

34. Nathenson, G., Schorr, J. B. and Litwin, S. D. (1971). Gm factor fetomaternal gamma globulin incompatibility. *Pediatr. Res.*, **5**, 2

3
Immunological Diagnosis of Early Pregnancy

J. K. FINDLAY

INTRODUCTION

Tests for pregnancy or non-pregnancy in animals have application both in the commercial and research fields. In general, an accurate diagnosis is required as soon as possible after mating has occurred. This enables special management procedures to be initiated to aid the pregnancy and to prevent wastage of valuable resources, such as re-insemination of pregnant animals or holding non-pregnant animals.

Table 3.1 Substances used for immunological diagnosis of early pregnancy

Stage of pregnancy	Substance	Species
Post-fertilization	early pregnancy factor	rodents, ruminants, humans
Pre-implantation	early pregnancy factor progesterone pregnancy proteins	rodents, ruminants, cow ruminants
Implantation	chorionic gonadotrophin progesterone	primates sheep, pig, horse
Post-implantation	pregnancy proteins oestrone sulphate PMSG	sheep, cow pig horse

The diagnosis of pregnancy relies on detecting a substance(s) specific to a certain stage of pregnancy or measuring changes specific to pregnancy in the level of a substance(s). In general, the best substances to measure are products of the conceptus or the uterus bearing a conceptus, and are detected in

63

maternal blood or urine. The ability to detect these substances will depend on the sensitivity and precision of the test used and the period when the substances are present in the mother.

The type of substance detected will depend on the stage of pregnancy (Table 3.1). There are no simple, routine tests for fertilization. Recent work suggests that an early pregnancy factor (EPF), present within 6–48 h of fertilization in mice[1] may be a potential test of this very early stage. The pre-implantation, blastocyst phase varies in length between species, from less than 10 days in primates to 16 days in sheep, 18 days in pigs and up to 45 days in cattle[2]. EPF may also be present during this phase[3]. In those species, e.g. cows, in which extension of corpus luteum (CL) function occurs during this phase, progesterone in plasma or milk may also be used as an indicator of pregnancy[4]. In non-human primates, implantation is associated with the production of a chorionic gonadotrophin, used to diagnose pregnancy[5]. Placental lactogen is first detected in the endometrium at implantation but is not detected in the circulation in measurable quantities until later in pregnancy[6]. Once the placenta has formed a number of pregnancy-associated substances[7], including steroids[8], can be detected in maternal blood or urine and used as tests for pregnancy.

Much of the success of the current methods of diagnosing pregnancy is due to the development and application of immunological methods to measure small quantities of test substances in blood and urine. The development of radioimmunoassays (RIA) and haemagglutination inhibition assays (HIA) for routine use has been of particular importance[9]. These tests have the sensitivity and precision to allow diagnosis of pregnancy at an earlier stage than methods previously used such as bioassays, palpation, X-ray, vaginal biopsies, etc.[10, 11]. Furthermore, the immunological tests involve procedures that are less traumatic to the animal and are more practical and relatively inexpensive.

This chapter reviews the current status of immunological tests for early pregnancy. The discussion is mostly confined to non-human primates, horses, cows, sheep and pigs, species in which there is widespread application of the tests. The basis for each test is described and the advantages, the limitations and future developments are discussed.

POLYPEPTIDES

Chorionic gonadotrophins (CG)

Non-human primates

All the non-human primates examined so far produce a CG, similar to HCG, during the early part of pregnancy[9, 12] (Table 3.2). In the human, CG is a glycoprotein of two subunits, α and β[13], and is secreted by the fetal

Table 3.2 Detection of chorionic gonadotrophin (CG) in plasma or urine of non-human primates by a non-human primate pregnancy test (NHPPT) based on a haemagglutination inhibition assay

Family	Species	Common name	Ovarian cycle length (Days)	Gestation length (Days)	Range of CG detection by NHPPT (Days)	Reference
NEW-WORLD MONKEYS						
Callithricidae	*Callithrix jacchus*	marmoset	15–18	142–150	28–70	114, 115*
Cebidae	*Cebus albifrons*	white-faced capuchin	16–20	180	30–60	22
	Saimiri sciureus	squirrel monkey	12	140–180	40–60	116
OLD-WORLD MONKEYS						
Cercopithecidae	*Macaca mulatta*	Rhesus monkey	28	144–197	18–23	5, 117
	Macaca speciosa	stump-tailed macaque	28–31	182	14–45	12
	Papio anubis *Papio cynocephalus*	baboon	32–36	175	17–30	118, 119
	Pygathrix nemaeus	Douc langur	25	180	21–31	22
Pongidae	*Pan troglodytes*	chimpanzee	36	216–260	{ 15–18 { 20–133	{ 120, 118* { 122
	Pongo pygmaeus	orangutan	27–29	275	21–275	22, 120, 123, 17, 124
	Gorilla gorilla gorilla	western gorilla	33	255	20–230	17

* Not detected by NHPPT

syncytiotrophoblast at or after implantation of the blastocyst and vascularization of the implantation site[14]. HCG is believed to be the luteotrophin responsible for maintenance of the CL in early pregnancy[14]. Evidence to date suggests that CG has a similar chemical structure, site of origin and role in non-human primates[12, 15, 16]. Thus, detection of primate CG can be regarded as a test for implantation.

In normal pregnancies, CG is found in urine and plasma of non-human primates[12]. The time of first detection and the period of production varies between species[17, 18], according to whether urine or plasma is tested and with the assay method used. The CG is generally found a few days after the time of implantation (Table 3.2). An HIA assay for pregnancy in non-human primates (NHPPT) has been developed for CG in urine[5] and evaluated in most of the species listed in Table 3.2. It is now distributed by NIAMDD, USA and has acceptable levels of accuracy and precision in those species for which sufficient numbers of samples have been assayed. HIA designed for diagnosing pregnancy in humans has been successfully applied to chimpanzee[19] but not to Rhesus monkeys[20, 21] or marmosets[18]. Specific antisera for β-HCG with improved sensitivity might allow detection of CG in plasma of primates nearer the time of implantation than the urine test. Alternatively, recent experience[22] suggests that an *in vitro* bioassay of LH/CG[23], using rodent testicular homogenates and measuring testosterone production by RIA, may be just as useful. This bioassay system is not species-specific for LH/CG and has good sensitivity and precision. The reagents for the bioassay are generally available in most laboratories and the use of iodinated rather than tritiated hormone in the steroid RIA will improve the sensitivity and capacity of the system and reduce the cost. The disadvantage of the *in vitro* bioassay for LH/CG is the lack of hormone specificity making it necessary to choose a discriminatory value above which CG is said to be detected. Recent studies suggest that the first detection of CG by the *in vitro* system is earlier or similar to the HIA test[22].

There are reports of CG being detected before implantation in the human[24, 25] which may represent synthesis by the blastocyst or an alternative source of CG-like immunoreactivity. The accuracy of diagnosis of pregnancy with CG can be reduced in the event of tumours producing CG or 'CG-like' immunoreactivity, as in the hydatidiform mole of human pregnancy[26]. There is also the possibility that trophoblast may continue to grow and secrete CG in the absence of a viable embryo, e.g. human tetraploidy[27]. Although such 'pregnancies' would end in abortion, they contribute to false positive tests early in pregnancy. There is evidence for HCG-like immunoreactivity in pituitary tissue and urinary extracts from non-pregnant subjects[28], but the levels detected in urine are unlikely to bias a pregnancy diagnosis unless a specific antisera to β-HCG is being used. The incidence of spontaneous placental tumours[29] in non-human primates is low and the spectrum of abnormalities of pregnancy is similar to the human[29, 30]. The extent to which

CG-like immunoreactivity exists in non-human primates and leads to errors in pregnancy diagnosis is not known at present.

Plasma and urine have been used as sources of CG measurement with equal success. Repeated plasma samples or total urinary output are not easy to obtain because some primates are difficult to handle. Also, long periods of restraint in special chairs or the use of indwelling catheters may not be desirable, for example, in zoos. To this end, successful attempts have been made to measure CG in urinary voidings and to relate CG concentration to urinary creatinine content[22, 31]. Total oestrogens have been measured in the same samples allowing daily hormone profiles of CG and oestrogen to be monitored during the reproductive cycle and early pregnancy of the orangutan, gorilla, capuchin, Douc langur and chimpanzee[22, 31].

Equidae

Pregnancy in horses is associated with the production of pregnant mares' serum gonadotrophin (PMSG) between days 40 and 130 of gestation[32, 33], well after the time of implantation (days 22–25). PMSG is a glycoprotein hormone with an α and β subunit[34] and possesses both LH and FSH activity[35]. It is secreted by the endometrial cups, formed by specialized trophoblast cells which migrate from the chorionic girdle deep into the adjacent endometrial stroma at about day 36–38[36]. The endometrial cup has no physical connection with the remaining fetal membranes and secretes PMSG into the maternal bloodstream via a complex network of lymph sinuses. Peak serum concentrations of 50–150 iu PMSG/ml are reached between days 50 and 70 and thereafter decline to non-detectable levels between days 120 and 130[36].

In 1963, Wide and Wide[37] applied the HIA developed for HCG[38], to PMSG and this test has been used extensively since its availability in kit forms. In 1967, Richards developed a more simple, but less sensitive test for PMSG which produces visible precipitation lines when PMSG and a specific antibody are allowed to diffuse in agar gel on Ouchterlony plates[39]. More recently, RIA[40] and radioreceptor assay (RRA)[41] methods for measuring PMSG have been described.

Several reports have compared the immunological methods with bioassays for PMSG[42, 43]. The HIA repeatedly gave an overall accuracy in excess of 90% except in the early phase (40–50 days) and during the decline in PMSG (100–130 days). It has been suggested[43] that at these times, the levels of PMSG fall below the sensitivity of the HIA assay (3 iu/ml: cf. mouse bioassay, 1 iu/ml; RIA 1 miu/ml[40]). Although the HIA test may lack sensitivity and sufficient accuracy to detect PMSG before day 50, it has found enormous popularity because of its simplicity and rapidity.

Of the many factors, e.g. size, parity and number of fetuses present, influencing both the amount of endometrial cup tissue which develops in individual mares and the concentration of PMSG in serum, fetal genotype is by far the most pronounced[44]. Peak serum concentrations of PMSG in mares mated to a jack donkey and therefore carrying a mule conceptus are generally 10-fold or more lower than in a mare carrying a normal intraspecific horse conceptus. Allen[36] concluded from this and other studies that hinney and mule endometrial cups thrive for longer and secrete larger amounts of PMSG in donkey compared to the mare because the donkey maternal leukocyte response is relatively ineffectual in destroying the endometrial cup.

Once PMSG production has been initiated at day 38–40, its continued production no longer requires the presence of the fetus[45]. Thus, in cases of abortion or resorption of the fetus after day 40, false positive tests may be encountered if the presence of PMSG is used to diagnose pregnancy without a rectal examination to confirm the result[43]. Testing for PMSG before day 40 cannot be used as a diagnostic method. This means that for the earliest, accurate diagnosis of pregnancy using PMSG, mating dates should be known precisely and the assay for PMSG be as sensitive as possible. There is a need to develop a test which will diagnose pregnancy before day 40 in the mare.

Other equidae produce PMSG-like activity at equivalent stages of gestation to the mare but, like CG in primates, the level and period of production differs between species. For example, zebras have lower levels of PMSG compared to horses during the peak period of production but PMSG production was maintained for longer in zebras and was still detected at 225 days of gestation[46]. PMSG has also been identified in urine of the giraffe[47].

Other species

Claims for chorionic gonadotrophins like HCG or PMSG in urine or blood of species other than primates and equidae have not been confirmed. There are reports of HCG-like activity in blastocysts of mice[48], rats[49], rabbits[50] and sheep[51] but there is no evidence that this activity is present in the circulation where its presence could be used as a test for pregnancy.

Placental lactogen (PL)

PL or chorionic somatomammotrophin is a product of the mammalian placenta and has been found in human and non-human primates, ruminants and rodents[52–54]. PL is first detected in placental tissue of sheep on day 16[6], when attachment of the blastocyst to the endometrium is initiated and when giant binucleate cells are first observed in the endometrium[55]. PL is thought to originate from these binucleate cells which are of fetal origin and migrate in-between the epithelial cells of the endometrium. PL has been detected in bovine conceptuses collected between 17 and 25 days *post coitum* (p.c.), at or shortly after the time of appearance of binucleate cells in the bovine trophectoderm, but before attachment or implantation[56].

PL is not detected in the maternal circulation until later in pregnancy, e.g.

day 40 in sheep[6], and therefore has limited appeal as a method of diagnosing early pregnancy. PL can be measured by RIA[57] or RRA[58], provided precautions are taken for cross-reaction with prolactin in the PL assays.

Pregnancy-associated substances

In addition to the hormones mentioned above, a number of antigenic, protein-like-substances have been identified using immunological techniques in the maternal circulation during pregnancy[7, 59–61]. Some of these antigens are specific to pregnancy and originate from the products of conception; others have an increased titre associated with pregnancy. Many of these antigens have no known physiological role, but can be used to diagnose pregnancy and embryonic or fetal loss.

Early pregnancy factor (EPF)

Morton and her co-workers have identified EPF in serum by a rosette inhibition test (RIT) within 6–48 h of fertilization in mice[1, 3] and women[62]. Subsequently, a factor(s) termed EPF because of similar activity in the RIT, has been described in serum of rats[63], cows[64] and adult[65, 66] and fetal sheep[67]. The factor(s) in mice was detected until 4–6 days prior to parturition[3] and biochemical evidence suggests it is a large peptide molecule[3]. There is evidence that EPF in sheep serum is immunosuppressive *in vivo*[68] and that its concentration decreases to non-pregnant levels within 6–48 h after the embryo is removed from the uterus[69]. It is interesting to note that uterine secretions from pregnant cows[70] and porcine fetal fluids[71] early in pregnancy have an immunosuppressive effect on PHA stimulation of lymphocyte activity, suggesting pregnancy-associated, immunosuppressive agents could be common to a number of species[72].

Detection of EPF offers a means of diagnosing pregnancy after fertilization and before implantation. It would be a test for fertilization and could be used to monitor embryonic losses during the pre-implantation stage, which would be a major advance. The current immunological RIT for EPF[1, 65] is laborious, has a small sample capacity and is subject to many non-specific effects. However, once EPF is purified it should be possible to develop an RIA which can be applied to determining the specificity of EPF to pregnancy and its usefulness as a method of diagnosis of pregnancy and early embryonic loss.

Pregnancy-associated antigens

Immunological studies have described antigens specific to pregnancy that are present in maternal tissues in a number of animals including rat, mouse[73], sheep[7], cow[74] and monkey[75]. Generally, these antigens are found during the second and third trimesters and few attempts have been made to exploit them as tests for pregnancy. Some of the antigens may be detected in tissues, particularly uterus, but not in blood or urine, and therefore are not suitable for use in pregnancy diagnosis.

(a) Non-human primates – In addition to HCG, the human placenta produces a number of other specific pregnancy proteins. Most of these proteins have no known biological function and their terminology is generally based on their physical and chemical characteristics and includes such substances as SP1-glycoprotein[59], pregnancy-associated macroglobulin[60] and α-fetoprotein[61]. Immunological techniques have often been used to identify these proteins and to characterize their patterns during pregnancy. Some of the substances are confined to placental tissue whilst others are secreted into the maternal blood with patterns of secretion which vary between the different proteins.

Proteins with similar antigenic activity have been described in the non-human primate. A rabbit antiserum to human SP1-glycoprotein cross-reacted with pregnancy serum of the baboon[54], cynomolgus monkey and Rhesus monkey[76]. Passive immunization of cynomolgus monkeys with rabbit antisera to SP1-glycoprotein resulted in termination of pregnancy[77], suggesting a role for this substance(s) in pregnancy. In the case of the baboon[54] the activity was first detected at around day 17 after fertilization and continued throughout the entire pregnancy and into the *post-partum* period. The decrease in immunoreactivity following birth was relatively slow and this could lead to errors if this particular substance is used to diagnose pregnancy in animals mated early in the *post-partum* period.

There have been no reports using these proteins to diagnose pregnancy in non-human primates. Although SP1-glycoprotein can be used as a method of diagnosing pregnancy in the human, it offers no advantage over HCG[78]. Placental proteins have been used more as a measure of placental function and fetal well-being rather than to diagnosis of pregnancy.

(b) Domestic animals – Initial studies in sheep described a species-specific, pregnancy-associated antigen (oPAA) in uterus, CL and conceptus tissue of seven pregnant ewes and on erythrocytes of 30 pregnant ewes from day 8 after mating to about day 50[79]. The oPAA on erythrocytes was detected by a haemagglutination test using a rabbit anti-sheep conceptus sera which had been absorbed with liver and kidney from non-pregnant ewes to remove non-specific antibodies. Erythrocytes from non-pregnant ewes did not agglutinate in the presence of these antisera. Subsequently, tests were done on 500 ewes up to 50 days pregnant[7, 80]. The absorbed rabbit antisera caused agglutination of 75% (range 50–92%) of samples of erythrocytes from pregnant ewes up to day 50 and did not cause agglutination of 75% (range 50–100%) of samples from non-pregnant ewes. This degree of discrimination was not statistically different due to day-to-day variations in accuracy, although individual tests on a day were often greater than 90% accurate in diagnosing pregnant and

non-pregnant ewes. The antisera were used at a low titre (1/8 to 1/16) and with limited amounts available, the supplies were quickly exhausted. Antisera obtained from the same rabbit late in the immunization schedule gave inconsistent results when haemagglutination tests were performed on 140 ewes.

Antisera against sheep conceptus were then raised in calves[81]. These antisera were also species-specific and detected immunoreactivity in a similar range of tissues to that of the rabbit antisera with two exceptions. The calf antisera detected activity in approximately 30% of non-pregnant uteri and there was no consistent evidence of activity on erythrocytes of pregnant ewes. In the presence of calf antisera, 35% of samples from pregnant ewes did not agglutinate and samples from non-pregnant ewes showed random agglutination[7].

Subsequent attempts to raise antisera against sheep conceptus in calves and rabbits have not produced antisera which detect pregnancy antigens on erythrocytes of pregnant ewes by immunofluorescence[82]. This does not preclude the possibility that antigens specific to pregnancy are present in the plasma of ewes. In the initial studies, Cerini[83] found evidence of a reduction in the haemagglutination reaction if the rabbit antisera were absorbed with plasma from pregnant ewes. On the other hand, absorption of the calf antisera by concentrates of pregnancy plasma did not alter the precipitation reaction against an extract of ovine conceptus in agar gel[84].

Two other immunological tests designed to detect pregnancy in ewes have been reported. Lam et al.[85] used an immunological test ('Wampole UCG-test') on blood from 25 ewe lambs. The accuracy of diagnosis of pregnancy was 66.7% at day 10, 68% at day 20, 78.3% at day 37, 91.3% at day 60 and 95.7% at day 120 after mating. The second test[86] was originally used to diagnose pregnancy in rats. Antisera were prepared by immunizing rabbits with rat placental extracts and dialysed, lyophilized powders of rat urine. These antisera were reacted in agar gel double diffusion against serum and urine from rats from day 12 of pregnancy onwards. 'Similar procedures to that used for the rat' were applied to the sheep and 'positive reactions were obtained with urine from pregnant ewes well within the first trimester of pregnancy'. When latex particles were coated with urine powder from pregnant sheep, only weak reactions were obtained between antisera and coated particles and the work was set aside. The stage of gestation at which placentas and urine were obtained from ewes was not mentioned.

The search for antigens specific to ovine pregnancy, and suitable to diagnose pregnancy, requires further work. Several possibilities exist. oPAA has been purified and is found in high- and low-molecular weight forms[7,87]. An antiserum has been raised against the low-molecular weight form[81]. This should allow development of an RIA for oPAA which can be used to determine its distribution in tissues and plasma and the potential of oPAA as a means of diagnosing pregnancy. Martal et al.[88] have recently extended our knowledge of the antiluteolysin of early pregnancy (days 12–25) in the ewe. This substance, called trophoblastin, was initially described by Moor and Rowson[89]. It is a protein produced by the ovine blastocyst, or by its presence in the uterus, and prevents the decline in CL function in early pregnancy. The site of action of trophoblastin is not known with certainty. If it is secreted into the peripheral circulation or is present in milk, saliva or urine, the measurement of trophoblastin as a diagnostic test for pregnancy has considerable potential in sheep and might also be applicable to cows, goats and mares in which the conceptus also produces an antiluteolysin to prevent the demise of the CL. Electrophoretic analysis of uterine secretions of ewes have revealed several bands of protein specific to pregnancy[90]. The identity of these proteins and their presence outside of the uterus is unknown. Protein bands specific to pregnancy have been noted in uterine secretions in cows[74] and Laster[91] has described a pregnancy-specific antigen in the uterine tissue of cows. As in the ewe, there is no evidence that these substances are present in blood, urine, milk or saliva of the cow, where samples could be taken for pregnancy testing.

There is preliminary evidence of pregnancy-associated antigen(s) in plasma of mares up to day 25 after mating[92]. Rabbit antisera against pregnant mare plasma (collected on day 15) or against equine blastocysts, form precipitin lines in agar gels against 20–30% of serum samples from pregnant mares between days 11 and 25 but not against any serum samples from non-pregnant mares. The precipitin test is a relatively insensitive method which may account for the low proportion of positive tests. The results are encouraging enough for the work to continue.

STEROIDS

Progesterone

Progesterone is essential for the maintenance of pregnancy in mammals[93]. In those species in which the length of gestation exceeds the length of the luteal phase of the cycle, the functional capacity of the CL to secrete progesterone must be maintained beyond the normal length of the luteal phase. The period of dependence on luteal progesterone varies between species, and is determined by the ability of the placenta to assume the function of producing progesterone and other hormones necessary for pregnancy[93].

The extension of luteal function beyond the life span of the CL of non-pregnancy has been exploited as a test for pregnancy, by measuring the levels of progesterone at a time when there would be declining levels in the non-pregnant animals[4]. This test has found particular application in sheep, cattle, pigs and horses, species which are not known to produce a chorionic protein early in pregnancy suitable for exploiting as a test for pregnancy.

The progesterone test only became practical with the development of adioligand assays for steroids in plasma during 1965–70. Robertson and Sarda[4] reported accuracies of greater than 87% for cows, 87% for sheep and 88% for pigs using a competitive protein-binding assay for progesterone in plasma. They recommended samples be taken 22–23 days p.c. in cows, 17–18 lays p.c. in sheep and 21 days p.c. in sows. Subsequent applications of the test are essentially variations on the method of Robertson and Sarda, with modifications using radioimmunoassays instead of competitive protein-binding assays and ways of automating the process, all improving specificity, accuracy and capacity of the test system.

The major practical application of the progesterone test has been its use in dairy herds, measuring progestagen concentrations in milk instead of plasma[94,95]. A number of studies had shown that the concentration of total progestagen activity in milk was similar to or higher than progesterone in peripheral plasma[94–96], and that the changes in plasma and milk concentrations of progesterone during the oestrous cycle were similar[95,97]. In their preliminary study, Heap *et al.*[95] suggested that 21, 24 and 28 days p.c. were the best times to test milk progestagen concentration as a method of diagnosing pregnancy. This method is now being used on commercial dairy herds in a number of areas including the UK[98,99], West Germany[97], France[100] and the USA[101]. A recent issue of the *British Veterinary Journal* (**132**(5), 1976) was devoted to an assessment of the method.

Table 3.3 Accuracy of diagnosis of pregnancy in dairy cows using the milk progestagen test

Day of sampling post coitum or post artificial insemination	Accuracy of diagnosis (%)		Reference
	Pregnancy	Non-pregnancy	
21	76	98	101
21	80	95–100	102
20	78	100	97
23	80	100	98
28 (21)	90	100	99

For the most accurate results, it is essential that the day of insemination is known, so that samples of milk (or plasma) can be collected on the day giving optimal results[4,98]. A consensus exists in the literature that this should be on days 21–24 p.c., on which the level of progestagen in a single milk sample will diagnose pregnancy with 76% accuracy and non-pregnancy with greater than 95% accuracy (Table 3.3). Because progestagen content is higher in afternoon than morning milk[98] and the steroid concentration is correlated with fat[97,100] and nitrogen content[100] of the milk, there have been opposing views about the optimum time of sampling and the necessity to correct for fat and nitrogen content. Some workers[101] have claimed equivalent accuracy of diagnosis in fat-free and whole milk. On balance, the afternoon whole milk sample appears preferable. The necessity for adding preservatives (e.g. potassium dichromate and mercuric chloride) to milk, analysing samples within 2 weeks of collection and the importance of standardized radioimmunoassay procedures have been emphasized[98].

The Editorial of the *British Veterinary Journal*, **132**(5), referring to the 80% accuracy of positive diagnosis of pregnancy in dairy cows using the milk progestagen test, stated that 'against a background of embryonic deaths and other pathological conditions of the reproductive tract this is not unexpected'. The problem of a persistent CL without a viable conceptus remains a major cause of false-positive diagnoses in cows using the milk progestagen test. Despite this limitation, the test has been well received by producers, judging by the number of services provided by the Milk Marketing Board in the UK[99].

More recently, the milk progestagen test was applied to beef cattle in an artificial insemination programme[103]. The test had a diagnostic accuracy comparable to that reported for dairy cattle. In contrast to the dairy cows, diagnostic errors were greater for non-pregnancy than pregnancy in beef cows, which the authors attributed to cows with short or extended cycle lengths. Because of this problem and the fact that the exact day of mating is not always known in beef herds in extensive operations, the authors recommended that analysis of sequential samples taken over a period may be necessary for a more accurate diagnosis.

The progesterone test has found application in intensive sheep-breeding systems where fertility control has been an essential component of the success of the venture[104]. Plasma samples are generally taken from ewes on days 17–19 p.c. Recently, the milk progestagen assay has been applied to Awassi sheep with some success, depending on season[105]. Diagnosis of non-pregnant ewes was only 50% during the non-breeding season, whereas more than 90% of ewes were diagnosed non-pregnant during the breeding season.

Limited use of the progesterone test has been made in the pig-breeding[4, 106] and horse-breeding[107] industries. A problem with pigs is the high incidence of persistent CL, leading to lower accuracy of diagnosing pregnancy. Attempts were made to combine progesterone analysis with oestradiol without a great deal of success[106].

Oestrone sulphate

Studies of the endocrine changes, particularly of steroids, associated with pregnancy have shown that oestrone sulphate (E_1S) is the major oestrogen of pregnancy in sheep[108, 109], cattle[110] and pigs[111] and that its major site of production is probably the trophoblast[2, 112]. Although E_1S is not detected readily in peripheral plasma until day 50 in the ewe[109] and day 72 in the cow[110], measurable quantities of E_1S are present in maternal plasma of the sow by day 16 and rise to peak levels between days 23 and 30 p.c.[111]. Robertson and his colleagues[8] subsequently showed that E_1S was present ($> 40 \, pg/ml$) in 50% of plasma samples taken on day 17 p.c. and that the logarithm of the concentration of E_1S plotted against time was linear over the period from days 20 to 26. E_1S was not detected in samples from non-pregnant gilts. These authors concluded that the presence of E_1S in the maternal plasma of the pig after day 20 of pregnancy can be considered indicative of pregnancy and may therefore be used as a pregnancy test.

Further evaluation of this test has not been reported to date. Measurement of E_1S offers considerable promise as a test for early pregnancy in the pig, particularly in view of the disappointing results with the progesterone test[106]. Efforts will be required to simplify the E_1S assay. At present the assay involves two extraction steps, solvolysis and re-extraction, and then RIA[111]. The possibility of using specific antisera to measure E_1S in plasma without extraction[113] should be examined.

CONCLUSIONS

Several conclusions can be made on immunological methods for diagnosis of pregnancy. First, the only simple and reliable tests currently available are those measuring chorionic gonadotrophins in non-human primates and horses. An exception to this is the milk progestagen test in cows. There is a need to develop better tests for pregnancy in those species which do not produce chorionic gonadotrophins, e.g. sheep, cattle and pigs. Secondly, there is a need to develop a test which will diagnose pregnancy in the mare before day 40 when PMSG appears. Thirdly, very little work has been done – let alone reported, on immunological methods for diagnosing pregnancy in those species such as dogs, in which the length of gestation does not exceed the length of the luteal phase, and cats, which are reflex ovulators. The development and application of the EPF test could help resolve this and the other deficiencies mentioned above. The EPF test offers considerable scope as a method of diagnosing pregnancy and embryonic loss, especially since it has been found in a number of species. Finally, continued use of steroid tests will require an advance in RIA technology to simplify the procedure and reduce the cost. One possibility is a solid-phase RIA using iodinated steroid as tracer. Such an advance would be particularly useful if E_1S proves a suitable steroid to test for pregnancy in pigs.

Acknowledgements

I am indebted to Noelene Colvin for editorial assistance, Jill Volfsbergs for typing, and to my colleagues at Werribee for their interest and collaboration in research on early pregnancy. The financial support of the Australian Wool Research Trust Fund and the National Health and Medical Research Council of Australia is gratefully acknowledged.

References

1. Morton, H., Hegh, V. and Clunie, G. J. A. (1974). Immunosuppression detected in pregnant mice by rosette inhibition test. *Nature (London)*, **249**, 459

2. Heap, R. B., Flint, A. P. and Gadsby, J. E. (1979). Role of embryonic signals in the establishment of pregnancy. *Br. Med. Bull.*, **35**, 129

3. Morton, H., Hegh, V. and Clunie, G. J. A. (1976). Studies of the rosette inhibition test in pregnant mice: evidence of immunosuppression? *Proc. R. Soc. Lond. B.*, **193**, 413

4. Robertson, H. A. and Sarda, I. R. (1971). A very early pregnancy test for mammals: its early application to the cow, ewe and sow. *J. Endocrinol.*, **49**, 407

5. Hodgen, G. D. and Ross, G. T. (1974). Pregnancy diagnosis by a haemagglutination inhibition test for urinary macque chorionic gonadotrophin (mCG). *J. Clin. Endocrinol. Metab.*, **38**, 927

6. Martal, J. and Djiane, J. (1977). The production of chorionic somatomammotrophin in sheep. *J. Reprod. Fertil.*, **49**, 285

7. Findlay, J. K., Cerini, M., Sheers, M., Staples, L. D. and Cumming, I. A. (1979). The nature and role of pregnancy-associated antigens and the endocrinology of early pregnancy in the ewe. In Whelan, J. (ed.) *Maternal Recognition of Pregnancy*, Ciba Foundation Symposium, **64**, 239–259. (Elsevier Press, Amsterdam)

8. Robertson, H. A., King, G. J. and Dyck, G. W. (1978). The appearance of oestrone sulphate in the peripheral plasma of the pig early in pregnancy. *J. Reprod. Fertil.*, **52**, 337

9. Hobson, B. M. (1974). Advances in human pregnancy testing. *Bibliogr. Reprod.*, **24**, 1

10. Forbes, T. R. (1957). Early pregnancy and fertility tests. *Yale J. Biol. Med.*, **30**, 16

11. Richardson, C. (1972). Pregnancy diagnosis in the ewe: a review. *Vet. Res.*, **90**, 264

12. Tullner, W. W. (1971). Chorionic gonadotrophin in non-human primates. In Diczfalusy, E. and Standley, C. C. (eds.) *The Use of Non-Human Primates in Research on Human Reproduction*, pp. 200–213. (Copenhagen: Bogtrykkeriet Forum)

13. Canfield, R. E., Morgan, F. J., Kammerman, S., Bell, J. J. and Agosto, G. M. (1971). Studies of human gonadotrophin. *Recent Progr. Horm. Res.*, **27**, 121

14. Ross, G. T. (1979). Human chorionic gonadotropin and maternal recognition of pregnancy. In Whelan, J. (ed.) *Maternal Recognition of Pregnancy*. Ciba Foundation Symposium, **64**, 191–208. (Elsevier Press, Amsterdam)

15. Knobil, E. (1973). On the regulation of the primate corpus luteum. *Biol. Reprod.*, **8**, 246

16. Hearn, J. P. (1979). Immunological interference with the maternal recognition of pregnancy in primates. In Whelan, J. (ed.) *Maternal Recognition of Pregnancy*. Ciba Foundation Symposium, **64**, 353–375. (Elsevier Press, Amsterdam)

17. Hobson, B. M. (1976). Evaluation of the sub-human primate tube test for pregnancy in primates. *Lab. Anim.*, **10**, 87 (In press)

18. Hobson, B. M., Hearn, J. P., Lunn, S. F. and Flockhart, J. H. (1977). Urinary excretion of biologically active chorionic gonadotrophin by the pregnant marmoset: *Callithrix jacchus jacchus*. *Folia Primatol.*, **28**, 251

19. Boorman, G. A., Speltie, T. M. and Fitzgerald, G. M. (1974). Urinary chorionic gonadotrophin excretion during pregnancy in the chimpanzee. *J. Med. Primatol.*, **3**, 269

20. Glass, R. H. and Van Wagenen, G. (1970). Immunological test for chorionic gonadotropin in serum of the pregnant monkey, *Macaca mulatta*. *Proc. Soc. Exp. Biol. Med.*, **134**, 467

21. Gribnau, A. A. M. (1975). Immunologic pregnancy test in the Rhesus monkey (*Macaca mulatta*). *J. Med. Primatol.*, **4**, 65

22. Czekala, N. M., Hodges, J. K. and Lasley, B. L. (1979). Pregnancy monitoring in diverse primate species by estrogen and bioactive luteinizing hormone determinations in small volumes of urine. *J. Med. Primatol.* (Submitted)

23. Dufau, M. L., Pock, R., Neubauer, A. and Catt, K. J. (1976). *In vitro* bioassay of LH in human serum: the rat interstitial cell testosterone (RICT) assay. *J. Clin. Endocrinol. Metab.*, **42**, 958

24. Saxtena, B. B., Hasan, S. H., Haour, F. and Schmidt-Gollwitzer, M. (1974). Radioreceptor assay of human chorionic gonadotrophin: detection of early pregnancy. *Science*, **8**, 349

25. Beling, C. G., Cederquist, L. L. and Fuchs, F. (1976). Demonstration of gonadotropin during the second half of the cycle in women using intra-uterine contraception. *Am. J. Obstet. Gynecol.*, **125**, 855

26. Ross, G. T. (1977). Clinical relevance of research on the structure of human chorionic gonadotropin. *Am. J. Obstet. Gynecol.*, **129**, 795

27. Carr, D. H. (1971). Chromosome studies in selected spontaneous abortions: polyploidy in man. *J. Med. Genet.*, **8**, 164

28. Chen, H.-C., Hodgen, G. D., Matsuura, S., Lin, L. J., Gross, E., Reichert, L. E. Jr., Birken, S., Canfield, R. E. and Ross, G. T. (1976). Evidence for a gonadotropin from non-pregnant subjects that has physical, immunological and biological similarities to human chorionic gonadotropin. *Proc. Natl. Acad. Sci. USA*, **73**, 2885

29. Myers, R. E. (1972). The pathology of the Rhesus monkey placenta. In Diczfalusy, E. and Standley, C. C. (eds.) *The Use of Non-Human Primates in Research on Human Reproduction*, pp. 221–257. (Copenhagen: Bogtrykkevert Forum)

30. Wilson, J. G. (1972). Abnormalities of intrauterine development in non-human primates. In Diczfalusy, E. and Standley, C. C. (eds.) *The Use of Non-Human Primates in Research on Human Reproduction*, pp. 261–292. (Copenhagen: Bogtrykkevert Forum)

31. Hodges, J. K., Czekala, N. M. and Lasley, B. L. (1979). Estrogen and luteinizing hormone secretion in diverse primate species from simplified urinary analysis. *J. Med. Primatol.* **8**, 349

32. Cole, H. H. and Hart, G. H. (1930). The potency of blood serum of mares in progressive stages of pregnancy in effecting the sexual maturity of the immature rat. *Am. J. Physiol.*, **93**, 57

33. Allen, W. R. (1969). The immunological measurement of pregnant mare serum gonadotrophin. *J. Endocrinol.*, **43**, 592

34. Papkoff, H. (1974). Chemical and biological properties of the subunits or pregnant mare serum gonadotrophin. *Biochem. Biophys. Res. Commun.*, **58**, 397

35. Cole, H. H. (1936). On the biological properties of mare gonadotropic hormone. *Am. J. Anat.*, **59**, 299

36. Allen, W. R. (1979). Maternal recognition of pregnancy and immunological implications of trophoblast-endometrium interactions in equids. In Whelan, J. (ed.) *Maternal Recognition of Pregnancy*. Ciba Foundation Symposium, **64**, 323–352. (Amsterdam: Excerpta Medica)

37. Wide, M. and Wide, L. (1963). Diagnosis of pregnancy in mares by an immunological method. *Nature (London)*, **198**, 1017

38. Wide, L. (1962). An immunological method on the assay of human chorionic gonadotrophin. *Acta Endocrinol.* Suppl., **70**

39. Richards, C. G. (1967). Simple immunological method for the diagnosis of pregnancy in mares. *Nature (London)*, **215**, 1280

40. Menzer, C. and Schams, D. (1979). Radioimmunoassay for PMSG and its application to *in vivo* studies. *J. Reprod. Fertil.*, **55**, 339

41. Stewart, F., Allen, W. R. and Moor, R. M. (1976). Pregnant mare serum gonadotrophin: ratio of follicle-stimulating hormone and luteinizing hormone activities measured by radioreceptor assay. *J. Endocrinol.*, **71**, 371

42. Jeffcott, L. B., Atherton, J. G. and Mingay, J. (1969). Equine pregnancy diagnosis. *Vet. Res.*, **84**, 80

43. Walker, D. (1977). Laboratory methods of equine pregnancy diagnosis. *Vet. Rec.*, **100**, 396

44. Allen, W. R. (1975). The influence of fetal genotype upon endometrial cup development and PMSG and progestagen production in equids. *J. Reprod. Fertil.*, **23** (Suppl.), 405

45. Allen, W. R. (1970). Endocrinology of early pregnancy in the mare. *Equine Vet. J.*, **2**, 64

46. Grosskopf, J. F. and Smuts, E. G. (1975). Activity of serum gonadotropins in pregnant zebras and mares. *J. S. Afr. Vet. Assoc.*, **46**, 367

47. Wilkinson, J. N. and Fremery, P. de (1940). Gonadotrophic hormones in the urine of the giraffe. *Nature (London)*, **146**, 491
48. Wiley, L. D. (1974). Presence of gonadotrophin on the surface of pre-implanted mouse embryos. *Nature (London)*, **252**, 715
49. Haour, F., Tell, G. and Sanchez, P. (1976). Mise en evidence et dosage d'une gonadotrophine chorionique chez le rat (rCG). *C.R. Acad. Sci. Paris (Ser. D.)*, **282**, 1183
50. Haour, F. and Saxena, B. B. (1974). Detection of gonadotropin in the rabbit blastocyst before implantation. *Science*, **185**, 444
51. Wintenberger-Torres, S. (1978). Role actif de l'embryon avant l'implantation. In du Mesnil du Buisson, F., Psychoyos, A. and Thomas, K. (eds.) *L'Implantation de L'oeuf*, pp. 181–192. (Paris: Masson)
52. Forsyth, I. A. and Hayden, T. J. (1977). Comparative endocrinology of mammary growth and lactation. In Peaker, M. (ed.) *Symposia of the Zoological Society of London*, No. 41, Comparative aspects of lactation, pp. 135–163. (London: Academic Press)
53. Kelly, P. A. (1977). Secretion and biological effects of placental lactogens. In *Endocrinology*, International Congress Series No. 238, p. 298. (Amsterdam and Oxford: Excerpta Medica)
54. Stevens, V. C., Bohn, H. and Powell, J. E. (1976). Serum levels of a placental protein during gestation in the baboon. *Am. J. Obstet. Gynecol.*, **124**, 51
55. Boshier, D. P. (1969). A histological and histochemical examination of implantation and early placentome formation in sheep. *J. Reprod. Fertil.*, **19**, 51
56. Flint, A. P. F., Henville, A. and Christie, W. B. (1979). Presence of placental lactogen in bovine conceptuses before attachment. *J. Reprod. Fertil.*, **56**, 305
57. Bolander, F. F., Ulberg, L. C. and Fellows, R. E. (1976). Circulating placental lactogen levels in dairy and beef cattle. *Endocrinology*, **99**, 1273
58. Shiu, R. P. C., Kelly, P. A. and Friesen, H. G. (1973). Radioreceptor assay for prolactin and other lactogenic hormones. *Science*, **180**, 968
59. Bohn, H. (1974). Characterization of the pregnancy associated glycoproteins as acute phase reactants. Their detection in sera from patients with tumours and other diseases. *Arch. Gynaekol.*, **213**, 54
60. Stimson, W. H. and Eubank-Scott, L. (1972). The isolation and partial characterization of a new α-macroglobulin from human pregnancy serum. *FEBS Lett.*, **23**, 298
61. Yachin, S. (1976). Demonstration of the inhibitory effect of human alphafetoprotein on *in vitro* transformation of human lymphocytes. *Proc. Natl. Acad. Sci. USA*, **73**, 2857
62. Morton, H., Rolfe, B., Clunie, G. J. A., Anderson, M. J. and Morrison, J. (1977). An early pregnancy factor detected in human serum by the rosette inhibition test. *Lancet*, **1**, 394
63. Heywood, L. H., Goodall, E. T. and Thornburn, G. D. (1979). Detection of early pregnancy in the rat using the rosette inhibition test. In *Proceedings of the Eleventh Annual Conference, Australian Society for Reproductive Biology*, p. 55
64. Nancarrow, C. D., Rigby, N. W., Evison, B. M., Wallace, A. L. C., Scaramuzzi, R. J. and Morton, H. (1978). A pregnancy test used for detection of induced embryo mortality in sheep and cattle. In *Proceedings of the 6th Asia and Oceania Congress of Endocrinology, Singapore*, Abstract 115
65. Morton, H., Nancarrow, C. D., Scaramuzzi, R. J., Evison, B. M. and Clunie, G. J. A. (1979). Detection of early pregnancy in sheep by the rosette inhibition test. *J. Reprod. Fertil.*, **56**, 75
66. Nancarrow, C. D. and Wallace, A. L. (1979). Distribution of an early pregnancy factor in the sheep. In *Proceedings of the Eleventh Annual Conference, Australian Society for Reproductive Biology*, p. 12
67. Goodall, E. T. and Thorburn, G. D. (1979). Evidence for immunosuppressive activity in ovine foetal serum. In *Proceedings of the Eleventh Annual Conference, Australian Society for Reproductive Biology*, p. 54
68. Noonan, F. P., Halliday, W. J., Morton, H. and Clunie, G. J. A. (1979). Early pregnancy factor is immunosuppressive. *Nature (London)*, **278**, 649

69. Nancarrow, C. D., Evison, B. M., Scaramuzzi, R. J. and Turnbull, K. E. (1979). Detection of induced death of embryos in sheep by the rosette inhibition test. *J. Reprod. Fertil.*, **57**, 385

70. Roberts, G. P. and Parker, J. M. (1974). Macromolecular components of the humoral fluid from the bovine uterus. *J. Reprod. Fertil.*, **40**, 291

71. Murray, F. A., Zurcher, V. and Grifo, A. P. J. (1979). Suppression of lymphocyte reactivity *in vitro* by porcine allantoic and amniotic fluids. *Theriogenology*, **11**, 217

72. Amoroso, E. C. and Perry, J. S. (1975). The existence during gestation of an immunological buffer zone at the interface between maternal and foetal tissues. *Phil. Trans. R. Soc. Lond.*, **271**, 343

73. Lin, T.-M., Halbert, S. P. and Kiefer, D. (1974). Pregnancy-associated serum antigens in the rat and mouse. *Proc. Soc. Exp. Biol. Med.*, **145**, 62

74. Roberts, G. P. (1977). Inhibition of lymphocyte stimulation by bovine uterine proteins. *J. Reprod. Fertil.*, **50**, 337

75. Behrman, S. J., Yoshida, T., Amano, Y. and Paine, P. (1974). Rhesus and squirrel monkey placental specific antigen(s). *Am. J. Obstet. Gynecol.*, **118**, 616

76. Bohn, H. and Ronnebeger, H. (1973). Immunologischer Nachweis von Schwanger-Schaftsproteinen des Menschen im serum trachtiger Tiere. *Arch. Gynaekol.*, **215**, 277

77. Bohn, H. and Weinmann, E. (1974). Immunologische Unterbrechung der Schwangerschaft bei Affen mit Antikorpern gegen das menschliche schwangerschaft-spezifische β_1-Glyko-protein (SP$_1$). *Arch. Gynaekol.*, **217**, 209

78. Grudzinskas, J. G., Gordon, Y. B., Jeffrey, D. and Chard, T. (1977). Specific and sensitive determination of pregnancy-specific β_1-glycoprotein by radioimmunoassay. *Lancet*, **1**, 333

79. Cerini, M., Findlay, J. K. and Lawson, R. A. S. (1976). Pregnancy-specific antigens in the sheep: application to the diagnosis of pregnancy. *J. Reprod. Fertil.*, **46**, 65

80. Findlay, J. K., Cerini, Mildred and Lawson, R. A. S. (1979). The use of rabbit anti-sheep conceptus sera to diagnose pregnancy by haemagglutination of erythrocytes from pregnant ewes. (In preparation)

81. Staples, L. D., Lawson, R. A. S. and Findlay, J. K. (1978). The occurrence of an antigen associated with pregnancy in the ewe. *Biol. Reprod.*, **19**, 1076

82. Staples, L. D., Borland, R., Chamley, W. A., Cumming, I. A., Lawson, R. A. S., Wilks, C. and Findlay, J. K. (1979). The failure of bovine anti-sheep conceptus sera to localize ovine pregnancy associated antigen on erythrocytes of pregnant ewes. (In preparation)

83. Cerini, M. (1976). The endocrinology and immunology of the transition to pregnancy in the ewe. *Thesis for the degree of Doctorate of Philosophy*, University of Melbourne

84. Staples, L. D. (1978). The biochemistry and physiology of ovine pregnancy associated antigens and the recognition of pregnancy. *Thesis for the degree of Master of Agricultural Science*, University of Melbourne

85. Lam, C. F., Godley, W. C., Kennedy, S. W. and Moore, S. L. (1968). An immunological test for pregnancy in the ewe. *J. Anim. Sci.*, **27**, 301

86. Geschwind, I. (1968). Early pregnancy diagnosis in the ewe. Presented by Ivan L. Lindahl at a *private symposium on the Physiology of Reproduction in Sheep*, Oklahoma, 1968. Personal communication

87. Staples, L. D., Lawson, R. A. S., Cerini, M. and Findlay, J. K. (1977). The characterization of an antigen(s) associated with pregnancy in the ewe. In Boettcher, B. (ed.) *Immunological Influence on Human Fertility*, pp. 139–152. (Sydney: Academic Press)

88. Martal, J., Lacroix, M. C., Loudes, C., Saunier, M. and Wintenberger-Torres, S. (1979). Trophoblastin, an antiluteolytic protein present in early pregnancy in sheep. *J. Reprod. Fertil.*, **56**, 63

89. Moor, R. M. (1968). Effect of embryo on corpus luteum function. *J. Anim. Sci.*, **27**, 97

90. Roberts, G. P., Parker, J. M. and Symonds, H. W. (1976). Macromolecular components of genital tract fluids from sheep. *J. Reprod. Fertil.*, **48**, 99

91. Laster, D. B. (1977). A pregnancy-specific protein in the bovine uterus. *Biol. Reprod.*, **16**, 682

92. Cerini, M., Wright, P. J., Murray, A., McColm, S. and Findlay, J. K. (1978). Pregnancy associated serum antigens in the mare. In *Proceedings of the Tenth Annual Conference, Australian Society for Reproductive Biology*, p. 41

93. Amoroso, E. C. and Finn, C. A. (1962). Ovarian activity during gestation, ovum transport and implantation. In Zuckerman, S. (ed.) *The Ovary*, Vol. 1, p. 451. (New York: Academic Press)

94. Laing, J. A. and Heap, R. B. (1971). The concentration of progesterone in the milk of cows during the reproductive cycle. *Br. Vet. J.*, **127**, xix

95. Heap, R. B., Gwyn, M., Laing, J. A. and Walters, D. E. (1973). Pregnancy diagnosis in cows: Changes in milk progesterone concentration during the oestrous cycle and pregnancy measured by a rapid radioimmunoassay. *J. Agric. Sci., Camb.*, **81**, 151

96. McCracken, J. A. (1963). The distribution of progesterone in body fluids and tissues of the dairy cow. *Ph.D. Thesis*, University of Glasgow

97. Hoffmann, B., Gunzler, O., Hamburger, R. and Schmidt, W. (1976). Milk progesterone as a parameter for fertility control in cattle; methodological approaches and present status of application in Germany. *Br. Vet. J.*, **132**, 469

98. Heap, R. B., Holdsworth, R. J., Gadsby, J. E., Laing, J. A. and Walters, D. E. (1976). Pregnancy diagnosis in the cow from milk progesterone concentration. *Br. Vet. J.*, **132**, 445

99. Booth, J. M. and Holdsworth, R. J. (1976). The establishment and operation of a central laboratory for pregnancy testing in cows. *Br. Vet. J.*, **132**, 518

100. Thibier, M., Fourbet, J. F. and Parez, M. (1976). Relationship between milk progesterone concentration and milk yield, fat and total nitrogen content. *Br. Vet. J.*, **132**, 477

101. Pennington, J. A., Spahr, S. L. and Lodge, J. R. (1976). Factors affecting progesterone in milk for pregnancy diagnosis in dairy cattle. *Br. Vet. J.*, **132**, 487

102. Pope, G. S., Majzlik, I., Ball, P. J. H. and Leaver, J. D. (1976). Use of progesterone concentrations in plasma and milk in the diagnosis of pregnancy in domestic cattle. *Br. Vet. J.*, **132**, 497

103. Thirapatsukun, T., Entwistle, K. W. and Gartner, R. J. W. (1978). Plasma progesterone levels as an early pregnancy test in beef cattle. *Theriogenology*, **9**, 323

104. Thibier, M. and Terqui, M. (1978). Les diagnostic de gestation et de non-gestation ches les mammiferes domestiques de ferme. In du Mesnil du Buisson, F., Psychoyos, A. and Thomas, K. (eds.) *L'Implantation de L'oeuf*, pp. 127–146. (Paris: Masson)

105. Shemesh, M., Ayalon, N. and Mazor, T. (1979). Early pregnancy diagnosis in the ewe, based on milk progesterone levels. *J. Reprod. Fertil.*, **56**, 301

106. Williamson, P., Hennessy, D. P. and Cutler, R. (1980). The use of progesterone and oestrogen concentrations in the diagnosis of pregnancy, and in the study of seasonal infertility in sows. *Aust. J. Agric. Res.*, **31**, 233

107. Shepherd, E., Findlay, J. K., Cooper, M. J. and Allen, W. R. (1976). Treatment of non-cycling mares with a synthetic prostaglandin analogue. *Aust. Vet. J.*, **52**, 345

108. Findlay, J. K. and Cox, R. I. (1970). Oestrogens in the plasma of the sheep foetus. *J. Endocrinol.*, **46**, 281

109. Carnegie, J. A. and Robertson, H. A. (1978). Conjugated and unconjugated estrogens in fetal and maternal fluids of the pregnant ewe: A possible role for estrone sulfate during early pregnancy. *Biol. Reprod.*, **19**, 202

110. Robertson, H. A. and King, G. J. (1979). Conjugated and unconjugated oestrogens in fetal and maternal fluids of the cow throughout pregnancy. *J. Reprod. Fertil.*, **55**, 463

111. Robertson, H. A. and King, G. J. (1974). Plasma concentrations of progesterone, oestrone, oestradiol-17β and of oestrone sulphate in the pig at implantation, during pregnancy and at parturition. *J. Reprod. Fertil.*, **40**, 133

112. Findlay, J. K. and Seamark, R. F. (1971). The occurrence and metabolism of oestrogens in the sheep foetus and placenta. In Pierrepoint, G. C. (ed.) *Symposium: The Endocrinology of Pregnancy and Parturition*, p. 54. (Tenovus Library Series)

113. Cox, R. I., Hodgkinson, R. M. and Wong, M. S. F. (1979). Antisera reactive directly to estrone sulfate. *Steroids*, **33**, 549

114. Hodgen, G. D., Wolfe, L. G., Ogden, J. D., Adams, M. R., Descalzi, C. C. and Hildebrand, D. F. (1976). Diagnosis of pregnancy in Marmosets: hemagglutination inhibition test and radioimmunoassay for urinary chorionic gonadotrophin. *Lab. Anim. Sci.*, **26**, 224

115. Chambers, P. L. and Hearn, J. P. (1979). Peripheral plasma levels of progesterone, oestradiol-17β, oestrone, testosterone, androstenedione, and chorionic gonadotrophin during pregnancy in the marmoset monkey, *Callithrix jacchus*. *J. Reprod. Fertil.*, **56**, 23

116. Hodgen, G. D., Stolzenberg, S. J., Jones, D. C. L., Hildebrand, D. F. and Turner, C. K. (1978). Pregnancy diagnosis in squirrel monkeys: Hemagglutination test, radioimmunoassay, and bioassay of chorionic gonadotropin. *J. Med. Primatol.*, **7**, 59

117. Hodgen, G. D., Niemann, W. H. and Tullner, W. W. (1975). Duration of chorionic gonadotropin production by the placenta of the rhesus monkey. *Endocrinology*, **96**, 789

118. Hodgen, G. D. and Niemann, W. H. (1975). Application of the subhuman primate pregnancy test kit to pregnancy diagnosis in baboons. *Lab. Anim. Sci.*, **25**, 757

119. Shaikh, A. A., Allen-Rowlands, C., Dozier, T., Kraemer, D. C. and Goldzieher, J. W. (1976). Diagnosis of early pregnancy in the baboon. *Contraception*, **14**, 391

120. Woodard, D. K., Graham, C. E. and McClure, H. M. (1976). Comparison of hemagglutination inhibition pregnancy tests in the chimpanzee and the orangutan. *Lab. Anim. Sci.*, **26**, 922

121. Clegg, M. T. and Weaver, M. (1972). Chorionic gonadotropin secretion during pregnancy in the chimpanzee, *Pan troglodyte*. *Proc. Soc. Exp. Biol. Med.*, **139**, 1170

122. Hodgen, G. D., Niemann, W. H., Turner, C. K. and Chen, H. (1976). Diagnosis of pregnancy in chimpanzees using the nonhuman primate pregnancy test kit. *J. Med. Primatol.*, **5**, 247

123. Davis, R. R. (1977). Pregnancy diagnosis in an orangutan using two prepared test kits. *J. Med. Primatol.*, **6**, 315

124. Hodgen, G. D., Turner, C. K., Smith, E. E. and Mitchell-Bush, R. (1977). Pregnancy diagnosis in the orangutan, *Pongo pygmaeus*, using the subhuman primate pregnancy test kit. *Lab. Anim. Sci.*, **27**, 99

4
Immunological Aspects of Eclampsia and Pre-eclampsia

C. W. G. REDMAN

INTRODUCTION

Pre-eclampsia/eclampsia is a disorder of the second half of human pregnancy, and a principal cause of both maternal and perinatal mortality and morbidity. Its cause is unknown and its investigation is constrained by the lack of any equivalent disorder in other mammalian species. The diagnosis of pre-eclampsia varies between different investigators – it may be a syndrome with several different aetiologies rather than a single disease entity.

The defining clinical feature is a rise in blood pressure reversed by delivery. This is accompanied by alterations in renal tubular and glomerular function, and proteinuria if the disorder is well advanced[1]. The clotting system is activated[2]. The usual cause of maternal death is cerebral haemorrhage[3] and at autopsy there is disseminated small vessel thrombosis[4]. The fetus is compromised indirectly by placental ischaemia which may be complicated by placental infarction or retro-placental bleeding[5,6].

The incidence of pre-eclampsia, like that of essential hypertension, depends entirely on how it is defined. A conservative estimate would be that it affects 5% of all pregnancies. Proteinuric pre-eclampsia is rarer with an incidence of about 0.5%. The development of effective prevention and treatment for this relatively common problem is unlikely while its pathological processes are so poorly understood. At the present time the only treatment available is ending the pregnancy by delivery.

Is pre-eclampsia a disturbance of the immune relationship between mother and fetus? The question has been asked many times and recently reviewed by several authors[7–14]. There is circumstantial but not direct evidence that the question is relevant, and it is possible that its further investigation may not only reveal the aetiology of pre-eclampsia but cast light on the immune mechanisms of mammalian pregnancy.

EPIDEMIOLOGICAL EVIDENCE

The protective effect of a first pregnancy

Severe pre-eclampsia occurs at least 10 times more commonly in first than in second or later pregnancies[15]. Even a single miscarriage has some effect on preventing the development of the disorder[15]. It is difficult to explain this first-pregnancy preponderance of pre-eclampsia without invoking immune mechanisms – that is by proposing that previous exposure to fetal antigens is in some way protective. It is usually assumed that a maternal immune reaction to the fetus will be harmful, as with rhesus isoimmunization. But if the first pregnancy phenomenon of pre-eclampsia points to an immune mechanism then in normal human pregnancy there must be a *beneficial* maternal immune reaction to fetal antigens, the absence of which causes pre-eclampsia. This would be most likely in a first pregnancy with a first-set immune response than in later pregnancies[11].

Pre-immunization

The concept that a maternal immune response to fetal or paternal antigens may prevent pre-eclampsia is supported by other studies. The protective effect of a first pregnancy may be nullified if a woman changes partners[16, 17]. It may be enhanced by pre-conceptual exposure to antigens of sperm and seminal fluid[18] and simulated by previous blood transfusions[19]. The latter observations parallel the disputed claims that prior blood transfusions prevent renal allograft rejection[20].

THE PLACENTA IN PRE-ECLAMPSIA

There is no known maternal immune response to the fetus which could explain these observations; and therefore neither are there antigens defined to which it might be directed. However these problems lead to consideration of the role of the placenta in pre-eclampsia, because it is the main maternal–fetal interface. Gross changes in its structure and vascular supply occur.

Vascular pathology of the placenta

In pre-eclampsia, the basal and spiral arteries which maintain the utero-placental circulation are obstructed by fibrinoid necrosis, infiltrating lipophages and secondary thrombosis, associated with a low-grade perivascular round-cell infiltrate[21]. The process has been called 'acute atherosis'[22]. The damaged vessel walls allow outward transudation of plasma proteins which include complement components; these are demonstrable by immuno-fluorescence.

The consequences of these lesions are placental changes characteristic of pre-eclampsia: reduced placental blood flow[23], with histological features ascribable to ischaemia – cytotrophoblast proliferation[24], syncytial budding[25] and placental infarction[5].

The cause of acute atherosis is not known, but the histological features are similar to those seen in the arteries of rejected renal allografts. The latter lesions were originally thought to be induced by hypertension[26] and only later was it realized that they resulted from immune injury[27]. Likewise acute atherosis is thought to result from raised blood pressure, but there is evidence against this.

If the lesions stem from hypertensive damage then the uterine arteries must be unusually sensitive to increases in blood pressure because the changes are not found elsewhere in the maternal arterial tree[21]. Furthermore, placental infarcts which are the consequence of uterine artery obstruction from acute atherosis occur in normotensive pregnancies[5]. Finally, the lesion has been found in pregnancies complicated by intra-uterine growth-retardation without hypertension[28]. Thus it is more likely that the hypertension is not the cause but a consequence of the problem, and that the vascular lesions result from other processes, possibly involving immune mechanisms.

This conclusion fits well with the evidence that placental ischaemia can cause some of the features of pre-eclampsia. Aortic hypoplasia may be associated with pre-eclampsia[29]. Experimentally placental ischaemia has been used to produce pre-eclamptic-like syndromes in baboons[30], dogs[31, 32], rabbits[33], or rats[34]. The uterus is a source of extra-renal renin, synthesized, for example, by the human chorionic membranes[35], and uterine renin may be released in response to hypotension in a comparable way to renal renin[36]. Angiotensin II levels may be increased in pre-eclampsia[37] although other investigators find the converse change[38]. However plasma renin activity seems to be higher in uterine compared to peripheral venous blood, and this is not true of normal pregnancy[39].

Hence the sequence of events: immune injury, causing uterine artery obstruction, causing placental ischaemia, causing maternal hypertension, might be explained in terms of the available evidence.

The placenta as an immune stimulus

Unusual presentations of pre-eclampsia occur with hydatidiform mole and hydrops fetalis with or without rhesus disease, including hydrops associated with chromosomal triploidy[40, 41]. These are all conditions with an unusually large placental mass. Pre-eclampsia is also three times more common in twin pregnancies[42]. Consequently it has been suggested that a relative excess of trophoblast tissue (hyperplacentosis) may precipitate pre-eclampsia. This could be by non-immune mechanisms (relative ischaemia) or via 'immuno- logical overload'[11] with an impaired maternal immune response generating pathogenic circulating immune complexes.

Normal pregnancy is characterized by 'deportation' of trophoblast into the maternal circulation. The trophoblast cells lodge in the pulmonary capillaries where they lyse without provoking an inflammatory reaction[43]. This process is exaggerated in pre-eclampsia[44, 45] and may cause antigenic overload in the absence of changes in placental size.

Does the placenta provoke an abnormal immune reaction in pre-eclampsia?

Trophoblast cell membrane does not contain histocompatibility antigens[46–48], and the absence of these antigens probably prevents direct rejection by the mother[49]. Other components of the placenta may stimulate maternal antibody production[50]. Pre-eclampsia may be associated with maternal antibodies to placental polysaccharide[51], to a placental microsomal fraction[52] or to trophoblast cells[53]. Pre-eclamptic placentas contain connective tissue proteins not present in normal placentas[54] which could be immunogenic. However it is unlikely that placental antibodies are a cause rather than a consequence of pre-eclampsia because their incidence should increase with parity, the con- verse pattern of pre-eclampsia.

Cell-mediated immunity to trophoblast preparations has been demon- strated in normal pregnancy[55–57] and the presence of autologous serum or plasma factors may block these reactions[58, 59]. However comparable studies in pre-eclamptic pregnancies have not been reported.

Cross-reactivity between placental and renal antigens

Human placentas and kidneys share common antigens[60] in basement membranes[61] and cytoplasmic structures, including microsomal and mito- chondrial fractions[62, 63]. This cross-reactivity explains the experimental nephritis caused by active or passive immunization to placental extracts[64–67]. The antigens include a non-collagenous glycoprotein[68] and lack species- specificity in that the nephritis can be induced both in sheep[61] and rats[68] by antisera to human placental extracts. Antisera to either placental or renal basement membranes cause similar and self-sustaining nephritides. The renal damage of pre-eclampsia is not self-sustaining, which argues against this being a model for the pre-eclamptic process.

ANTIGENIC RELATIONSHIP BETWEEN MOTHER AND FETUS

Histocompatibility antigens

Maternal immunization to fetal HLA antigens occurs during normal pregnancy, despite their absence from trophoblast. These antigens are the main determinants of allograft rejection[69]. Consequently if pre-eclampsia represents maternal rejection of the fetus[70] the antigenic relationship between mother and fetus with respect to HLA should be critical.

Earlier reports suggested that pre-eclampsia is associated with *increased* maternal–fetal incompatibility, in that a higher incidence was found in out-bred compared to in-bred populations[71], in dizygous compared to monozygous twins[72], and with male compared to female fetuses[73]. The latter two claims have not been confirmed[42, 74].

The contrary claims of *less* incompatibility between mother and fetus emerged from a study of the HLA types of mothers with severe pre-eclampsia and their partners compared with control couples[75]. Eighteen out of 20 A and B antigens were shared more commonly than expected, although for no single antigen was the increased sharing statistically significant (Figure 4.1).

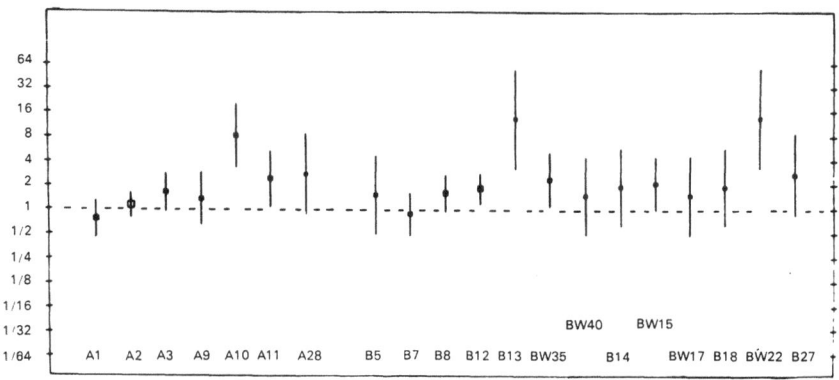

Figure 4.1 Sharing of HLA-A and B antigens in 38 couples with pre-eclampsia compared with estimates from general population data. The vertical axis marks increased incidence of sharing, above dotted line, and reduced incidence below. Eighteen of the 20 antigens were more commonly shared in the pre-eclamptic pairs than predicted from the control data. (Reproduced by permission from the *British Medical Journal*, see reference 75.)

In a second pregnancy by the same partner a woman has a 50% chance of being exposed to a completely new HLA haplotype. If exposure to HLA alloantigens were the entire cause of pre-eclampsia then its incidence would be halved in a second pregnancy, whereas the observed reduction is much greater[15]. Thus other factors such as other antigens or immune responses must be involved.

HLA antibodies

Even though fetal trophoblast is devoid of HLA antigens, maternal leuko-cytotoxic antibodies directed against fetal HLA specificities are found in normal pregnancy, more often in parous than primigravid women[76]. If maternal HLA antibody production (increasing with parity) were linked to pre-eclampsia (decreasing with parity) a *negative* association would be predicted. This has been found in one study[77] but not in others which were, however, less well controlled[78-82]. These all relate to HLA-A and B anti-bodies; nothing is yet published concerning DR_w antibodies whose role may be more to block rather than augment cellular immune reactions[83].

Histocompatibility complex and immune responses

The human histocompatibility complex on the short arm of the sixth chromosome regulates many immune functions[84]. The association of some human diseases, particularly autoimmune diseases, with particular HLA types, probably stems from the close relationship between HLA genes and neighbouring but undefined genes controlling immune responses[85].

Table 4.1   Incidence of presumed HLA-A and B homozygosity in 80 pre-eclamptic women compared with 83 women with normal pregnancies (see reference 74)

		Mother homozygous at	
		Locus A	Locus B
Pre-eclamptic pregnancies	(80)	22 (27.5%)	18 (22.5%)
Fetal survival in pre-eclampsia			
Dead	(48)	14 (29%)	14 (29%)*
Alive	(32)	8 (25%)	4 (13%)
Controls	(83)	13 (15.7%)	5 (6.0%)
Time of delivery in pre-eclampsia			
≤ 28 weeks	(16)	4 (25%)	5 (31%)†
29–32 weeks	(23)	6 (26%)	6 (26%)
> 32 weeks	(41)	12 (29%)	7 (17%)
Controls	(83)	13 (15.7%)	5 (6.0%)

* $\chi^2 = 11.62, p < 0.01$; with significant linear trend $p < 0.01$
† $\chi^2 = 8.35, p < 0.05$; with significant linear trend $p < 0.01$

Three separate studies agree that pre-eclampsia is not associated with particular HLA-A or B antigens[74, 75, 86]. In the largest study, an unpredicted but significant association was found with maternal homozygosity at the A and B loci, particularly locus B (Table 4.1) which correlated with the severity of the disease[74]. Although homozygosity may be the result of consanguinity, there was no evidence for this from the patients' family histories. These data were tentatively interpreted as evidence for homozygosity for one or several neighbouring immune response genes which, on general genetic grounds, would be predicted to be recessive and therefore associated with absent or defective function.

Could pre-eclampsia be caused by a single recessive gene?

The first genetic theories of pre-eclampsia assumed that a *dominant* gene for an antigen which generated maternal–fetal incompatibility caused the disease. If the mother had this gene then the fetus had to be homozygous for the recessive allele, or vice-versa[87–89]. Either alternative required that both the mothers and daughters of pre-eclamptic women never got pre-eclampsia themselves which several studies have clearly shown *not* to be true[90–92].

In Chesley's study, for example[91], the incidence of eclampsia in daughters of eclamptic women was increased eight-fold. However a modification of the proposal by Kalmus, of maternal homozygosity for a recessive gene, without the requirement that the fetus be heterozygous, is not only consistent with the HLA observations[74] but can explain the familial incidence of pre-eclampsia. The frequency of the hypothetical recessive immune-response gene would need to be 24%, and would explain the familial incidence equally well operating either as a maternal or a fetal gene[93].

The concept of a single recessive gene does not fit with the claim that pre-eclampsia is commoner in out-bred populations[71] but explains the very high incidence of eclampsia in one in-bred family[94].

Evidence of involvement of other antigen systems

Associations between maternal blood groups and pre-eclampsia have been claimed[95–97] but not confirmed[98,99]. Earlier reports that pre-eclampsia was increased with a male fetus[73,100] would have implied that Y chromosome determined products were implicated, but other studies have not confirmed these[75,101].

MATERNAL CELLULAR IMMUNE FUNCTION IN PRE-ECLAMPSIA

Although there are no data to implicate a genetically controlled immune response in the aetiology of pre-eclampsia, there are several reports which have started the complicated process of mapping maternal cellular immune function in this disorder. Total lymphocyte counts and the relative proportions of T and B lymphocytes are similar when pre-eclamptic and normal pregnant women are compared[102]. Spontaneous lymphocyte transformation, which is increased during allograft rejection[103], is also increased in normal pregnancy, and may be reduced in mild but not severe pre-eclampsia[104,105].

In vitro lymphocyte transformation with phytohaemagglutinin (PHA) is depressed in normal pregnancy[105–107]. However contrary results are reported in pre-eclamptic patients, either of diminished PHA responsiveness compared with normal pregnancy[107] or of increased responsiveness[108], particularly in the pre-clinical phase of the disorder. The two groups used different culture techniques and Need[107] was investigating patients with more severe pre-eclampsia. Even so the discordant results are difficult to explain.

In a serial study, using stored lymphocytes, an early depression of PHA responsiveness was found in one patient who later developed pre-eclampsia[109]. One-way mixed-lymphocyte reactivity (MLR), either between mother and fetus or mother and father, has been reported to be higher in pre-eclampsia[110–112], or depressed[75]. In the latter study there was increased histocompatibility between patients and their partners, which would account for the observed hyporeactivity in MLR.

Pre-eclamptic women produce a cellular immune response to cultured cells infected with primate oncornavirus more frequently than normal pregnant women[113]. This intriguing observation stands alone and its significance is unknown.

These studies are difficult to do. They are even more difficult to interpret; not only because of the contradictory results but because the relation between *in vitro* tests of cellular immune functions and the *in vivo* situation is still poorly understood. A further compounding factor is the possible effects, specific and otherwise, of factors in pregnancy plasma which may alter lymphocyte function.

IMMUNOSUPPRESSIVE FACTORS, IMMUNOGLOBULINS, IMMUNE COMPLEXES

The pregnancy hormones, oestrogens, progesterone or placental lactogen, may inhibit cellular immune function[114–116]. Plasma levels of oestriol and placental lactogen, but probably not progesterone are reduced in pre-eclampsia[117–119]. These changes might diminish non-specific immune suppression.

Other possible non-specific immune suppressive factors include pregnancy-associated α_2-macroglobulin and the acute phase reactant seromucoid. Pregnancy-associated α_2-macroglobulin is reduced in pre-eclampsia and inhibits lymphocyte transformation initiated by allogeneic cells or mitogens[121].

A correlation has been claimed between maternal seromucoid levels, which are raised during and after pre-eclampsia, and depression of mixed lymphocyte reactions between patient and partner[122].

There is evidence that an immunosuppressive maternal IgG directed against fetal B cell alloantigens is present in normal pregnancy plasma and absent with pregnancy abnormalities such as recurrent abortion[56, 58]. IgG with similar properties can be acid-eluted from placental homogenates[123]. Faulk has identified a placental antigen which seems to powerfully inhibit mixed lymphocyte reactions and may be present in pregnancy plasma[59, 124]. However there is no information available with respect to the levels of these factors in pre-eclampsia.

Immunoglobulins

Total serum IgG is depressed in the disorder[125–127], whereas IgA and IgM levels are maintained. The same changes are characteristic of nephrotic syndrome and are ascribed to selective losses of IgG in the urine, rather than any specific immune phenomenon[128].

Circulating immune complexes have been detected in normal human pregnancy[129] which has led to speculation about their possible role in pre-eclampsia, either as immunosuppressive factors or as mediators of 'immune complex' disease.

Is pre-eclampsia an immune complex disease?

The evidence is conflicting, almost certainly because the different assays which have been used for detecting immune complexes cannot be expected to give comparable results[130]. Immune complexes have not been detected in normal pregnancies using the Raji cell assay[131] nor in normal or pre-eclamptic pregnancies using either the Raji cell assay or radiolabelled C1q binding[132]. By polyethylene-glycol precipitation, complexes were not found in normal pregnancy, but were found in two of 10 women with pre-eclampsia[133]. The latex agglutination inhibition assay, however, not only detects circulating immune complexes in normal pregnancy[129] but even higher levels of C1q binding, and IgG complexes in pre-eclampsia[134] (Figure 4.2).

Evidence for immune complex deposition in the renal glomeruli during pre-eclampsia has been claimed[135–137]. Although there are IgG deposits, IgM deposits in either the mesangium or capillary loops associated with complement are more consistent features. Others dispute these findings[138, 139], and the reasons for the disagreement are not clear.

If pre-eclampsia were an immune complex disease we could expect to find systemic changes in the complement system. But the available data about complement do not give convincing evidence in favour of an immune complex aetiology.

THE COMPLEMENT SYSTEM AND PRE-ECLAMPSIA

Increased conversion of C3 (third component of complement) would be expected in pre-eclampsia. Not only are there higher levels of C1q binding

IgG complexes[134] but there is activation of the coagulation system[140]. Both thrombin and plasmin can cleave C3[141] and the two systems, coagulation and complement, interact at several different levels[142]. But there is not unequivocal evidence of complement activation in pre-eclampsia, although there is increased anti-complementary activity, a non-specific change which could be caused by soluble immune complexes, aggregated IgG or other undefined factors[143]. Total haemolytic complement and C1q levels remain unchanged[144–147], and C3 and C3PA (C3-pro-activator) conversion products are not found[143]. Two of four studies have reported increased C3 levels[143, 147–149]. But the increase was only significant in the third study cited. C4 was also measured in the latter two studies, and decreased in pre-eclamptic patients. Analysis of the data of Tedder[147] shows the decrease to be significant at a 5% level but this was not claimed by the authors themselves. C3PA is increased in pre-eclampsia[143]. Overall the pattern of changes is not similar to that seen in an immune complex disorder such as disseminated lupus

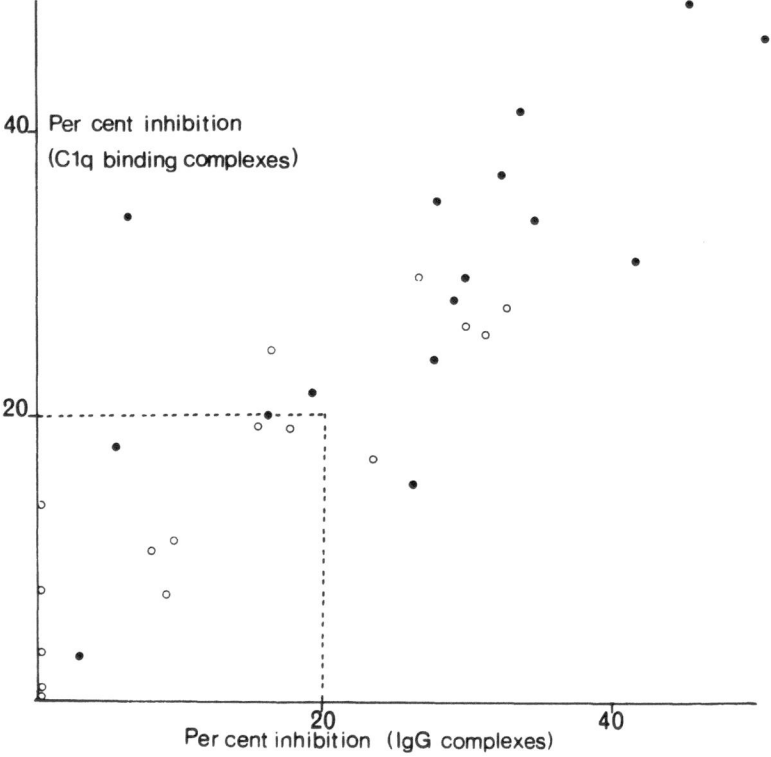

Figure 4.2   IgG and Clq-fixing immune complexes in pregnant women with pre-eclampsia (●) and normal women (○) matched for parity and gestational maturity. Inhibition of less than 20% is normal for non-pregnant individuals (see reference 134)

erythematosus. This leaves an unresolved paradox with, on one hand, good reason for expecting complement activation and on the other hand, no good evidence that it is occurring.

Three factors need to be considered in examining this problem. First the complement system, like the clotting system, functions locally and systemic changes will reflect these events poorly or not at all. Secondly many complement components are acute-phase reactants[150] and therefore may be non-specifically increased in response to the stress of pre-eclampsia. Thirdly the function of the system is the product not only of its active components but of inhibitors whose action might also be altered in pre-eclampsia.

Local activation of complement – evidence for vasculitis in pre-eclampsia

Complement deposition in renal glomeruli is not a uniform feature of pre-eclampsia, whereas its presence is much more consistent in the arterioles of kidneys[135, 151], liver[152], and the utero-placental circulation[153, 154]. However in the spiral arteries the pattern of immunofluorescent staining is not directly related to particular structures in the arterial wall but has the bland appearance of non-specific transudation of plasma constituents, i.e. plasmatic vasculosis[154]. The blood pressures quoted by Petrucco[135] were not in all instances high enough for the vasculitis to result from hypertensive damage. It is therefore possible that the hypertension is a *consequence* of vascular injury, possibly mediated by immune complexes or other immunological factors.

Acute phase reactants and the complement system

Seromucoid, its principal component α_1-acid glycoprotein, ceruloplasmin, α_1-antitrypsin, but not haptoglobin, are all increased in pre-eclampsia[155–159]. The seromucoid content of pre-eclamptic placentas is also increased[160]. All these proteins are classified as acute-phase reactants[161]. In addition, pre-eclamptic sera show the acute-phase property of an enhanced capacity to generate $\overline{C56}$[162]. Fibrinogen, another acute-phase reactant, is consumed by the disseminated intravascular coagulation of advanced pre-eclampsia or eclampsia but is probably increased in the early stages of the disease[163]. Persistence of high α_1-acid glycoprotein for a long time after an acute-phase reaction has been noted[164], and it also occurs after pre-eclampsia[157]. It is clear that pre-eclampsia stimulates an acute-phase reaction. Therefore any interpretation of alteration in the concentrations of these proteins, particularly of complement components, needs to take account of this non-specific stimulus. The rises in pre-eclampsia of C3 and C3PA can therefore be ascribed to an acute-phase reaction. The tendency for C4 to be lower may provide some evidence for early consumption.

CHRONIC HYPERTENSION AS AN IMMUNE DISORDER

The immune system may be involved in the development of hypertension, not associated with pregnancy. It has been postulated that long-term progressive vascular damage might be caused by circulating immune complexes formed, either with self-antigens, or with exogenous antigens such as food or tobacco proteins[165]. The evidence is summarized by Mathews[166]. Permanent hypertension can be produced in rats by infarction of one kidney and removal of the other. The hypertension can be transferred using lymphocytes from such animals, injected into tolerant recipients[167]. Hypertension induced in mice by the same technique or by loading with salt and desoxycorticosterone acetate seems to progress in two phases, the later phase is characterized by inflammatory vascular injury and is thymus-dependent in that athymic mice show a lesser response which is restored to normal by thymic transplantation[168, 169].

Pre-eclampsia and essential hypertension are closely related disorders. Hypertension preceding pregnancy increases the risk of developing pre-eclampsia five-fold[170]. Women who develop pre-eclampsia recurrently in several pregnancies have a higher incidence of vascular disease in later life[171, 172]. In contrast, those who develop pre-eclampsia only in the first pregnancy do not have an abnormal incidence of later vascular disease[171]. These observations have been used to justify the suggestion that pre-eclampsia confined to a first pregnancy is a different disorder from recurrent pre-eclampsia. However it can equally well be argued that the differences are not between two diseases, but between two susceptibilities to the same disease. Both pre-eclampsia and essential hypertension are familial conditions, so there is the tantalizing possibility that there are genes for both, which are either the same or closely linked.

CONCLUSIONS

The evidence that pre-eclampsia is an immune disorder is not only circumstantial but contradictory. Thus, different investigators claim that maternal HLA antibodies are increased, decreased or unchanged in the disorder; that maternal lymphocyte responses to PHA are increased or decreased; that maternal–fetal histoincompatibility is increased or decreased; and so on.

But it is not disputed that a first pregnancy changes a mother so that the risk of pre-eclampsia in later pregnancies, *by the same partner*, is reduced. If this results from the development of an immune response, it must be protective and presumably normally developed in all unaffected pregnancies. What sort of response it might be (humoral or cellular), to what antigens it is directed (trophoblast, HLA or other), and how it might be classified (active, blocking or suppressor) are all completely undefined. Furthermore how the classical signs of pre-eclampsia might develop in the absence of this hypothetical immune response is also poorly delineated, but requires that we postulate a second immune reaction, normally suppressed, which is active and damaging. The possibilities (all hypothetical) can be summarized as follows.

Immune complex disease

A normal pregnancy exposes the mother to an increasing influx of fetal antigens which have to be cleared by complexing with maternal antibodies and removal by the reticuloendothelial system. If the antibody response is inadequate, or the antigenic burden excessive, pathological immune complexes are formed, causing vasculitis, glomerular damage and abnormal activation of the clotting system, from which the outward signs of pre-eclampsia result.

Uteroplacental vascular disease

The lesions of 'acute atherosis' in the uterine spiral arteries are the consequence of an allograft rejection reaction between mother and fetus. Who is rejecting whom? The distal ends of the spiral arteries are lined by fetal trophoblast cells so it is not clear if these should be considered to be fetal vessels, with the mother rejecting the fetus, or maternal vessels, with the fetus rejecting the mother. In either case the ultimate development of the clinical signs of pre-eclampsia would be mediated by placental ischaemia; for example through the release of uterine renin.

If we postulate maternal rejection of the fetus then the protective immune response of a first pregnancy is likely to be a blocking (humoral) or suppressor (T-cell) function. If fetal rejection of the mother is proposed, then the response could be the ability to destroy fetal immune cells entering the maternal circulation by cellular or humoral cytotoxic reactions. Thus this model encompasses two opposite proposals about the nature of the *protective* maternal immune response, one inhibitory and one active.

Antigenic cross-reactivity

Maternal antibodies to placental or other fetal antigens form aberrantly and cross-react with renal or other maternal tissues. This hypothesis classifies pre-eclampsia as a maternal autoimmune disease with the implication that the protective maternal immune response is the suppression of autoantibody synthesis.

It is a reflection of our lack of knowledge that these hypotheses cannot be further developed at present.

References

1. Sims, E. A. H. (1970). Pre-eclampsia and related complications of pregnancy. *Am. J. Obstet. Gynecol.*, **107**, 154
2. Bonnar, J., McNichol, G. P. and Douglas, A. S. (1971). Coagulation and fibrinolytic systems in pre-eclampsia and eclampsia. *Br. Med. J.*, **2**, 12
3. Department of Health and Social Security (1979). *Report on Confidential Enquiries into Maternal deaths in England and Wales 1973–1975*, p. 21. (London: HMSO)
4. McCartney, C. P. (1964). Pathological anatomy of acute hypertension of pregnancy. *Circulation*, **29** (Suppl. II), 37
5. Little, W. A. (1960). Placental infarction. *Obstet. Gynecol.*, **15**, 109
6. Hibbard, B. M. and Jeffcoate, T. N. A. (1966). Abruptio placentae. *Obstet. Gynecol.*, **27**, 155
7. Scott, J. R. and Beer, A. A. (1976). Immunologic aspects of pre-eclampsia. *Am. J. Obstet. Gynecol.*, **125**, 418
8. Jenkins, D. M. (1977). Immunological aspects of the pathogenesis of pregnancy hypertension. *Clin. Obstet. Gynaecol.*, **4**, 665
9. Kitzmiller, J. L. (1977). Immunologic approaches to the study of pre-eclampsia. *Clin. Obstet. Gynaecol.*, **20**, 717
10. Willems, J. (1977). The etiology of pre-eclampsia. *Obstet. Gynecol.*, **50**, 495
11. Scott, J. S., Jenkins, D. M. and Need, J. A. (1978). Immunology of pre-eclampsia. *Lancet*, **1**, 704
12. Beer, A. E. (1978). Possible immunologic bases of pre-eclampsia/eclampsia. *Semin. Perinatol.*, **2**, 39
13. Rocklin, R. E., Kitzmiller, J. L. and Kaye, M. D. (1979). Immunobiology of the maternal–fetal relationship. *Ann. Rev. Med.*, **30**, 375
14. Need, J. A. (1979). Immunological phenomena in pre-eclamptic toxaemia. *Clin. Obstet. Gynaecol.*, **6**, 443
15. MacGillivray, I. (1958). Some observations on the incidence of pre-eclampsia. *Br. J. Obstet. Gynaecol.*, **65**, 536
16. Need, J. A. (1975). Pre-eclampsia in pregnancies by different fathers: immunological studies. *Br. Med. J.*, **1**, 548
17. Feeney, J. G. (1980). Pre-eclampsia and changed paternity. *Proceedings of 1st Congress of the International Society for the Study of Hypertension in Pregnancy*. (In press)
18. Marti, J. J. and Herrman, U. (1977). Immunogestosis. A new concept of 'essential' EPH gestosis, with special consideration of the primigravid patient. *Am. J. Obstet. Gynecol.*, **128**, 489
19. Feeney, J. G., Tovey, L. A. D. and Scott, J. S. (1977). Influence of previous blood transfusion on incidence of pre-eclampsia. *Lancet*, **1**, 874
20. Stiller, C. R., Sinclair, N. R., Sheppard, R. R., Lockwood, B. L., Ulan, R. A., Sharpe, J. A. and Hayman, P. (1978). Beneficial effect of operation-day blood transfusions on human renal-allograft survival. *Lancet*, **1**, 169
21. Robertson, W. B., Brosens, I. and Dixon, H. G. (1967). The pathological response of the vessels of the placental bed to hypertensive pregnancy. *J. Pathol. Bacteriol.*, **93**, 581
22. Zeek, P. M. and Assali, N. S. (1950). Vascular changes in decidua associated with eclamptogenic toxemia of pregnancy. *Am. J. Clin. Pathol.*, **20**, 1099
23. McClure Browne, J. C. and Veall, N. (1953). The maternal placental blood flow in normotensive and hypertensive women. *Br. J. Obstet. Gynaecol.*, **60**, 141
24. Fox, H. (1964). The villous cytotrophoblast as an index of placental ischaemia. *Br. J. Obstet. Gynaecol.*, **71**, 885
25. Cibils, L. A. (1974). The placenta and newborn infant in hypertensive conditions. *Am. J. Obstet. Gynecol.*, **118**, 256
26. Hume, D. M., Merrill, J. P., Miller, B. F. and Thorn, G. W. (1955). Experiences with renal homotransplantation in the human: report of nine cases. *J. Clin. Invest.*, **34**, 327

27. Porter, K. A., Thomson, W. B., Owen, K., Kenyon, J. R., Mowbray, J. F. and Peart, W. S. (1963). Obliterative vascular changes in four human kidney homotransplants. *Br. Med. J.*, 2, 639

28. Sheppard, B. L. and Bonnar, J. (1976). The ultrastructure of the arterial supply of the human placenta in pregnancy complicated by fetal growth retardation. *Br. J. Obstet. Gynaecol.*, 83, 948

29. Clemetson, C. A. B. (1960). Aortic hypoplasia and its significance in the aetiology of pre-eclamptic toxaemia. *Br. J. Obstet. Gynaecol.*, 67, 90

30. Cavanagh, D., Papineni, S., Cheng Tsai, C. and O'Connor, T. C. (1977). Experimental toxemia in the pregnant primate. *Am. J. Obstet. Gynecol.*, 128, 75

31. Kumar, D. (1962). Chronic placental ischemia in relation to toxemias of pregnancy. *Am. J. Obstet. Gynecol.*, 84, 1323

32. Abitbol, M. M. (1977). Hemodynamic studies in experimental toxemia of the dog. *Obstet. Gynecol.*, 50, 293

33. Wardle, E. N. and Wright, N. A. (1973). Role of fibrin in a model of pregnancy toxaemia in the rabbit. *Am. J. Obstet. Gynecol.*, 115, 17

34. Douglas, B. H. and Langford, H. G. (1969). Post-term blood pressure elevation produced by uterine wrapping. *Am. J. Obstet. Gynecol.*, 97, 231

35. Skinner, S. L., Lumbers, E. R. and Symonds, E. M. (1968). Renin concentration in human fetal and maternal tissues. *Am. J. Obstet. Gynecol.*, 101, 529

36. Ferris, T. F., Stein, J. H. and Kauffman, J. (1972). Uterine blood flow and uterine renin secretion. *J. Clin. Invest.*, 51, 2827

37. Symonds, E. M., Broughton-Pipkin, F. and Craven, D. J. (1975). Changes in the renin–angiotensin system in primigravidae with hypertensive disease of pregnancy. *Br. J. Obstet. Gynaecol.*, 82, 643

38. Weir, R. J., Fraser, R., Lever, A. F., Morton, J. J., Brown, J. J., Kraszewski, A., McIlwaine, G. M., Robertson, J. I. S. and Tree, M. (1973). Plasma renin, renin substrate, angiotensin II and aldosterone in hypertensive disease of pregnancy. *Lancet*, 1, 291

39. Kokot, F. and Cekánski, A. (1972). Plasma renin activity in peripheral and uterine vein blood in pregnant and non-pregnant women. *J. Obstet. Gynaecol. Br. Commonw.*, 79, 72

40. Jeffcoate, T. N. A. and Scott, J. S. (1959). Some observations on the placental factor in pregnancy toxaemia. *Am. J. Obstet. Gynecol.*, 77, 475

41. Niebuhr, E. (1974). Triploidy in man. *Humangenetik*, 21, 103

42. McFarlane, A. and Scott, J. S. (1976). Pre-eclampsia/eclampsia in twin pregnancies. *J. Med. Genet.*, 13, 208

43. Thomas, L., Douglas, G. W. and Carr, M. C. (1959). The continual migration of syncytial trophoblasts from the fetal placenta into the maternal circulation. *Trans. Assoc. Am. Physicians*, 72, 140

44. Attwood, H. D. and Park, W. W. (1961). Embolism to the lungs by trophoblast. *Br. J. Obstet. Gynaecol.*, 68, 611

45. Jaameri, K. E. U., Koivuniemi, A. P. and Carpén, E. O. (1965). Occurrence of trophoblasts in the blood of toxaemic patients. *Gynaecologia*, 160, 315

46. Faulk, W. P. and Temple, A. (1976). Distribution of β_2-microglobulin and HLA in chorionic villi of human placentae. *Nature (London)*, 262, 799

47. Goodfellow, P. N., Barnstable, C. J., Bodmer, W. F., Snary, D. and Crumpton, M. J. (1976). Expression of HLA system antigens on placenta. *Transplantation*, 22, 595

48. Stirrat, G. M., Mason, D. and Redman, C. W. G. (1979). Absence of HLA on human trophoblasts demonstrated by immunofluorescence with a monoclonal anti-HLA antibody. (Unpublished observations)

49. Barnstable, C. J. and Bodmer, W. F. (1978). Immunology and the fetus. *Lancet*, 1, 326

50. Hulka, J. F., Hsu, K. C. and Beiser, S. M. (1961). Antibodies to trophoblasts during the post-partum period. *Nature (London)*, 191, 510

51. Kaku, M. (1953). Placental polysaccharide and the aetiology of the toxaemia of pregnancy. *J. Obstet. Gynaecol. Br. Commonw.*, **60**, 148

52. Gaugas, J. M. and Curzen, P. (1974). Complement fixing antibody against solubilised placental microsomal fraction in pre-eclampsia sera. *Br. J. Exp. Pathol.*, **55**, 570

53. Hulka, J. F. and Brinton, V. (1963). Antibody to trophoblast during early post-partum period in toxemic pregnancies. *Am. J. Obstet. Gynecol.*, **86**, 130

54. Vardi, I. and Halbrecht, I. (1974). Toxemia of pregnancy: 1. Antigens associated with toxemia of pregnancy in placental connective tissue. *Am. J. Obstet. Gynecol.*, **118**, 552

55. Youtananukorn, V., Matangkasombut, P. and Osathanondh, V. (1974). Onset of human maternal cell-mediated immune reaction to placental antigens during the first pregnancy. *Clin. Exp. Immunol.*, **16**, 593

56. Stimson, W. H., Strachan, A. F. and Shepherd, A. (1979). Studies on the maternal immune response to placental antigens: absence of a blocking factor from the blood of abortion-prone women. *Br. J. Obstet. Gynaecol.*, **86**, 41

57. Taylor, P. V. and Hancock, K. W. (1975). Antigenicity of trophoblast and possible antigen-masking effects during pregnancy. *J. Immunol.*, **28**, 973

58. Rocklin, R. E., Kitzmiller, J. L., Carpenter, C. B., Garovoy, M. R. and David, J. R. (1976). Maternal fetal relation. Absence of an immunologic blocking factor from the serum of women with chronic abortions. *N. Engl. J. Med.*, **295**, 1209

59. McIntyre, J. A. and Faulk, W. P. (1979). Maternal blocking factors in human pregnancy are found in plasma not serum. *Lancet*, **2**, 821

60. Baxter, J. H. and Goodman, H. C. (1956). Nephrotoxic serum nephritis in rats. *J. Exp. Med.*, **104**, 467

61. Steblay, R. W. (1962). Localisation in human kidney of antibodies formed in sheep against human placenta. *J. Immunol.*, **88**, 434

62. Curzen, P. (1968). The antigenicity of human placenta. *Br. J. Obstet. Gynaecol.*, **75**, 1128

63. Boss, J. H. (1965). Antigenic relationships between placenta and kidney in the human. *Am. J. Obstet. Gynecol.*, **93**, 574

64. Seegal, B. C. and Loeb, E. N. (1946). The production of chronic glomerulonephritis in rats by the injection of rabbit anti-rat-placenta serum. *J. Exp. Med.*, **84**, 211

65. McCaughy, W. T. E. (1955). The nephrotoxic action of anti-placenta serum in rats. *Br. J. Obstet. Gynaecol.*, **62**, 863

66. Okuda, T. and Grollman, A. (1966). Renal lesions in rats following injection of placental extracts. *Arch. Pathol.*, **82**, 246

67. Irino, T., Okuda, T. and Grollman, A. (1967). Changes induced in the glomeruli of the kidney of rats by placental extracts as observed with the electron microscope. *Am. J. Pathol.*, **50**, 421

68. Gang, N. F., Schwarz, E. S., Majerovics, A., De Champlain, M.-L. and Trachtenberg, E. (1974). Studies on the placenta. II. Nephrotoxicity of antibodies produced against a chorionic glycoprotein. *Am. J. Obstet. Gynecol.*, **120**, 73

69. Singal, D. P., Mickey, M. R. and Terasaki, P. I. (1969). Serotyping for homotransplantation. XXIII. Analysis of kidney transplants from parental versus sibling donors. *Transplantation*, **7**, 246

70. Robertson, W. B., Brosens, I. and Dixon, G. (1976). Maternal uterine vascular lesions in the hypertensive complications of pregnancy. *Perspect. Nephrol. Hyperten.*, **5**, 115

71. Stevenson, A. C., Davison, B. C. C., Say, B., Ustuoplus, L. D., Einen, M. A. and Toppozada, H. K. (1971). Contribution of fetal/maternal incompatibility to aetiology of pre-eclamptic toxaemia. *Lancet*, **2**, 1286

72. Stevenson, A. C., Say, B., Ustaoglu, S. and Durmus, Z. (1976). Aspects of pre-eclamptic toxaemia of pregnancy, consanguinity and twinning in Ankara. *J. Med. Genet.*, **13**, 1

73. Toivanen, P. and Hirvonen, T. (1970). Sex ratio of newborn; preponderance of males in toxaemia of pregnancy. *Science*, **170**, 187

74. Redman, C. W. G., Bodmer, J. G., Bodmer, W. F., Beilin, L. J. and Bonnar, J. (1978). HLA antigens in severe pre-eclampsia. *Lancet*, **2**, 397
75. Jenkins, D. M., Need, J. A., Scott, J. S., Morris, H. and Pepper, M. (1978). Human leukocyte antigens and mixed lymphocyte reaction in severe pre-eclampsia. *Br. Med. J.*, **1**, 542
76. Terasaki, P. I., Mickey, M. R. and Yamazaki, J. N. (1970). Maternal–fetal incompatibility. I. Incidence of HLA antibodies and possible association with congenital anomalies. *Transplantation*, **9**, 538
77. Jenkins, D. M., Need, J. and Rajah, S. M. (1977). Deficiency of specific HLA antibodies in severe pregnancy pre-eclampsia/eclampsia. *Clin. Exp. Immunol.*, **27**, 485
78. Fingleton, A. M. (1971). Leucocytotoxic antibodies and pre-eclampsia of pregnancy. *Transplantation*, **12**, 319
79. Tiilikainen, A. (1971). Fetomaternal histoincompatibility in toxaemia of pregnancy. In Grubb, R. and Samuelsson, G. (eds.) *Human Anti-Human Gammaglobulins*, pp. 223–277. (Oxford: Pergamon Press)
80. Caretti, N., Chiaramonte, P., Pasini, C., Zenetti, M. and Fagiolo, U. (1974). Association of anti-HLA antibodies with toxaemia of pregnancy. In Centaro, A., Caretti, N. and Addison, G. M. (eds.) *Immunology in Obstetrics and Gynecology*, pp. 221–225. (Excerpta Medica)
81. Nymand, G. (1975). Complement-fixing and lymphocytotoxic antibodies in serum of pregnant women at delivery. *Vox. Sang.*, **28**, 101
82. Harris, R. E. and Lordon, R. E. (1976). The association of maternal lymphocytotoxic antibodies with obstetric complications. *Obstet. Gynecol.*, **48**, 302
83. Davies, D. A. L. and Staines, N. A. (1976). A cardinal role for I-region antigens (Ia) in immunological enhancement, and the clinical implications. *Transplant. Rev.*, **30**, 18
84. Festenstein, H. and Démant, P. (1978). *HLA and H-2. Basic immunogenetics, Biology and Clinical Relevance*, pp. 16–89. (London: Edward Arnold)
85. McDevitt, H. O. and Bodmer, W. F. (1972). Histocompatibility antigens, immune responsiveness and susceptibility to disease. *Am. J. Med.*, **52**, 1
86. Scott, J. R., Beer, A. E. and Stastny, P. (1976). Immunogenetic factors in pre-eclampsia and eclampsia. *J. Am. Med. Assoc.*, **235**, 402
87. Kalmus, H. (1946). Genetical antigenic incompatibility as a possible cause of the toxaemias occurring late in pregnancy. *Ann. Eugen.*, **13**, 146
88. Penrose, L. S. (1946). On the familial appearances of maternal and fetal incompatibility. *Ann. Eugen.*, **13**, 141
89. Platt, R. (1947). The problem of Bright's disease. *Practitioner*, **159**, 159
90. Adams, E. M. and Finlayson, A. (1961). Familial aspects of pre-eclampsia and hypertension in pregnancy. *Lancet*, **2**, 1375
91. Chesley, L. C., Annitto, J. E. and Cosgrove, R. A. (1968). The familial factor in toxaemia of pregnancy. *Obstet. Gynaecol.*, **32**, 303
92. Humphries, J. O'Neal (1960). Occurrence of hypertensive toxemia of pregnancy in mother–daughter pairs. *Bull. Johns Hopkins Hosp.*, **107**, 271
93. Cooper, D. W. and Liston, W. A. (1979). Genetic control of severe pre-eclampsia. *J. Med. Genet.*, **16**, 409
94. Brocklehurst, J. C. and Ross, R. (1960). Familial eclampsia. *J. Obstet. Gynaecol. Br. Emp.*, **67**, 971
95. Pike, L. A. and Dickins, A. M. (1954). ABO blood groups and toxaemia of pregnancy. *Br. Med. J.*, **2**, 321
96. May, D. (1973). Maternal blood group A and pre-eclampsia. *Br. Med. J.*, **4**, 738
97. Harlap, S. and Davies, A. M. (1974). Maternal blood group A and pre-eclampsia. *Br. Med. J.*, **3**, 171
98. Pearson, M. G. and Pinker, G. D. (1956). ABO blood groups and toxaemia of pregnancy. *Br. Med. J.*, **1**, 777

99. Andrews, G. S. (1959). Blood groups and toxaemia of pregnancy. *Br. Med. J.*, **2**, 806
100. Salzmann, K. D. (1955). Do transplacental hormones cause eclampsia? *Lancet*, **2**, 953
101. Juberg, R. R., Gaar, D. G., Humphries, J. R., Cenac, P. L. and Zambie, M. F. (1976). Sex ratio in the progeny of mothers with toxemia of pregnancy. *J. Reprod. Med.*, **16**, 299
102. Gusdon, J. P., Heise, E. R. and Herbst, G. A. (1977). Studies of lymphocyte populations in pre-eclampsia/eclampsia. *Am. J. Obstet. Gynecol.*, **129**, 255
103. Hersh, E. M., Butler, W. T., Rossen, R. D. and Morgen, R. O. (1970). Lymphocyte activation; a rapid test to predict allograft rejection. *Nature (London)*, **226**, 757
104. Gaugas, J. M., Jones, E. and Curzen, P. (1975). Spontaneous lymphocyte transformation in pregnancies complicated by pre-eclampsia. *Am. J. Obstet. Gynecol.*, **121**, 542
105. Petrucco, O. M., Seamark, R. F., Holmes, K., Forbes, I. J. and Symonds, R. G. (1976). Changes in lymphocyte function during pregnancy. *Br. J. Obstet. Gynaecol.*, **83**, 245
106. Purtilo, D. T., Hallgren, H. M. and Yunis, E. J. (1972). Depressed maternal lymphocyte response to phytohaemagglutinin in human pregnancy. *Lancet*, **2**, 769
107. Need, J. A., Jenkins, D. M. and Scott, J. S. (1976). The response of lymphocytes to phytohaemagglutinin in women with pre-eclampsia. *Br. J. Obstet. Gynaecol.*, **83**, 438
108. Griffin, J. F. T. and Wilson, E. M. (1979). Lymphocyte response to phytohaemagglutinin in pre-eclampsia. *Int. J. Lab. Clin. Immunol.* (In press)
109. Birkeland, S. A. and Kristofferson, K. (1979). Pre-eclampsia – a state of mother–fetus immune imbalance. *Lancet*, **2**, 720
110. Halbrecht, I. G. and Komlos, L. (1974). Mixed wife–husband leukocyte cultures in disturbed and pathological pregnancies. *Isr. J. Med. Sci.*, **10**, 1100
111. Curzen, P., Jones, E. and Gaugas, J. M. (1977). Maternal–fetal mixed lymphocyte reactivity in pre-eclampsia. *Br. J. Exp. Pathol.*, **58**, 500
112. Gille, J., Williams, J. H. and Hoffman, C. P. (1977). The feto-maternal lymphocyte interaction in pre-eclampsia and in uncomplicated pregnancy. *Eur. J. Obstet. Gynaecol. Reprod. Biol.*, **7**, 227
113. Thiry, L., Sprecher-Goldberger, S., Bossens, M. and Neukay, F. (1978). Immune response to primate oncornaviruses in pre-eclampsia. *Lancet*, **1**, 1268
114. Ablin, R. M., Bruns, G. R. and Guinan, P. (1974). The effect of estrogen on the incorporation of 3H-thymidine by PHA-stimulated human peripheral blood. *J. Immunol.*, **113**, 705
115. Simmons, R. L., Price, A. L. and Ozerkis, A. J. (1968). The immunologic problems of pregnancy. V. The effect of estrogen and progesterone on allograft survival. *Am. J. Obstet. Gynecol.*, **100**, 908
116. Contractor, S. F. and Davies, H. (1973). Effect of human chorionic somatomammotrophin and human chorionic gonadotrophin on phytohaemagglutinin-induced lymphocyte transformation. *Nature (New. Biol.)*, **243**, 284
117. Masson, G. M. (1973). Plasma oestriol in pre-eclampsia. *J. Obstet. Gynaecol. Br. Commonw.*, **80**, 206
118. Letchworth, A. T. and Chard, T. (1972). Human placental lactogen levels in pre-eclampsia. *J. Obstet. Gynaecol. Br. Commonw.*, **79**, 680
119. Eton, B. and Short, R. V. (1960). Blood progesterone levels in abnormal pregnancies. *J. Obstet. Gynaecol. Br. Commonw.*, **67**, 785 ·
120. Horne, C. H. W., Briggs, J. D., Howie, P. W. and Kennedy, A. C. (1972). Serum α-macroglobulins in renal disease and pre-eclampsia. *J. Clin. Pathol.*, **25**, 590
121. Stimson, W. H. (1975). Immunosuppressive effect of pregnancy-associated α_2-macroglobulin. *Lancet*, **2**, 989
122. Jenkins, D. M., Good, W. and Good, S. (1973). Serum seromucoid and the materno-paternal mixed lymphocyte reaction following previous severe pre-eclampsia. *Br. J. Obstet. Gynaecol.*, **80**, 19

123. Revillard, J. P., Brochier, J., Robert, M., Bonneau, M. and Traeger, J. (1975). Immunologic properties of placental eluates. *Transplant. Proc.*, **VIII**, 275

124. Faulk, W. P., Temple, A., Lovins, R. E. and Smith, N. (1978). Antigens of human trophoblasts: a working hypothesis for their role in normal and abnormal pregnancies. *Proc. Natl. Acad. Sci.*, **75**, 1947

125. Horne, C. H. W., Howie, P. W. and Goudie, R. B. (1970). Serum alpha$_2$-macroglobulin, transferrin, albumin and IgG levels in pre-eclampsia. *J. Clin. Pathol.*, **23**, 514

126. Benster, B. and Wood, E. J. (1970). Immunoglobulin levels in normal pregnancy and pregnancy complicated by hypertension. *Br. J. Obstet. Gynaecol.*, **77**, 518

127. Kelly, A. M. and McEwan, H. P. (1973). Proteinuria in pre-eclamptic toxaemia of pregnancy. *J. Obstet. Gynaecol. Br. Commonw.*, **80**, 520

128. Studd, J. W. W. (1971). Immunoglobulins in normal pregnancy, pre-eclampsia and pregnancy complicated by the nephrotic syndrome. *J. Obstet. Gynaecol. Br. Commonw.*, **78**, 786

129. Masson, P. L., Delire, M. and Cambiaso, C. L. (1977). Circulating immune complexes in normal human pregnancy. *Nature (London)*, **266**, 542

130. McLaughlin, P. J., Stirrat, G. M., Redman, C. W. G. and Levinsky, R. J. (1979). Immune complexes in normal and pre-eclamptic pregnancy. *Lancet*, **1**, 934

131. Gleicher, N., Theofilopoulous, A. N. and Beers, P. (1978). Immune complexes in pregnancy. *Lancet*, **1**, 1108

132. Knox, G. E., Stagno, S., Volanakis, J. E. and Huddleston, J. F. (1978). A search for antigen–antibody complexes in pre-eclampsia; further evidence against immunologic pathogenesis. *Am. J. Obstet. Gynecol.*, **132**, 87

133. D'Amelio, R., Bilotta, P., Pachi, A. and Aiuti, F. (1979). Circulating immune complexes in normal pregnant women and in some conditions complicating pregnancy. *Clin. Exp. Immunol.*, **37**, 33

134. Stirrat, G. M., Redman, C. W. G. and Levinsky, R. J. (1978). Circulating immune complexes in pre-eclampsia. *Br. Med. J.*, **1**, 1450

135. Petrucco, O. M., Thomson, N. M., Lawrence, J. R. and Weldon, M. W. (1974). Immunofluorescent studies in renal biopsies in pre-eclampsia. *Br. Med. J.*, **1**, 473

136. Tribe, C. R., Smart, G. E. and Mackenzie, J. C. (1974). Pre-eclampsia and the kidney. *Br. Med. J.*, **2**, 335

137. Seymour, A. E., Petrucco, O. M., Clarkson, A. R., Haynes, W. D. G., Lawrence, J. R., Jackson, B., Thompson, A. J. and Thomson, N. M. (1976). Morphological and immunological evidence of coagulopathy in renal complications of pregnancy. *Perspect. Nephrol. Hyperten.*, **5**, 139

138. Spargo, B. H., Lichtig, C., Luger, A. M., Katz, A. I. and Lindheimer, M. D. (1976). The renal lesion in pre-eclampsia. *Perspect. Nephrol. Hyperten.*, **5**, 129

139. Kincaid-Smith, P. and Fairley, K. F. (1976). The differential diagnosis between pre-eclamptic toxemia and glomerulonephritis in patients with proteinuria during pregnancy. *Perspect. Nephrol. Hyperten.*, **5**, 157

140. Redman, C. W. G., Denson, K. W. E., Beilín, L. J., Bolton, F. J. and Stirrat, G. M. (1977). Factor-VIII consumption in pre-eclampsia. *Lancet*, **2**, 1249

141. Bokisch, V. A., Müller-Eberhard, H. J. and Cochrane, C. G. (1969). Isolation of a fragment (C3a) of the third component of human complement containing anaphylatoxin and chemotactic activity and the description of an anaphylatoxin inactivator of human serum. *J. Exp. Med.*, **129**, 1109

142. Zimmerman, J. S. (1976). The coagulation mechanism and the inflammatory response. In Miescher, P. A. and Müller-Eberhard, H. J. (eds.) *Textbook of Immunopathology*, pp. 95–116. (New York: Grune & Stratton)

143. Thomson, N. C., Stevenson, R. D., Behan, W., Sloan, D. and Horne, C. (1976). Immunological studies in pre-eclamptic toxaemia. *Br. Med. J.*, **1**, 1307

144. Prall, R. H. and Kantor, F. S. (1966). Serum complement in eclamptogenic toxemia. *Am. J. Obstet. Gynecol.*, **95**, 530
145. Kitzmiller, J. L., Stoneburner, L., Yelenosky, P. F. and Lucas, W. E. (1973). Serum complement in normal pregnancy and pre-eclampsia. *Am. J. Obstet. Gynecol.*, **117**, 312
146. Fadel, H. E., Soliman, M. D. E. and El-Mehairy, M. M. (1974). Serum complement activity in pre-eclamptic pregnancies. *Int. J. Gynecol. Obstet.*, **12**, 6
147. Tedder, R. S., Nelson, M. and Eisen, V. (1975). Effects on serum complement of normal and pre-eclamptic pregnancy and of oral contraceptives. *Br. J. Exp. Pathol.*, **56**, 389
148. Millar, K. G. and Mills, P. (1972). C13 and IgG levels in mothers and babies at delivery. *Obstet. Gynecol.*, **39**, 527
149. Yang, S.-L., Kleinmann, A. and Wei, P.-Y. (1973). Immunologic aspects of term pregnancy toxemia. *Am. J. Obstet. Gynecol.*, **122**, 727
150. Mak, L. W. (1978). The complement profile in relation to the 'reactor' state: a study in the immediate *post-partum* period. *Clin. Exp. Immunol.*, **31**, 419
151. Naish, P. F., Aber, G. and Boyd, W. N. (1975). C3 deposition in renal arterioles in the loin pain and haematuria syndrome. *Br. Med. J.*, **3**, 746
152. Arias, F. and Mancilla-Jimenez, R. (1976). Hepatic fibrinogen deposits in pre-eclampsia. *N. Engl. J. Med.*, **295**, 578
153. Kitzmiller, J. L. and Benirschke, K. (1973). Immunofluorescent study of placental bed vessels in pre-eclampsia of pregnancy. *Am. J. Obstet. Gynecol.*, **115**, 248
154. Weir, P. (1979). *MD Thesis*. Belfast
155. Clarke, H. G. M., Freeman, T. and Pryse-Phillips, W. (1971). Serum proteins in normal pregnancy and mild pre-eclampsia. *J. Obstet. Gynaecol. Br. Commonw.*, **78**, 105
156. Good, W. (1975). Maternal serum sialomucins during pregnancy and post-partum in patients with pre-eclampsia. *Br. J. Obstet. Gynaecol.*, **82**, 907
157. Good, W., Jenkins, D. M., Collins, M. C. and Cumberbatch, K. N. (1973). Serum seromucoid levels in women with previous severe pre-eclampsia or eclampsia. *Br. J. Obstet. Gynaecol.*, **80**, 22
158. Fattah, M. M., Ibrahim, F. K., Ramadan, M. A. and Sammour, M. B. (1976). Ceruloplasmin and copper levels in maternal and cord blood and in the placenta in normal pregnancy and in pre-eclampsia. *Acta Obstet. Gynecol. Scand.*, **55**, 383
159. Redman, C. W. G., Adinolfi, M. and Stirrat, G. M. (1979). Acute phase reactants in pre-eclampsia. (Unpublished observations)
160. Scandrett, F. J. (1963). Studies of the mucoprotein content of serum and placental tissue in toxaemia of pregnancy. *Br. J. Obstet. Gynaecol.*, **70**, 78
161. Koj, A. (1974). Acute phase reactants. Their synthesis, turnover and biological significance. In Allison, A. C. (ed.) *Structure and Function of Plasma Proteins*, pp. 73–125. (London: Plenum Press)
162. Stark, J. M., Johansen, K. A., Rees, J. A. and Williams, J. H. (1977). Acute-phase sera in pre-eclampsia and latent hypertension of pregnancy. *Lancet*, **2**, 299
163. Galton, M., Merritt, K. and Beller, F. K. (1971). Coagulation studies on the peripheral circulation of patients with toxemia of pregnancy; a study for the evaluation of disseminated intravascular coagulation in toxemia. *J. Reprod. Med.*, **6**, 78
164. Dobryszycka, W., Zeineh, R., Ebroon, E. and Kukral, J. C. (1969). Metabolism of plasma proteins in injury state. *Clin. Sci.*, **36**, 231
165. Poston, R. N. and Davies, D. F. (1974). Immunity and inflammation in the pathogenesis of atherosclerosis. *Atherosclerosis*, **19**, 353
166. Mathews, J. D., Whittingham, S. and Mackay, I. R. (1974). Autoimmune mechanisms in human vascular disease. *Lancet*, **2**, 1423
167. Okuda, T. and Grollman, A. (1967). Passive transfer of autoimmune induced hypertension in the rat by lymph node cells. *Tex. Rep. Biol. Med.*, **25**, 257
168. Svendsen, U. G. (1976). Evidence for an initial, thymus independent and a chronic thymus

dependent phase of doca and salt hypertension in mice. *Acta Pathol. Microbiol. Scand.*, Sect. A, **84**, 523

169. Svendsen, U. G. (1977). The importance of thymus in the pathogenesis of the chronic phase of hypertension in mice following partial infarction of the kidney. *Acta Pathol. Microbiol. Scand.*, Sect. A, **85**, 539

170. Butler, N. R. and Bonham, D. G. (1963). Toxaemia in pregnancy. In *Perinatal Mortality*, p. 87. (Edinburgh: E. & S. Livingstone)

171. Chesley, L. C., Annitto, J. E. and Cosgrove, R. A. (1976). The remote prognosis of eclamptic women. Sixth periodic report. *Am. J. Obstet. Gynecol.*, **124**, 446

172. Adams, E. M. and MacGillivray, I. (1961). Long-term effect of pre-eclampsia on blood pressure. *Lancet*, **2**, 1373

5
Immunological Factors in Male and Female Infertility

W. R. JONES

INTRODUCTION

Theoretically, immunological factors may operate at any step in the human reproductive process leading up to implantation since the gametes and the fertilized egg, as well as the hormones, tissues and other secretions in their invironment are all potentially antigenic and capable of eliciting an immune response. Cells and proteins with a foreign (in this context, male) genetic constitution may cause isoimmunization in the female partner. On the other hand autoimmunization against components ('self'-antigens) of the reproductive process may occur in both the male and the female.

This chapter is concerned with the immunology of spontaneous infertility in the human male and female, and aims to review current knowledge arising from experimental models and from the study of immunological infertility as a clinical entity. The reader is also referred to representative reviews in references 1–15.

EXPERIMENTAL IMMUNITY TO SPERM ANTIGENS

Sperm antigens develop relatively late in ontogenesis, they are immunologically secluded in the reproductive tract in the male, and they are potentially foreign to the female. They may therefore be autoantigens (antigenic within an individual) or isoantigens (antigenic in the female) but they may equally include alloantigens (antigenic in any other genetically distinct member of the same species). The alloantigens of sperm include blood group, histocompatibility and differentiation antigens, and will be discussed in detail below.

An extensive literature has accumulated concerning the experimental immunization of animals against male reproductive tract antigens[2, 3, 12, 16–18]. Selected aspects only of autoimmunization and isoimmunization in experimental animals will be considered here.

Autoimmunization

The best characterized model is that of experimental allergic orchitis (EAO) which is an organ-specific autoimmune syndrome produced experimentally in animals (notably the guinea-pig) by the injection of autologous or homologous testis or sperm mixed with Freund's complete adjuvant[19, 20]. Immunized animals develop autoimmune testicular damage which culminates in germinal cell destruction and azoospermia. The pathogenesis of these changes probably involves a complex interplay of both humoral and cellular immunity.

Although sperm clearly possess multiple intracellular and surface antigens that are capable of eliciting autoantibodies, only some of the antigens (aspermatogenic) have the capacity to induce EAO. Several investigators have attempted to purify the aspermatogenesic antigens from guinea-pig testis or epididymal sperm.

Voisin et al.[16] isolated and characterized three preparations of aspermatogenic antigen from the guinea-pig. The antigens, designated S, T and P, were characterized respectively as glycoprotein, lipoprotein and simple protein. The T antigen is plasma membrane-associated and induces the formation of a spermatoxic antibody which has properties similar to sperm-immobilizing antibodies in rabbits and infertile women. The S and P antigens are in the acrosomal apparatus and the first of these provokes antibodies which react with sperm of rabbits, rats and mice.

Other investigators have isolated antigenic preparations of guinea-pig sperm[21–23] and although some of these may be identical with the fractions described by Voisin et al.[16] there is now strong evidence that sperm may have multiple aspermatogenic antigens. Eylar and his colleagues[24, 25] have isolated three highly purified antigens (GP1, GP2, AP1) which have been shown capable of eliciting EAO at sub-microgram doses. As Tung[26] points out, this finding stresses the importance of establishing purity in presumed EAO-inducing immunogens since contamination by these highly potent antigens could impart immunogenicity to a preparation yet remain undetectable on standard immunochemical analysis. Using an immunofluorescence technique with monospecific antisera Eylar and colleagues[24, 25] showed that the three antigens occupied similar positions in the sperm acrosome. On the other hand, they isolated a third glycoprotein antigen, GP2, which elicited antibody to acrosome but did not provoke EAO. These findings highlight the potential problems involved in correlating serum antibodies and immunopathological events in orchitis induced by impure antigens.

It is surprising that, in the many years since EAO was first described in guinea-pigs, there have been very few comprehensive studies of experimental sperm autoimmunization in higher animals. Certainly the essential features of EAO have been reduplicated in many species, including birds, mice, rats, rabbits and bulls, and some studies have been performed in the monkey, but these have done little beyond confirming the crude association between immune orchitis and infertility. In a unique human study[27], male volunteers with prostatic carcinoma, who were awaiting orchidectomy, were immunized with testicular extracts in adjuvant. A proportion of these men developed a classical, though mild, form of allergic orchitis with low titre antibody levels, positive skin reactions and focal destruction of germinal cells.

Many other procedures have been shown to provoke immunological aspermatogenesis in animals[6]. In essence they all involve the disruption of the blood–testis barrier in one way or another. Exposure of one testis to a variety of insults, including mechanical trauma, heat, cold, injected turpentine or Freund's complete adjuvant results in an EAO syndrome with lesions in the contralateral gland. Immunization with antigenic material from adrenal glands or seminal plasma may also lead to immune orchitis. However, the possibility of cross-reactivity is raised by reports of the induction of EAO in guinea-pigs following immunization with non-reproductive tract tissues such as brain and parotid gland.

In a series of human experiments[27], unilateral testicular infusion with hot (80 °C) water produced autoimmune lesions detectable in the contralateral testis on examination following orchidectomy 60 days later. Chemicals such as α-chlorohydrin and cadmium also cause lesions in the rete testis and efferent duct system which result in immune aspermatogenesis and infertility[28,29]. With α-chlorohydrin, granuloma formation and fibrosis in the caput epididymis cause destruction with back-pressure and disruption of the seminiferous tubules. This allows phagocytosis of spermatozoa and their precursors with exposure of normally secluded antigens to the body's immune system.

Bilateral experimental occlusion of the vasa deferentia has similar effects. In some species this may be augmented by concurrent systemic injection of Freund's adjuvant. Tung[26] has demonstrated immune complex orchitis following vasectomy in rabbits, the antibody involved being directed against acrosome. There was also histochemical evidence of immune complex deposition in the kidneys of some animals. Cell-mediated immunity (CMI) to sperm without testicular pathology has been demonstrated post-vasectomy in other rodents, particularly when extravasation of sperm occurs at the operation site[30].

Vasectomy in man can be considered as an immunological 'experiment' and the autoimmune concomitants have been studied extensively[31]. There is controversy regarding the occurrence of CMI following human vasectomy[32,33] but there is no evidence of immunological testicular damage (see below).

Except in experimental models where a direct assault is made on the testis, it appears to be necessary to use strong adjuvants to induce experimental autoimmunity in males. When native testicular antigen is used without adjuvant, a prolonged immunization regime is necessary to provoke infertility and EAO lesions in guinea-pigs[34]. Effective immunogenicity and subsequent aspermatogenesis and infertility can be induced in guinea-pigs by up to three injections of testicular antigen chemically modified by conjugation to a hapten diazsulphanilic acid[35]. In one sense it is surprising that this approach has not been pursued with more enthisiasm in higher animals as a possible fertility-regulating method. On the other hand, the broad message from experimental sperm autoimmunization is that some degree of allergic orchitis is a necessary accompaniment of the infertility so produced.

Isoimmunization

Varying degrees of immunity and infertility can be induced in female experimental animals by the injection of homologous male reproductive tract antigens. The responses obtained depend on the preparation of the antigen, the use of adjuvants and 'carriers', the species studied, the method and route of immunization and the immunological techniques used to evaluate results.

Table 5.1 indicates the sequelae of active immunization against homologous sperm antigens in several species. In these studies, the antigenic preparation required the addition of an adjuvant in order to provoke immunity and an anti-fertility effect. It is therefore surprising that there were at least 12 studies of immunological contraception in women[36], and that in some of these reports infertility and humoral antibody formation were achieved by repeated injections of semen without adjuvant. The implications of these early studies are considerable and their main findings will be summarized.

Table 5.1 Experimental isoimmunization against semen or testicular extracts in several animal species. (Data summarized from references 2, 4 and 5)

Species	Route of active immunization	Immunological response			Effect on fertility	
		Humoral antibody response	Local antibody response	Cellular immunity	Decreased fertilization	Early embryo mortality
Guinea-pig	Intradermal	+	+	+		+
	Transvaginal	+	+	+		+
Mouse	Systemic (prolonged)	+			+	
	Transvaginal	−			−	
Rabbit	Combined systemic and transvaginal	+	+	+	+	+
Bovine	Systemic	+	+		+	+
	Transvaginal	+	+		+	+

Following isolated reports from birth-control clinics on contraceptive effects of up to 20 months duration following injections of semen, Rosenfeld[37] attempted to immunize two women with multiple subcutaneous injections of human semen. Mild local reactions were noted on two occasions but no systemic disturbance occurred; nor, however, was there serological evidence of immunity to spermatozoa.

Baskin[38] reported on 20 women who had received three intramuscular injections, 7 days apart, of between 5 and 20 ml of fresh human semen. The injections appeared harmless and, in all cases but one, humoral sperm cytotoxicity was induced and persisted for up to 12 months. No pregnancies occurred while positive serology persisted, and although the follow-up period was too short to allow assessment of subsequent fertility, one patient became pregnant 3 months after her serum reverted to negative following 9 months' immunity. Cervical secretions exhibited sperm cytotoxicity in 50% of cases but this showed no consistent relationship to serum reactivity.

Subsequent studies confirmed the induction of temporary infertility, without overt side-effects, in women injected with human spermatozoa[39, 40] and bovine sperm phospholipid[1]. Although in 1937 a United States Government patent was awarded to Baskin for the development of a spermatozoal vaccine, ethical restrictions apparently proscribed further attempts at parenteral immunization against semen in man.

The mechanisms involved in the induction of immunological infertility in female animals is complex. Immobilization and death of sperm, interference with sperm penetration of mucus and sperm transport, increased phagocytosis and interference with sperm–ovum contact probably all contribute to the decreased fertilization rate. Local immune responses, both afferent and efferent, are pre-eminent in these mechanisms. Evidence from experimental isoimmunization in animals (Table 5.1) suggests that it is extremely difficult to provoke a local immune response in the female genital tract in the absence of a systemic response. The immunological investigation of infertile females, however, indicates that this may not be so in nature[41]. The nature and significance of locally produced anti-sperm antibodies in cervical mucus must be clarified in studies of infertile women in order to identify antigens which might be relevant to the induction of a local block to fertility.

An additional anti-fertility mechanism involving early embryonic mortality is apparent in animals, and this can also be reproduced *in vitro* by exposing rabbit blastocysts to immune (anti-sperm) antisera, resulting in decreased embryo survival on transfer to recipient animals[2]. Female guinea-pigs immunized against the S antigen of Voisin et al.[16] and rabbits immunized against the spermatozoal enzyme lactic dehydrogenase-X (LDH-X)[42] also suffer embryo loss.

The complexity of the biological sequelae of sperm isoimmunization has been highlighted by an intriguing series of experiments conducted by Beer and Billingham[43]. When female rats were primarily immunized against the tissue antigens of a genetically foreign donor strain by means of an intra-uterine challenge with epididymal sperm, the uterus acquired the capacity to respond to local re-challenge with the same antigen by a striking recall flare reaction. Thus each subsequent mating with the donor strain provoked a local hypersensitivity response but had no effect on fertility; indeed reproductive efficiency appeared to be enhanced in the immunized animals. These experiments serve to emphasize that the sequelae of sperm isoimmunization may vary with the site and nature of the afferent and efferent pathways of immunization.

Another major area of interest in experimental isoimmunization relates to the potential behaviour of spermatozoal enzymes as isoantigens. Over 20 enzymes have been identified in mammalian sperm. Those of interest as potential target antigens include acrosomal hyaluronidase[44, 45], acrosin[45] and LHD-X (also known as LDH-C$_4$)[42]. The significance of these enzymes as immunogens in naturally occurring infertility is ill-defined (see below). There is now clear evidence from animal studies that active or passive immunization against sperm hyaluronidase and acrosin, either separately or combined, has no anti-fertility effect[45].

On the other hand there is evidence that LDH-X is a relevant antigen for the induction of immunological infertility. This enzyme is specific to the sperm mid-piece, being distinct from the LDH isoenzymes found in other tissues and possessing many characteristic enzyme properties. It has both iso- and autoantigen properties and antibodies to LDH-X block sperm penetration. Female animals show a reduced fertilization rate, but in rabbits this effect is embellished by a significant embryonic mortality in animals in which fertilization occurs. This effect has not been seen in a preliminary trial of active immunization against LDH-X in female baboons in which a significant anti-fertility effect has been demonstrated (V. C. Stevens and E. Goldberg, personal communication, 1979). LDH-X lacks species-specificity and this has allowed great flexibility in experimental studies as well as favouring its potential utility in the development of a fertility control vaccine.

The role of seminal plasma antigens in isoimmune infertility is difficult to define. These antigens may coat sperm within the male tract (even in the epididymis) and their incomplete removal by washing procedures may cause confusion in the characterization of antigens that are intrinsic to the gamete. Furthermore, there is evidence in the rabbit that sperm-coating antigen(s) are removed within the female tract as part of the capacitation process[46]. The immunization of female animals against seminal plasma or extracts of accessory male reproductive glands, although it may elicit a humoral antibody response, usually has little effect on fertility. There is evidence from human studies, however, to suggest that bacterially modified seminal plasma antigens provoke the production of sperm-immobilizing antibodies which may be related to infertility[47].

An additional complexity in relation to sperm isoimmunization has been raised by Cohen[48] who has data in many species which indicate the presence of two genetically selected populations of sperm with distinct antigenic properties. Of these, a minor population comprises 'fertile' sperm, whereas a majority appear to be biologically redundant. The immunological identification and manipulation of the 'fertile' sperm population has interesting implications in immunological infertility.

THE ANTIGENIC SPECTRUM OF HUMAN SEMEN

It is clear from studies of heterologous immunization that human spermatozoa, their precursor cells and seminal plasma contain antigens capable of provoking strong heteroantibody formation.

Sensitive immunological precipitation methods such as agar gel diffusion and immunoelectrophoresis have demonstrated up to 30 antigens in human semen[3, 49]. Some of these are unique to sperm or seminal plasma (tissue-specific) but others are shared with human serum, milk, saliva, nasal secretions, gastric fluid, urine, vagina, cervical mucus, cervix, endometrium, Fallopian tube, ovary, kidney, and liver, as well as with alcohol extracts of testis, corpus luteum and brain and with certain ubiquitous micro-organisms. Semen-specific antigens may exhibit genetic polymorphism (variation) within individuals and some show an identity with antigens in the semen of other species. Alloantigens are also present in seminal plasma and on sperm, and will be discussed in some detail below.

Antigens identified by naturally occurring immune reactions in man

The significance in human reproduction of antigens detected by hetero-immunization in animals is difficult to establish. The use of iso- and autoantibodies developed in infertile humans to identify antigens of potential relevance to fertility control is an important exercise. Many of the data accumulated are confusing owing to a lack of standardization of methodology and the use of poorly-defined clinical-study groups. These aspects will be dealt with in more detail in the section on 'The Investigation of Immunological Infertility'.

Studies of antibody responses in infertile humans have been extensively reviewed; see references 6, 14, 17, 47, 50 and 51.

Biological tests involving the agglutination and complement-dependent immobilization of sperm have been used extensively in blood and genital tract secretions to demonstrate antibodies directed against cell-surface (membrane) antigens. These studies have been complemented by antibody-localization techniques (mainly immunofluorescence) applied to fixed sperm. Using these methods infertile individuals have been shown to possess antibodies directed variously against the sperm acrosome, equatorial segment, postnuclear cap, nucleus, mid-piece, main tail-piece and tail end-piece (Figure 5.1). Of these surface antigens of acrosome and main tail-piece appear to provoke antibodies of special relevance to infertility both in males and females. These antigens are best recognized by circulating sperm-immobilizing antibodies in women and by immobilizing and agglutinating antibodies in men. They also appear to be recognized by antibodies secreted locally into cervical mucus and seminal plasma, where a major part of the block to fertility occurs.

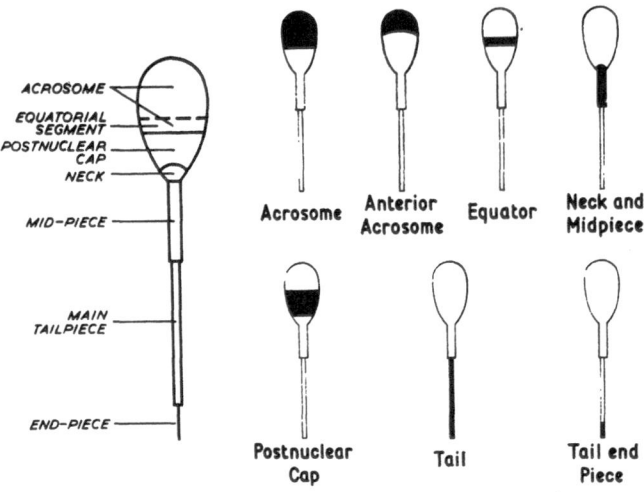

Figure 5.1 Diagrammatic representation of the principal structures of the spermatozoon and staining patterns obtained by immunofluorescence

The best characterized sperm-specific autoantigens were identified by serum antibodies in infertile and vasectomized males which reacted against sperm heads swollen by treatment with dithiothiestol and trypsin[52]. Sera with anti-nuclear activity, especially those with anti-DNA, may localize on nuclei of normal or swollen sperm heads. A further autoantigen exposed in the sperm mid-piece by detergent treatment was described by Tung[54] and shown to have a similar association with male infertility.

Studies in infertile and fertile individuals suggest that some sperm antigens may be ubiquitous and associated with the formation of 'natural' and heterophile antibodies which may cross-react with other antigens. Tung and co-workers[55, 56] demonstrated that antibodies giving homogeneous immuno-fluorescent staining of the acrosome are present in up to 60% of normal adults. This finding presumably reflects exposure to foreign antigens including ubiquitous micro-organisms which provoke antibodies cross-reactive with spermatozoa. These workers described a second 'speckled' acrosome pattern associated with antibodies found more specifically in infertile individuals. Another source of complexity is the demonstration that antibodies against smooth muscle cross-react with the contractile protein actin in the post-acrosomal region of the sperm[57]. Anti-smooth muscle antibodies are relatively common in adults and are present in high incidence in infertile women both with and without sperm antibodies present (W. R. Jones, unpublished data, 1978). Data such as these explain at least part of the confusion surrounding the incidence and significance of circulating anti-sperm antibodies detected by immunofluorescence techniques.

Antibodies reacting against native seminal plasma antigens do not appear to be relevant to infertility. Some of these antigens adhere to sperm and can either modify or contribute to its antigenicity. One sperm-coating antigen called SCA, or Scaferrin, is a β-globulin derived from the seminal vesicle and is immunologically identical with lactoferrin. It is located on the whole or multiple areas of the sperm surface and may serve to mask more important antigens. Absorption of spermagglutinating or immobilizing sera with seminal plasma or testicular homogenate and affinity chromatography using columns containing seminal plasma, showed that the antibodies producing these activities in the sera were directed against intrinsic sperm components and not at coating antigens from seminal plasma[58].

Despite these findings relating to native seminal plasma antigens, there is recent evidence that these antigens may be significantly modified by bacteria both *in vitro* and *in vivo*, and may provoke an immune response causing infertility in humans[47, 59, 60]. This phenomenon requires further examination since the isolation and characterization of seminal plasma antigens has technical advantages over the preparation of solubilized membrane antigens from sperm for the purposes of the development of a fertility control vaccine. A further problem however is associated with the potential use of seminal plasma antigens in fertility control. Acute hypersensitivity and local allergic reactions to semen have been reported and the offending antigens identified in seminal plasma. These bizarre clinical phenomena dictate caution in use of antigens from this source in immunizing vaccines.

A search for naturally occurring antibodies against sperm hyaluronidase and acrosin has produced confusing results[58] and, as pointed out previously, these antigens appear to have little relevance to infertility. On the other hand, isoantibodies to LDH-X have been demonstrated in infertile women using antigen from both mouse and human sources.

While there is no clear evidence that incompatibility of reproductive partners in the ABO blood group and HLA systems is related to infertility, these and other alloantigens are part of the antigenic profile of semen and therefore are relevant to the induction of immunity to sperm. For example untoward sensitization against these antigens or more subtle mechanisms of gamete selection might accompany induced anti-sperm immunity. At the very least they are important genetic markers on sperm cells and at most it is possible that differentiation alloantigens, by their transient nature, may be used as target molecules for immunological contraception.

Alloantigens of mammalian sperm

The following section is a brief review of this important area and is summarized in Table 5.2. For further information the reader is referred to references 61–65.

Table 5.2 Alloantigens of sperm

	Man	*Mouse*
Blood group antigens	ABO ? Rh ?MNS ?P	
Histocompatibility antigens	HI-A (incl. HLA D) β_2 microglobulin (H Y)	H-2 D and K Ia β_2 microglobulin (H Y)

Differentiation antigens:
  Teratoma
  t-locus
  Sperm/brain shared
	
	$+t^{12}$
		F9
		t-allelic antigens
		G^{lx}, NS-4, SIKR

Blood group antigens

The presence of ABO blood group substances on human spermatozoa was demonstrated by Landsteiner and Levine in 1926[66] and confirmed more recently by Kerek[67]. There is continuing controversy as to whether those substances are intrinsic to sperm with haploid-expression or are sperm-coating; the balance of evidence favours the latter but the matter awaits resolution. There is a similar controversy regarding the Rh, MNS and P antigen systems, all of which are present in semen.

Histocompatibility antigens

The serologically detected antigenic components of the major histocompatibility locus appear to be present on sperm in mice and men but there is as yet no convincing evidence for their haploid expression[65]. H-2 D and K antigens appear on mouse sperm at the primary spermatocyte stage; the Ia antigen appears at the same stage and the question arises as to whether this represents haploid expression or a reflection of low turnover and persistence from pre-meiotic stages.

   HLA A antigens have been detected on human spermatozoa by cyto-toxicity, absorption and immunofluorescence and there is also evidence in man for antigens (HLA D) which are equivalent to Ia antigens[65]. β_2 microglobulin is also present on sperm at the same location (post-acrosomal region) as the HLA antigens. As with H-2 antigens in the mouse, it has been suggested strongly that human sperm express haploid HLA A antigens. Alternative explanations are available for the data underlying this proposition and once again the matter remains to be resolved.

Sensitization to transplantation antigens has been provoked experimentally in rats, mice and hamsters by the intra-uterine instillation of washed homologous spermatozoa[43]. This procedure stimulates hypertrophy of draining lymph nodes and sensitizes the host to skin allografts from the donor strain. Despite these clear-cut findings there have been variable results using sperm to stimulate allogeneic lymphocytes directly[68–71], and the suggestion has been made[71] that the allogeneic stimulation observed in mixed cultures is due to non-spermatozoal cells, probably lymphocytes.

Although it is not strictly an alloantigen, it is relevant to mention here the presence on sperm of the H-Y antigen, a histocompatibility antigen regulated by the Y chromosome. This antigen may have a role in the primary determination of sex[72].

Differentiation antigens

Differentiation antigens are alloantigens specific to particular groups of differentiating tissues and are not normally associated with graft rejection. Differentiation antigens on spermatozoa fall into three categories: teratoma antigens, t-allele antigens and antigens shared by sperm and brain[65].

The F-9 teratoma antigen is present (along with β_2 microglobulin) on gonocytes and spermatozoa in the mouse and its relationship with H-2 antigens, which succeed it, is under intense study. The t-locus of mice consists of a series of alleles linked to the major histocompatibility locus, H-2, which have major effects on development. One of the t-allelic antigens, $+t^{12}$, is common to mouse and man and is located in the post-acrosomal region along with HLA A antigens and β_2 microglobulins[73].

It is a well-established and curious observation that alcohol extracts of brain and testis possess cross-reactive antigens[65] (Table 5.2). The implications of these studies remain to be studied and extended to man.

ISOIMMUNIZATION IN THE HUMAN FEMALE AGAINST SPERM ANTIGENS

In nature, the introduction of sperm into the female genital tract may evoke an isoimmune response. The afferent and efferent limbs of this response are depicted in Figure 5.2

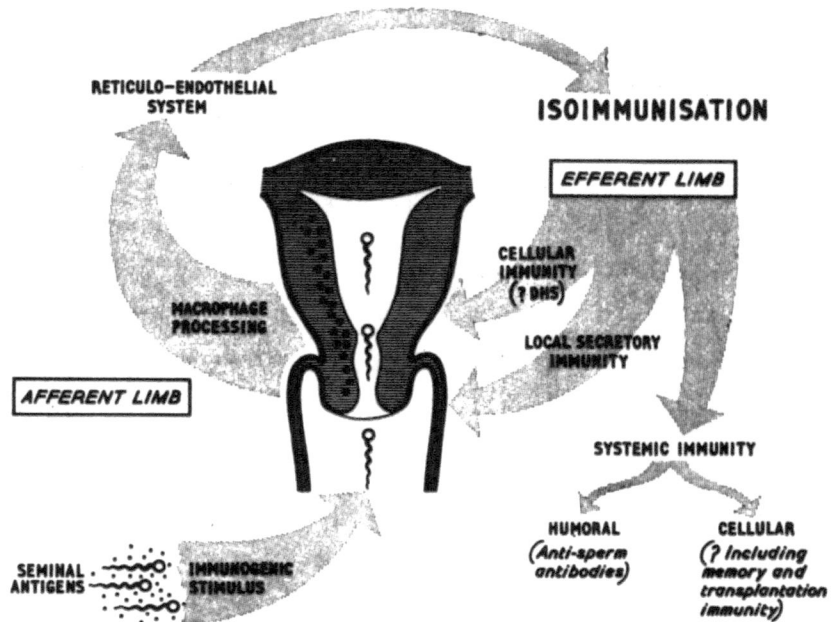

Figure 5.2 Immunological pathways involved in isoimmunization to antigens of semen. Antigens are processed by macrophages and presented to the reticuloendothelial system in the afferent pathway. The efferent responses may be both local and systemic and involve antibody formation and cell-mediated immunity

Immunological pathways

In the human female the genital tract, particularly the uterus, is well endowed with immunologically competent cells. These phagocytose spermatozoa and process their antigens for recognition by the host's immune defences. The operation of these isoimmune mechanisms following coitus may be influenced by several factors.

(1) The large numbers of biologically redundant sperm introduced into the vagina[48]. It is possible that only a genetically selected minority gain access to the Fallopian tube and that these are immunologically different from the residual majority.

(2) The phagocytosis of sperm by somatic cells of the uterine cervix, as well as by macrophages, and the chemotactic attraction of semen for macrophages and neutrophils.

(3) The possible adjuvant effects of other foreign antigens gaining access to the genital tract. In other words, immune responses to sperm antigens may be exaggerated in the presence of vaginal infections[74, 75].

(4) The contribution of lymphocytes in semen to the induction in the female of sensitization to histocompatibility antigens of the male partner[71].

(5) The presence of factors which might modify the immune response to sperm. These include prostaglandin E which is immunosuppressive, and an ill-defined glycoprotein fraction of seminal plasma which also has immunosuppressive properties[76]. In addition seminal plasma exerts an anticomplementary effect[77] at least part of which may be due to the presence of precipitins directed against the first component of complement (C1q)[78].

Isoimmune responses to sperm in the female may be antibody- or cell-mediated, each of these may have a predominantly local, rather than a systemic, effect. Humoral anti-sperm antibodies have been detected by a variety of techniques in infertile women, and their clinical significance will be discussed below. Experimental studies in humans involving chemical and microbial antigens indicate that the effector pathways of local immunization in the female genital tract mediate both systemic and local cell-mediated immune responses. These include transplantation immunity and immunological memory with secondary responses and local hypersensitivity reactions. There is also clinical evidence which suggests that coitally introduced antigens may initiate cellular immunity and in rare cases provoke systemic and local hypersensitivity reactions.

Local immunity in the female genital tract

The immunological characteristics of genital tract secretions are important in our understanding of immune mechanisms in female infertility[13, 79]. The uterine cervix is the major site of secretory immunological activity in the female genital tract; the uterine endometrium and the Fallopian tubes may also participate to a limited extent but the vagina is probably inactive.

Local (intra-vaginal) immunization with experimental antigens results in a specific antibody response in the cervical mucus. Usually an antigenic stimulus to a mucous membrane results in the formation of both local and circulating antibodies but in some circumstances antigen may not reach the circulation in immunogenic quantities at any one time and therefore a systemic response may not occur. The immunological characteristics of the cervix and its secretions have been reviewed by Jones[80] and Menge et al.[41].

The cervix is adequately equipped with plasma cells and cervical mucus contains immunoglobulins at least some of which are locally secreted. This can be demonstrated by finding secretory immunoglobulin A (SIgA) as well as serum immunoglobulin A (IgA) and immunoglobulin G (IgG) in the mucus. SIgA is formed locally at mucous surfaces and is composed of two serum IgA molecules and a non-immunoglobulin peptide called secretory component

(SC) (Figure 5.3). Immunoglobulin and C3 complement levels in cervical mucus vary during the menstrual cycle, tending to be lowest at ovulation time. Total complement levels appear to be low in cervical mucus but require further study. Schumacher and Yang[81] found mean levels at mid-cycle of 1.3 mg/ml for IgG and 0.5 mg/ml for IgA. Lower concentrations were present in endometrial secretions.

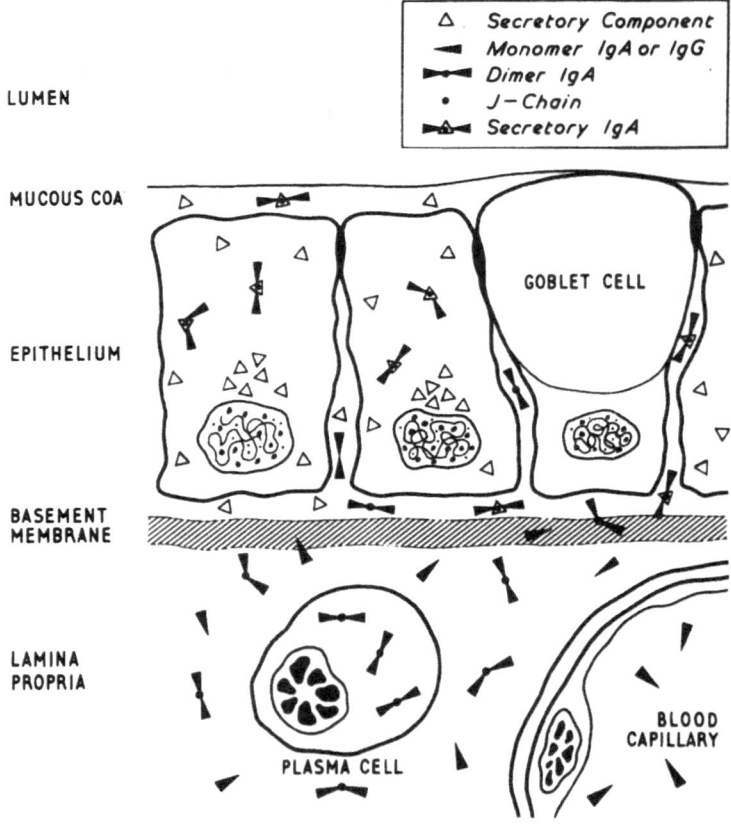

Figure 5.3 Mechanisms of IgA secretion at a mucosal surface. Monomeric IgA and IgG do not pass beyond the epithelial basement membrane. Dimeric IgA combines with secretory component (SC) receptor on the epithelial cell membrane to form SIgA which then passes to the lumen. For clarity IgM is not represented

Specific antibodies may also appear in oviductal and follicular fluid. In man, Lippes et al. [82,83], have demonstrated IgG, IgA and SC in tubal epithelium and the presence of IgG or IgA in tubal fluid in concentrations 10% and 20% respectively of serum levels. C3, but not total complement, activity is detectable in tubal fluid. The potential ubiquity of sperm antibodies is suggested by the presence of IgG and IgA in human follicular fluid in mean concentrations of 1026 mg/dl and 88 mg/dl respectively and the demonstration of specific antibodies in this fluid at titres only slightly lower than those in serum (W. R. Jones, J. McBain and G. Clark, unpublished data, 1978). The potential importance of follicular fluid in the mediation of local immunity in the reproductive tract is further enhanced by evidence that it contains only slightly less complement activity than is present in serum (G. F. B. Schumacher, personal communication, 1979).

In summary, local antibodies might interfere with the reproductive process in the following ways:[14]

(1) They could arm macrophages and enhance phagocytic clearance of spermatozoa from the genital tract.

(2) They could be cytotoxic (immobilizing) to sperm if adequate levels of complement cascade components are present.

(3) They could prevent sperm from adequately penetrating cervical mucus by agglutination or more subtle mechanisms.

(4) They could interfere with sperm capacitation.

(5) They could influence sperm selection within the female genital tract.

AUTOIMMUNIZATION AGAINST GENITAL TRACT COMPONENTS IN THE HUMAN MALE

As reviewed above, it has been known for many years that male experimental animals can be rendered sterile by active or passive immunization against testicular or seminal antigens. This causes an allergic orchitis with immunological disruption of testicular tissue. This disruption involves the 'blood–testis' barrier which normally maintains a degree of immunological seclusion of the seminiferous tubules. The Sertoli cells, and their junctions in the testes and the intercellular epithelial junctions in the efferent duct system, form the basis of this barrier. The barrier, however, can be breached in the region of the rete testis and efferent tubules and it is here that the opening assault of autoimmune allergic orchitis occurs. Immune lymphocytes cause the initial damage, allowing the entry of cytotoxic antibodies and complement. Disruption and blockage of the efferent duct system then leads to secondary immune lesions within the seminiferous tubules involving cell-specific antigens in all of the maturation stages from spermatogonia to spermatozoa.

In experimental animals disruption of the testis on one side by a variety of means may result in autoimmune orchitis with lesions in the contralateral organ. Procedures used to produce this effect have included freezing, needling and injecting Freund's adjuvant, turpentine or boiling water. Autoimmune allergic orchitis has also been produced experimentally in humans by active immunization or by unilateral testicular disruption.

These situations have their counterparts in clinical medicine (Figure 5.4). Dissruption of testicular tissue by surgical or accidental trauma, infection of the testis or accessory glands (particularly the prostate and seminal vesicles) and occlusion of the reproductive tract may compromise the blood–testis barrier and cause autoimmunity to testicular and seminal antigens[6, 17]. Of particular interest is the possibility that at least part of the pathology and clinical sequelae of mumps orchitis has an autoimmune basis.

The most studied example of immunological disruption of the reproductive tract in man is vasectomy[31, 84, 85]. Current knowledge of the immunological concomitants of vasectomy can be summarized as follows:

(1) Following the operation there is leakage of sperm antigens at the weak points in the immunological 'barrier' of the testis. These are the epididymis, rete testis and efferent ductules. Macrophages enter the tract and phagocytose sperm for 'processing' in regional lymph nodes.

(2) A patchy orchitis may occur in monkeys and has been described on occasions in man. Cell-mediated immune reactions are provoked by vasectomy in rodents but there is no clear evidence that this occurs in primates.

(3) Circulating anti-sperm antibodies develop in 50% of vasectomised men within 6–12 months of the operation. The propensity to antibody formation is greater in men with initially high sperm counts and in those

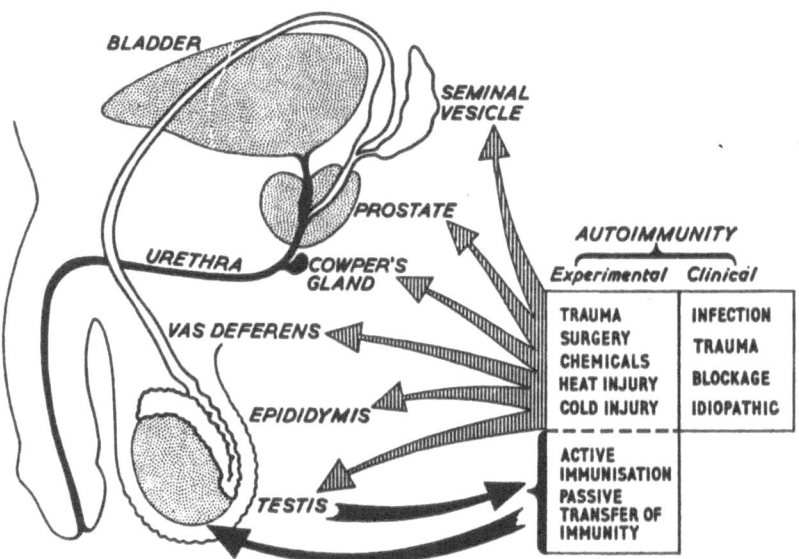

Figure 5.4 Schematic representation of the pathogenesis of experimental and clinical auto-immunity developed against reproductive tract components (antigens)

where granuloma formation occurs at the operation site (suggesting sperm leakage). The initial characteristics of the antibody response indicate that it is a primary immune reaction.

(4) Anti-sperm antibodies seldom appear in seminal plasma following vasectomy. If they do they are in low titre and appear to represent transudation of serum antibodies mostly in the region of the prostate. Local antibody production occurs proximal to the operation site and there is evidence of high titre activity in epididymal fluid.

(5) Following vaso-vasostomy in previously vasectomized men high levels of anti-sperm antibodies may appear in the semen due to re-establishment of communication with the site of antibody production. Both serum and semen anti-sperm antibodies may persist following vaso-vasostomy, presumably due to continued leakage at the anastomosis site or permeability of the genital tract to sperm antigens. There is some evidence that the persistence of antibodies modifies the success of vasectomy reversal.

In a relatively small proportion of infertile males, humoral and local immunity to sperm occurs without demonstrable organic lesions in the reproductive tract. The clinical significance of these phenomena will be discussed in detail below. Cellular immunity to sperm can also accompany immunological disruption of the male genital tract but its extent and significance require further study.

Serum IgG and IgA, but not IgM, appear in the seminal plasma of normal men by transudation mainly in the prostate. The levels are of the order of 1% of those in serum and this is reflected in correspondingly low levels of seminal anti-sperm antibodies in autoimmunized males. In addition, however, local SIgA is found in semen and this, together with the demonstration of complement components in semen, completes the armamentarium necessary for the mediation of a variety of anti-sperm activity both within the male tract and in the ejaculate[86]. It should be reiterated, however, that these activities may represent a balance of immune mechanisms and a variety of immuno-suppressive and anti-complementary factors known to be present in seminal plasma.

It is also clear that the environment of the female genital tract into which semen containing anti-sperm antibodies may be delivered will influence the ultimate effect of such antibodies on fertility.

THE INVESTIGATION OF IMMUNOLOGICAL INFERTILITY

A bewildering variety of methods have been used to detect anti-sperm antibodies which is a reflection of a generally held concern about the immunological validity, interpretation and standardization of many of the tests. In addition, there has been considerable confusion regarding the clinical significance of some of the commonly used methods for the detection of circulating anti-sperm antibodies. This has placed a major and evolving emphasis on the development and application of tests of local immunity to sperm.

This section deals with the commonly used methods in the investigation of immunological infertility and examines the clinical significance of some of these tests in both males and females.

Methodology

Many of the problems of standardization have been overcome by a WHO-sponsored international collaborative programme which produced a definitive review of methodology for anti-sperm antibody detection[87]. The reader is referred to this and subsequent publications (Boettcher et al.[58,88]) for details of the various techniques and their reproducibility. Beer and Neaves[14] also provide a detailed critical review of anti-sperm antibody tests.

Since there is no epidemiological or serological evidence that the HLA or ABO systems are involved in immunological infertility, donor sperm may be used as an antigen source in anti-sperm antibody testing. The reactions, therefore, are tissue- rather than individual-specific.

Sperm microagglutination

The agglutination of sperm may be observed microscopically on slides or in the wells of a micro-chamber. The author's experience, and that of many other workers, indicates a perplexing variation in the incidence of sperm micro-agglutination in the blood of both infertile and control subjects. Several reasons may account for this and should dictate caution in the immunological and clinical interpretation of this test. Human sperm may agglutinate in the presence of microbial agents, chemicals and even homologous serum. Technical variations in quantitation and the omission of appropriate control experiments have tended to exaggerate the effects of these non-specific factors in many published studies.

The relevance of microagglutination tests to immunological infertility has also been questioned by the demonstration that the activity may be in the β-globulin rather than the γ-globulin fraction. Furthermore head-to-head sperm agglutination can be induced by test serum containing sex steroids (progesterone and testosterone) of endogenous or exogenous origin and this activity resides in the steroid binding β-lipoprotein fraction. These findings explain many of the vagaries of the sperm microagglutination test in different groups of patients, including the occurrence of positive tests in pregnancy sera. Notwithstanding these considerations, there are some sera exhibiting strong anti-sperm activity in other immunological tests which show positive sperm microagglutination due to IgG and IgM antibodies. It has also been a consistent finding that positive activity in female sera tends to be of the head-to-head type and that in male sera of the tail-to-tail type. This suggestion of a divergence of antibody specificity in males and females is reflected in the results of other tests for both circulatory and local anti-sperm antibodies (see below).

Gelatin agglutination

In this test, motile spermatozoa are suspended in a gelatin medium and the serum or fluid under study is added in serial dilution to small test tubes containing sperm suspensions. Agglutination is observed macroscopically. This method has been used extensively in the investigation of infertile males but its use in females has been limited. One reason for this might be that head-to-head sperm agglutination, which appears to be mediated more commonly by antibodies developed in the female, is not readily detected by the gelatin technique. Although there is no doubt that gelatin agglutination activity resides in the IgG and IgM fractions, the method requires careful control and interpretation under consistent laboratory conditions. This may account for the disturbingly high incidence of positive tests in unmarried and fertile control groups in some reports.

Sperm immobilization

Complement-dependent sperm immobilization forms the basis of a simple reproducible test for sperm antibodies. The interaction of antibody molecules with sperm antigens activates the complement system and disrupts the permeability and integrity of the cell membrane of the sperm acrosome and mid-piece. The ultimate effect on the sperm can be microscopically detected as a loss of motility followed by cell death. Sperm-immobilizing activity has been shown to reside in the IgG and IgM factions of positive sera and appears to provide the most reliable method of detecting humoral anti-sperm activity with possible clinical significance. Sera with immobilizing activity usually show sperm-agglutinating activity but the converse does not apply. The sperm-immobilization test is the method of choice for screening females for serum antibodies, and may also be applied to cervical mucus. It appears to exhibit relatively low titre activity in male sera which are strongly positive in gelatin agglutination. It is simpler to perform, however, and may be used as a screening test on blood to detect subjects requiring further investigation for seminal plasma antibodies. For this purpose, however, the gelatin agglutination test appears to have a clear advantage in sensitivity over the immobilization test.

Spermatozoa used in immobilization tests have to be freshly obtained from ejaculates of high quality. Serum used as a source of complement should be freshly obtained and stored frozen in small aliquots. Sera from humans, guinea-pigs and rabbits appear to be equally suitable sources of complement but activity must be checked and titrated periodically.

Several sperm-immobilization techniques have been devised. Most are based on the initial method described by S. Isojima (see Rose et al.[87]) but where large numbers of sera are to be tested a microtechnique based on the principle of lymphocyte tissue typing[77] has certain advantages, particularly in ease of titration. The test end-point may be extended from sperm immobilization to cytotoxicity by the use of dye exclusion; however this neither improves the validity nor the sensitivity of the method.

Immunofluorescence techniques

The sensitive indirect immunofluorescent antibody technique has been applied to the study of anti-sperm antibodies. Early unsatisfactory results were obtained using unfixed sperm as substrate but subsequent refinements in technique[89], notably the use of methanol-fixation of spermatozoal smears, have led to widespread use of the test in the investigation of infertility.

The method involves three basic steps. The antigenic substrate is prepared by making an air-dried and fixed smear of spermatozoa. The smear is then exposed successively to test serum (or cervical mucus or seminal plasma) and to fluorescent labelled antibody against immunoglobulins. Antigen–antibody reactions between the test fluid and sperm cells may then be visualized and localized by microscopy under appropriate illumination and their surface representation related to the anatomy of the spermatozoon (see Figure 5.1). The staining patterns obtained on fixed sperm involve sub-surface antigens which are presumably less important than surface antigens in the provocation of antibodies with potential clinical significance. This fact is borne out by the generally poor correlation of immunofluorescent sperm antibodies with fertility status and with antibodies detected by immobilization and gelatin agglutination techniques.

The immunofluorescence technique presents a number of difficulties in this context. Background fluorescence and unevenness of staining on individual spermatozoa cannot be avoided. Staining patterns vary with the quality of the substrate semen and there is usually a heterogeneity of staining in which up to 30% of the spermatozoa fail to exhibit the predominant pattern. A particular problem is that the animal sera from which the fluorescent conjugates are prepared often contain small amounts of antibodies reactive against spermatozoa of other species. To overcome this it is important to use conjugates of such a strength that this potential source of unwanted staining can be diluted out. Non-specific staining is common and dictates the careful use of control slides. Despite precautions the high incidence and ubiquitous nature of weakly reactive antibodies has caused problems at test serum titres less than 1:16. Specificity can be reasonably assured by using Fab preparations of antibodies to exclude Fc binding but the complexity of such an approach is not compatible with the use of the method as a routine screening test.

Weak staining reactions of uncertain significance are often seen with undiluted serum and positive results should only be reported on titres greater than 1:16. Some regions of the sperm such as the equatorial segment, neck and mid-piece are common sites of non-specific staining patterns. Anti-sperm antibodies in blood react in the immunofluorescence technique mainly against antigens in the acrosome and tail. Acrosome staining occurs with both IgM and IgG antibodies and staining of the main tail-piece appears to be almost exclusively due to IgG. Staining of the tail end-piece is occasionally observed and is due to IgM antibodies.

The treatment of normal human spermatozoa with trypsin in the presence of dithiothreitol causes swelling of the head and exposes DNA and nuclear proteins[53]. Some of the sera of infertile or post-vasectomy males with high titres of sperm-agglutinating antibodies contain IgG antibodies which localize on the swollen sperm heads (Kolk et al.[52]). This reaction is rare in female sera and may reflect autoimmunity to somatic nuclear antigens. The antibodies appear to be directed against a strongly basic human protein – protamine. Sera with anti-nuclear antibody activity, especially those with anti-DNA, may stain the nuclei of normal or swollen sperm heads.

Antibodies in cervical mucus

Local isoimmunity to sperm is likely to operate throughout the uterus and Fallopian tubes and even at an ovarian level since sperm-immobilizing antibodies can be detected in follicular fluid. The cervix, however, is both the most accessible and potentially important site of local immunity in the female genital tract. Largely because of logistic difficulties in collection and technical processing problems, cervical mucus has remained somewhat neglected in the investigation of immunological infertility. More recently, however, the realization that sperm antibodies may appear in the mucus in the absence of readily detectable serum levels, or may be locally secreted in the SIgA class, has led to attempts to establish routine methods for their measurement.

In general terms, cervical mucus is most easily and appropriately collected at mid-cycle. For the specific purpose of sperm antibody measurement, the time of collection is less important since there tends to be an inverse relationship between the amount of cervical mucus and its immunoglobulin concentration. Various techniques have been devised to prepare cervical mucus for sperm antibody testing:

(1) Ultracentrifugation to produce a water supernatant. This tends to exclude a large proportion of the antibodies.

(2) Liquefaction with Bromelin, a proteolytic enzyme. The introduction of such an agent into a test system involving sperm surface antigens is not advisable.

(3) Extraction with a physiological buffer followed by centrifugation to produce an antibody-containing supernatant.

In the author's laboratory, mucus is aspirated into a syringe with 0.5 ml phosphate buffered saline at pH 7.6. After storage at 4 °C for 24 h, it is liquefied by repeated passage through a 25G needle. It may be stored at −20 °C in this state before centrifugation for 5 min at 12 000 rev./min in a microfuge. The resultant supernatant contains the immunoglobulin fraction and is suitable for use in a sperm micro-immobilization method. This appears to be the most suitable test for use on cervical mucus. Both the indirect immunofluorescence test and sperm microagglutination have proved unreliable and lacking in correlation with infertility.

Antibodies in seminal plasma

Sperm antibodies in the IgG and IgA class may appear in seminal plasma when they are present in relatively high titre in serum. When high titres are present in seminal plasma this is usually due to a significant contribution from locally secreted (SIgA) antibodies. When head-to-head agglutinins are present in serum, being mostly IgM antibodies, these are unlikely to appear in seminal plasma. Tail-to-tail antibodies (IgG) appear in the semen but only when serum titres are greater than 1:64.

The direct measurement of seminal plasma antibodies is of uncertain value since serum titres can usually be used to predict the likely local situation and additional information on SIgA antibodies can be obtained in the SCMC test (see below). It has also been claimed[90] that when sperm-agglutinating titres reach 1:64 in serum in infertile men, the ejaculated semen shows spontaneous sperm agglutination.

Cell-mediated immunity (CMI)

The *in vitro* assessment of cell-mediated immunity to spermatozoal or testicular antigens has proved fraught with technical and interpretational difficulties[91]. There is little doubt that CMI may be part of the autoimmune response to genital tract disruption in the male. In the female, however, there is little evidence that CMI to sperm is a specific accompaniment of immunological infertility. The final answer awaits improvement in techniques, particularly the preparation of purified soluble sperm antigens for use in the testing of both the recognition and effector arms of the cellular immune response.

Methods involving both partners

Post-coital test – Despite its shortcomings and its dependence on multiple factors, a properly performed post-coital test serves as a reasonable guide to the presence of sperm antibodies either in seminal plasma or (more likely) in cervical mucus[92,93]. It is equally clear that there is little correlation between the post-coital test and the presence of circulating antibodies as determined by a variety of methods.

Sperm–cervical mucus penetration test – This may be performed in a tube or on a slide and allows for a more controlled *in vitro* type of post-coital test, but again, non-antibody factors may operate. The method does allow crossed-hostility testing[94] in which combinations of male partner/male donor sperm and female partner/female donor mucus are used to identify the site of local anti-sperm activity.

Sperm–cervical mucus contact test (SCMC) – This test was devised by Kremer and Jager[95] to demonstrate the presence of local antibodies in either partner. A positive test indicating anti-sperm antibodies in either semen or cervical mucus or both is associated with characteristic shaking movements of the sperm when they come into contact with the cervical mucus on a slide. It was originally hypothesized that the phenomenon was mediated by 'stickiness' of the Fc fragment of IgA antibody molecules which adhered to the glycoprotein micelles of cervical mucus. Newer evidence suggests that the 'shaking' phenomenon can be mediated by $F(ab)_2$ fragments of anti-sperm antibodies in both IgA and IgG classes (T. Hjort, personal communication, 1979). Nonetheless, the SCMC test is a valuable method for the detection of local antibodies and is also suitable for cross-over testing.

The need for new methodology

There remains an urgent need for the development of radioimmunoassays for the precise detection and quantitation of antibodies to specific sperm antigens. Several investigators have moved towards meeting this need with the development of radiolabelling methods involving whole sperm. Sung *et al.*[96] have used radiolabelled actinomycin D in a microassay for sperm cytotoxicity and its value has been confirmed by Boettcher and Boettcher[97]. Other potential test systems involve radiolabelled staphylococcal protein A binding to antibody–sperm complexes and double antibody techniques with radio-labelled rabbit anti-human globulin detecting antibody binding to sperm.

Other approaches, yet to be fully developed, involve the use of *in vitro* fertilization systems to assess the biological activity of anti-sperm antibodies. Such tests may utilize human sperm and zona-free rodent eggs or an isologous system using human gametes.

CLINICAL SIGNIFICANCE OF ANTI-SPERM ANTIBODIES

In the female

The complement-dependent sperm immobilization test appears to be a reliable index of immunological infertility in the female. In a study of 539 women with 'unexplained' infertility, the author found this test to be positive in 7.6%. A prospective evaluation of reproductive patterns in women with anti-sperm antibodies was undertaken to compare the significance of the sperm-immobilization test with the immunologically suspect sperm-micro-agglutination test. A form of treatment was undertaken by a small group of these women (see below) but the majority either refused or were not offered treatment for a variety of reasons.

In order to assess subsequent fertility in untreated women with positive tests, and in those without antibodies, questionnaires were sent to 430 consecutive patients who had been investigated between 1 and 6 years previously. Replies were received from 391 patients, a return rate of 91%, and details of these patients are shown in Table 5.3. The mean follow-up period since investigation was 45 months, with a range of 12–73 months.

Table 5.3 Reproductive performance subsequent to anti-sperm antibody testing in 391 infertile couples (follow-up period 12–73 months; mean 45 months)

Infertility category	Mean age (range) (years)	Number of patients	Duration of infertility (years) Mean	Range	Number of patients who became pregnant
Unexplained (primary and secondary)	28.5 (20–45)	281	3.2	1–15	142 (50.5%)
Organic (minor)	28.4 (22–37)	51	3.5	1–9	29 (56.9%)
Organic (major)	29.7 (18–39)	59	4.1	1–13	14 (23.7%)

So that a more meaningful analysis might be made of the clinical significance of anti-sperm antibodies, the group of patients with major organic lesions was excluded and data were analysed in 332 women with unexplained or minor organic pathology (Table 5.4). Although pregnancy rates were higher in those patients with negative tests compared to those with positive tests, none of the differences approached statistical significance. The pregnancy rates in all groups appear surprisingly high, but are compatible with the figure of 51% for subsequent fertility in patients with unexplained infertility of at least 12 months' duration in the large and comprehensive study of Southam[98].

In the face of this lack of clear evidence of an association of anti-sperm antibodies with subsequent fertility, a sub-group of 156 patients with relatively long-term infertility was analysed (Table 5.5). These were women with unexplained and minor organic infertility of 3 or more years' duration at the time of testing. In this group there were lower pregnancy rates in patients with positive tests compared to those with negative tests. These results indicate that the clinical significance of these tests may be restricted to those patients with relatively long-term infertility of an unexplained nature.

Table 5.4 Reproductive performance subsequent to investigation in 332 infertile couples, primary and secondary

Sperm antibody test in female partner	Number of patients	Number of patients who became pregnant
Microagglutination		
Negative	274	147 (53.6%)
Positive	58	24 (41.4%)
Immobilization		
Negative	309	163 (52.8%)
Positive	23	8 (34.8%)

Unexplained, 281; minor organic, 51

Table 5.5 Subsequent fertility in 156 couples previously infertile for 3 or more years

Sperm antibody test in female partner	Number of patients	Number of patients who became pregnant
Microagglutination		
Negative	124	55 (44.4%)
Positive	32	12 (37.5%)
Immobilization		
Negative	141	64 (45.4%)
Positive	15	2 (13.3%)

A superior clinical significance of sperm-immobilization over sperm micro-agglutination was evident when serum titres were analysed in selected patients (Table 5.6). The advantages of sperm immobilization as a screening test in women for circulatory anti-sperm antibodies, compared with both micro-agglutination and gelatin agglutination, have now been stressed by many workers.

The indirect immunofluorescence test appears to correlate with infertility when performed by certain experienced workers at appropriate serum dilutions. Despite this, there is an undercurrent of concern about the value of this method as a screening test for anti-sperm antibodies in both men and women. Certainly there is a poor correlation with other screening tests, which is not surprising in view of the different antigen–antibody systems involved.

Another major source of confusion has stemmed from the demonstration by Tung and co-workers[55,56], that naturally occurring antibodies giving homogeneous immunofluorescent staining of the acrosome are present in up to 60% of normal adults. This finding presumably reflects exposure to foreign antigens, including ubiquitous micro-organisms, which provokes antibodies cross-reactive with spermatozoa.

Table 5.6 Reproductive performance subsequent to sperm antibody testing in 20 couples with unexplained infertility

Sperm antibody test in female partner	Result	Number of test results	Number of patients who became pregnant
Microagglutination	Negative	2	0
	Undiluted positive	10	3
	> 1:16	8	2
Immobilization	Negative	6	3
	Undiluted positive	9	2
	> 1:16	5	0

Mean follow-up period 3 years; range 1–6 years

The application of anti-sperm antibody testing to cervical mucus should become an integral part of the investigation of immunological infertility. The sperm-immobilization test appears suitable for this purpose, although long-term follow-up studies will be necessary to elucidate its ultimate clinical significance in this situation. The value to be obtained from antibody testing of cervical mucus hinges on the incidence of local secretory activity in the absence of a positive serum test. Data from experimental model systems suggest that it is extremely difficult to provoke local immunity in the female without a concurrent systemic response; there is evidence, however, that this is not so in nature, and this provides the rationale for cervical mucus testing. On the other hand serum anti-sperm antibodies may on occasions be present in the absence of activity in cervical mucus and may exert an anti-fertility effect by transudation into the reproductive tract at a higher level. It is necessary therefore to best both blood and cervical mucus to obtain a comprehensive profile.

In the male

Many large groups of infertile males have been investigated for the presence of circulating anti-sperm antibodies using the gelatin agglutination test. Positive results are obtained in between 3 and 8% compared with up to 2% in fertile males. Rumke et al.[99] studied the reproductive history of 254 men, originally infertile, who had been tested for gelatin agglutination sperm antibodies between 2 and 16 years previously. In those with normal sperm counts initially there was a close positive correlation between high serum titres of antibodies and continuing infertility; low titres were compatible with fertility.

Using a different test, complement-dependent sperm immobilization, the author found that 2.7% of 409 infertile males showed positive serum tests compared with 0% in 65 fertile men. There appears to be a correlation between positive sperm immobilization and high titre ($> 1:64$) reactivity in the gelatin agglutination test in the blood of infertile males. This finding is consistent with the concept that immobilization is mostly mediated by IgM or IgG antibodies directed against the sperm head and tail respectively, and that gelatin agglutination in male serum is usually due to IgG agglutinins against the sperm tail. High titre gelatin agglutinins or sperm-immobilizing activity in serum usually indicate the concurrent presence of antibodies in seminal plasma.

Immunofluorescence antibody tests in men show a poor correlation with fertility status and with other tests of anti-sperm antibodies. There are two exceptions to this generalization. The autoantibody which was mentioned above, which is directed against swollen sperm heads[52], and an antibody described by Tung[55] which causes speckled acrosomal fluorescence, both seem to reflect true autoimmunity and correlate with the infertile status.

The fact that phagocytosis of spermatozoa within the male genital tract is probably a common event but is associated with the appearance of anti-sperm antibodies in the blood of so relatively few males, may be related to the following factors:

(1) Immunological tolerance induced by continuous resorption of seminal antigens.

(2) Blocking of the formation of anti-sperm antibodies by other antibodies.

(3) Individual variation in antibody-forming capacity.

Depending on the population under study, up to two-thirds of men with anti-sperm antibodies demonstrate genital tract pathology. This may include the aftermath of trauma or surgical damage, prostatitis, seminal vesiculitis, epididymo-orchitis, and testicular atrophy following infection. In these cases antibody formation presumably is secondary to disruption or obstruction of the genital tract with sperm extravasation and resorption into interstitial tissue. The exact pathogenic relationship between genital tract obstruction and the appearance and persistence of circulating anti-sperm antibodies is unclear, since 75% of males with obstructive lesions fail to develop sperm agglutinins. Also some patients with sperm agglutinins in whom an obstruction is relieved surgically continue to maintain positive titres. Studies of males with primary or secondary endocrine atrophy of testicular function have established that impaired spermatogenesis *per se* is not related to the presence of anti-sperm antibodies.

The possible presence of occult genital tract lesions in men with anti-sperm antibodies must be considered. Notwithstanding this, in infertile males without demonstrable organic lesions, there is a close association between sperm antibodies in serum and the presence in semen of agglutinated or sluggish sperm with a poor capacity for cervical mucus penetration. It is likely that, in men who remain fertile in spite of relatively high titres of circulating antibodies, these fail to enter the seminal plasma in sufficient concentration to impair sperm efficiency.

ASPECTS OF TREATMENT

Attempts at treatment of immunological infertility have proved disappointing and the benefits derived from the detection of a presumptive immunological aetiology have been somewhat intangible. The results of immunological investigations may provide both doctor and patient with the largely academic satisfaction of finding 'something wrong' and if properly performed and interpreted they may form the basis of a helpful prognosis[47].

In the female

Occlusion therapy

Over the years there have been enthusiastic claims for the success of occlusion therapy (male partner using condom for 6–9 months) in women with evidence of an immunological basis for their otherwise unexplained infertility. However a review of the results of occlusion therapy[17] indicated that they compare unfavourably with the outcome in patients with circulating anti-sperm antibodies who remain untreated. The somewhat more rational selection of patients for this treatment on the basis of local immunity demonstrable in the cervical mucus might lead to improved results. It must be stressed, however, that local immunity to sperm is not confined to the cervix and the 'block' may occur at a higher level.

Immunosuppression

Immunosuppressive therapy with corticosteroids has been attempted and has led to anecdotal reports of lowered antibody levels and the occurrence of pregnancies. The use of high dosage immunosuppressive treatment for a non-life-threatening disorder on tenuous theoretical grounds may be difficult to justify.

Intra-uterine insemination

In women with evidence of local anti-sperm antibodies in their cervical mucus causing poor or absent sperm penetration the intra-uterine insemination of semen from the husband has an attractive theoretical basis. Several workers have attempted this approach. Kremer reported four pregnancies in 20 patients (see Boettcher[11]) and the present author has achieved four pregnancies in seven cases. Controlled studies are required to establish the validity of this therapeutic approach. Also in this, as in other treatment methods in the female, it is impossible to distinguish therapeutic success from pregnancies occurring during one of the many nadirs of the sperm antibody titre which have been recorded in long-term studies by S. Isojima (personal communication, 1979).

It should be remembered that the insemination of whole semen into the uterine cavity is unphysiological, and improved results might be obtained by technical modifications such as sperm concentration.

In the male

Immunosuppression

Therapy with ACTH or corticosteroids has proved disappointing in men with circulating anti-sperm antibodies. However there is some evidence that this treatment may have a place in immunological aspermatogenesis where cellular immunity is operative and where irreversible testicular changes have not occurred.

Spermatogenesis suppression

On the hypothesis that anti-sperm antibodies are formed as a result of resorption of spermatozoa, interruption of this process by suppression of spermatogenesis could lead to a decline in antibody levels. Suppression has been attempted by several workers using long-term testosterone treatment, but the results were unconvincing.

Sperm washing

Another approach has been adopted in which sperm from males with immunological infertility are washed several times in a physiological buffer supplemented with 5–10% human serum or albumen. They are then inseminated into the cervical canal or uterine cavity of the female partner. Good-quality semen is an essential starting point of this procedure. Pregnancies have been reported but there is no clear evidence yet of a specific therapeutic benefit from this method.

OTHER IMMUNOLOGICAL CONSIDERATIONS IN INFERTILE WOMEN

The reciprocal clinical relationship between the thymus and certain endocrine glands, such as the anterior pituitary and the gonads, is well established but little is known about possible intrinsic immunological influences on reproduction in the female. The existence of some form of immunological control of gonadal function is suggested by the inhibition of ovarian development and germ cell maturation which occurs in neonatally thymectomized mice and which may be reversed by thymic replacement.

Autoimmune ovarian failure

There is now persuasive clinical evidence that some cases of ovarian failure, both primary and secondary, belong to a spectrum of autoimmune disease involving primarily endocrine glands[17]. Such cases usually exhibit organ-specific autoantibodies which react against ovarian granulosa and theca internal cells, as well as against steroid-producing cells in other organs such as testis, adrenal and placenta. There is also evidence in some women for autoimmunity directed against gonadotrophin receptor molecules in the ovary. Ovarian failure and amenorrhoea with a possible autoimmune basis have now been reported in association with a number of immunological disorders. These include Addisonian adrenal disease, Hashimoto's thyroiditis, thyrotoxicosis, hypoparathyroidism, diabetes mellitus, pernicious anaemia, idiopathic thrombocytopenia purpura, autoimmune haemolytic anaemia, the immune deficiency disorders, mucocutaneous candidiasis and ataxia telangiectasia, and alopecia and vitiligo. This association appears closest with autoimmune disorders which involve the adrenal, thyroid and parathyroid glands and the stomach.

Women with secondary ovarian failure (premature menopause) but without other immunological disorders fail to exhibit ovarian autoantibodies but have a high incidence of other tissue autoantibodies. Despite this observation, there is no evidence that the majority of cases of uncomplicated premature menopause have an immunological basis. Ovarian autoimmunity may be associated with primary as well as secondary ovarian failure, underlining the fact that these two syndromes, though often clinically discrete, may emerge imperceptibly to form a spectrum in which similar aetiological factors may operate.

In addition to the association of primary ovarian failure (pure ovarian dysgenesis) with autoimmunity, there have been a number of reports of the coexistence of Turner's syndrome and other chromosomally determined cases of ovarian dysgenesis, with autoimmune disease. An abnormal incidence of tissue autoantibodies (especially against the thyroid) has been reported in some but not all studies of such patients. It is an intriguing fact that ovarian embryogenesis is initially normal in Turner's syndrome but that the primordial follicles disappear some time during fetal and prepubertal development. There may be an immunological basis for this phenomenon which should be examined further by histological and immunological study of appropriate fetal material.

Ovarian involvement in mumps virus infection is a rare but well-recognized occurrence. It is likely that this involvement, as well as causing primary tissue destruction, may also provoke an autoimmune reaction similar to that seen in mumps orchitis and in the apparently very rare condition of mumps adrenalitis.

Antibodies to zona pellucida

The zona pellucida contains cell-specific antigens which may be susceptible to immunological reactions causing infertility[58, 100]. Heterologous antibodies raised against zona pellucida, and also certain lectins, specifically coat the outer surface of the zona, block sperm attachment and fertilization and prevent its dissolution by enzymes[101]. This reaction is mostly species-specific; however there is cross-reactivity of antibodies to primate and porcine zona[102]. The pig, therefore, may act as a source of antigen for vaccine development should the zona pellucida be considered a feasible target for immuno-contraception. Isolated porcine zonae can also be used as substrate for the detection of anti-zona antibodies in biological fluids. Methods used include the indirect immunofluorescence antibody technique and the ability of antibodies to coat the zona and alter its light-scattering properties. These tests are difficult to control and interpret, and many of the data obtained to date are open to methodological criticism, In addition, anti-zona antibodies may cross-react with homologous erythrocyte antigens so that an appropriate absorption step must precede any assay procedure. Many of the problems will probably only be overcome when zona antigens are isolated and purified to allow radioimmunoassays to be developed. Using the current methods, autoantibodies to zona pellucida have been demonstrated in the blood of a proportion of infertile women; however they have also been found in fertile women and in a significant number of peri- and post-menopausal subjects. The latter findings suggest that their presence in some circumstances could be an epiphenomenon of ovarian follicular resorption.

Conclusions

The author makes no apology for the air of therapeutic nihilism pervading this section. There is an important need for prospective controlled assessment of the therapeutic manoeuvres currently in use to establish whether they offer any advantage over nature. The other major problems in the field which confuse our understanding of immunological infertility and make treatment prospects disappointing are the role of cell-mediated immunity and the precise significance and distribution of local antibody-mediated immunity, especially in the female.

References

1. Katsh, S. (1959). Immunology, fertility and infertility: a historical survey. *Am. J. Obstet. Gynecol.*, **77**, 949

2. Menge, A. C. (1970). Immune reactions and infertility. *J. Reprod. Fertil.* (Suppl. 10), 171

3. Shulman, S. (1971). Antigenicity and autoimmunity in sexual reproduction: a review. *Clin. Exp. Immunol.*, **9**, 267

4. Behrman, S. J. and Menge, A. C. (1973). Immunological aspects of reproduction. In Hafez, E. S. E. and Evans, T. N. (eds.) *Human Reproduction: Conception and Contraception*, pp. 237–256. (New York: Harper & Row)

5. Behrman, S. J. (1975). The immune response and infertility. In Behrman, S. J. and Kistner, R. W. (eds.) *Progress in Infertility*, 2nd Edn, pp. 793–815. (Boston: Little Brown & Co.)

6. Rumke, P. and Hekman, A. (1975). Auto- and isoimmunity to sperm in infertility. *Clin. Endocrinol. Metabol.*, **4**, 473

7. Jones, W. R. (1979a). Immunological factors in infertility. In Pepperell, B. J., Hudson, B. and Woods, C. (eds.) *The Infertile Couple*. (London: Churchill-Livingstone.) (In press)

8. Diczfalusy, E. (ed.) (1974). *Immunological Approaches to Fertility Control*. 7th Karolinska Symposium. (Stockholm: Karolinska Institute)

9. Hafez, E. S. E. (ed.) (1976). *Human Semen and Fertility Regulation in Men*. (St Louis: C. V. Mosby Co.)

10. Scott, J. S. and Jones, W. R. (eds.) (1976). *Immunology of Human Reproduction*. (London: Academic Press)

11. Boettcher, B. (ed.) (1977). *Immunological Influence on Human Fertility*. (Sydney: Academic Press)

12. Edidin, M. and Johnson, M. H. (eds.) (1977). *Immunobiology of Gametes*. (Cambridge: Cambridge University Press)

13. Insler, V. and Bettendorf, G. (eds.) (1977). *The Uterine Cervix and Reproduction*. (Stuttgart: Geo. Thième)

14. Beer, A. E. and Neaves, W. B. (1978). Antigenic status of semen from the viewpoint of the male and female. *Fertil. Steril.*, **29**, 3

15. Jones, W. R. (ed.) (1979b). Immunological aspects of reproduction. *Clin. Obstet. Gynaecol.*, **6**, No. 3

16. Voisin, G. A., Toullet, F. and D'Almeida, M. (1974). Characterisation of spermatozoal auto-, iso- and alloantigens. In Diczfalusy, E. (ed.) *Immunological Approaches to Fertility Control*, pp. 173–201. 7th Karolinska Symposium. (Stockholm: Karolinska Institute)

17. Jones, W. R. (1976a). Immunological aspects of infertility. In Scott, J. S. and Jones, W. R. (eds.) *Immunology of Human Reproduction*, pp. 375–414. (London: Academic Press)

18. Mancini, R. E. (1976). Immunopathology of animal and human testis. In Hafez, E. S. E. (ed.) *Human Semen and Fertility Regulation in Men*, pp. 287–307. (St Louis: C. V. Mosby Co.)

19. Voisin, G. A., Delauncay, A. and Barber, M. (1951). Sur des lesions testiculaires provoquees chez le cobaye par iso-et autosensibilisation. *Ann. Inst. Pasteur.*, **81**, 48

20. Freund, J., Lipton, M. M. and Thompson, G. E. (1953). Aspermatogenesis in the guinea-pig induced by testicular tissue and adjuvants. *J. Exp. Med.*, **87**, 711

21. Freund, J., Thompson, G. E. and Lipton, M. M. (1955). Aspermatogenesis, anaphylaxis and cutaneous sensitisation induced in the guinea-pig by homologous testicular extract. *J. Exp. Med.*, **101**, 591

22. Brown, P. C., Holborrow, E. J. and Glynn, L. E. (1969). The early lesion of experimental allergic orchitis in guinea pigs. *Immunology*, **9**, 255

23. Katsh, S., Aquirre, A. R., Leaver, F. W. and Katsh, G. F. (1972). Purification and partial characterisation of aspermatogenic antigen. *Fertil. Steril.*, **23**, 644

24. Jackson, J. J., Hagopian, A., Carlo, D. J., Limfuco, G. A. and Eylar, E. H. (1975).

Experimental allergic orchitis. I. Isolàtion of a spermatozoal protein (API) which induces aspermatogenic orchitis. *J. Biol. Chem.*, **250**, 614

25. Hagopian, A., Jackson, J. J., Carlo, D. J., Limfuco, G. A. and Eylar, E. H. (1975). Experimental allergic orchitis. III. Isolation of spermatozoal glycoproteins and their role in allergic aspermatogenic orchitis. *J. Immunol.*, **115**, 1731

26. Tung, K. S. K. (1977). The nature of antigens and pathogenic mechanisms in autoimmunity to sperm. In Edidin, M. and Johnson, M. H. (eds.) *Immunobiology of Gametes*, pp. 157–186. (Cambridge: Cambridge University Press)

27. Mancini, R. E. (1971). Immunological approaches to fertility control. In Diczfalusy, E. and Borell, U. (eds.) *Control of Human Fertility, Nobel Symposium No. 15*, p. 159. (Stockholm: Almqvist & Wiksell)

28. Johnson, M. H. (1969). The effect of cadmium chloride on the blood-testis barrier of the guinea pig. *J. Reprod. Fertil.*, **19**, 551

29. Ericsson, R. J. and Andress, J. M. (1973). Chemically induced autoimmunisation in the male rat. In Bratanov, K., Edwards, R. G., Vulchanov, V. H., Dikov, V. and Samlev, B. (eds.) *Immunology of Reproduction*, pp. 123–124. (Sofia: Bulgarian Academy of Sciences Press)

30. Tumboh-Qeri, A. G. and Roberts, T. K. (1977). Cell mediated immunity to spermatozoa following vasectomy. In Boettcher, B. (ed.) *Immunological Influence on Human Fertility*, pp. 100–204. (Sydney: Academic Press)

31. Anderson, D. J. and Alexander, N. J. (1979). Consequences of autoimmunity to sperm antigens in vasectomised men. In Immunological aspects of reproduction, *Clin. Obstet. Gynaecol.*, Vol. 6, No. 3. (London: W. B. Saunders)

32. Nagarkatti, P. S. and Rao, S. S. (1976). Cell mediated immunity to homologous spermatozoa following vasectomy in the human male. *Clin. Exp. Immunol.*, **26**, 239

33. Muir, V. Y., Turk, J. L. and Hanley, H. C. (1977). Comparison of allergic aspermatogenesis with that induced by vasectomy. *Clin. Exp. Immunol.*, **28**, 461

34. Bishop, D. W. (1961). Aspermatogenesis induced by testicular antigen uncombined with adjuvant. *Proc. Soc. Exp. Biol. Med. (N.Y.)*, **107**, 116

35. Pokorna, Z. and Vojtiskova, M. (1964). Autoimmune damage of the testes induced with chemically modified organ-specific antigen. *Folia Biol. (Praha)*, **10**, 261

36. Joel, C. A. (1971). Historical survey of research on spermatozoa from antiquity to the present. In Joel, C. A. (ed.) *Fertility Disturbances in Men and Women*, p. 3. (Basel: S. Karger)

37. Rosenfield, S. S. (1926). Semen injections with serologic studies. *Am. J. Obstet. Gynaecol.*, **12**, 385

38. Baskin, M. J. (1932). Temporary sterilisation by the injection of human spermatozoa – a preliminary report. *Am. J. Obstet. Gynecol.*, **24**, 892

39. Escudar, D. J. (1936). La esterilizacion biologica temporaria la mujer por esperma humano. *Arch. Urug. Med.*, **8**, 484

40. Rodriguez-Lopes, M. M. (1936). Esterilizacion biologica temporaria de la mujer. *Arch. Urug. Med.*, **121**, 373

41. Menge, A. C., Schwarz, R. L., Riolo, R. L., Breenberg, V. N. and Meda, T. (1977). The role of the cervix and cervical secretions in immunologic infertility. In Insler, V. and Bettendorf, G. (eds.) *The Uterine Cervix in Reproduction*, p. 221. (Stuttgart: Geo. Thième)

42. Goldberg, E. (1974). Effects of immunisation with LDH-X on fertility. In Diczfalusy, E. (ed.) *Immunological Approaches to Fertility Control*, p. 202. 7th Karolinska Symposium. (Stockholm: Karolinska Institute)

43. Beer, A. E. and Billingham, R. E. (1974). Host responses to intra-uterine tissue, cellular and fetal grafts. *J. Reprod. Fertil.*, **21**, 59

44. Metz, C. B. (1972). Effects of antibodies on gametes and fertilisation. *Biol. Reprod.*, **6**, 358

45. Morton, D. B. (1977). Immunoenzymatic studies on acrosin and hyaluronidase in ram spermatozoa. In Edidin, M. and Johnson, M. H. (eds.) *Immunobiology of Gametes*, pp. 115–156. (Cambridge: Cambridge University Press)

46. Johnson, W. L. and Hunter, A. G. (1972). Seminal antigens: their alteration in the genital tract of female rabbits and during partial *in vitro* capacitation with beta amylase and beta glucuronidase. *Biol. Reprod.*, **7**, 332

47. Chen, C. (1979). Immunological infertility. In Immunological aspects of reproduction. *Clin. Obstet. Gynaecol.*, Vol. 6, No. 3

48. Cohen, J. (1974). Gametic diversity within an ejaculate. In Afzelius, B. (ed.) *The Functional Anatomy of the Spermatozoon*, p. 329. (Oxford: Pergamon Press)

49. de Fazio, S. R. and Ketchel, M. M. (1972). The occurrence of seminal plasma antigens in the tissues of women. *J. Reprod. Fertil.*, **30**, 125

50. Hjort, T. (1975). Iso- and autoantibodies to human sperm as reactants for the study of immunogenic components of human sperm. In *Development of Vaccines for Fertility Regulation* (WHO Symposium), p. 37. (Copenhagen: Scriptor)

51. Boettcher, B. (1979). Immunity to spermatozoa. In Immunological aspects of reproduction. *Clin. Obstet. Gynaecol.*, Vol. 6, No. 3

52. Kolk, A. H. J., Samuel, T. and Rumke, P. (1974). Autoantigens of human spermatozoa. *Clin. Exp. Immunol.*, **16**, 63

53. Kolk, A. H. J. and Samuel, T. (1975). Isolation, chemical and immunological characterisation of two strongly basic nuclear proteins from human spermatozoa. *Biochem. Biophys. Acta*, **333**, 307

54. Tung, K. S. K. (1975). Human sperm antigens and anti-sperm antibodies. I. Studies on vasectomy patients. *Clin. Exp. Immunol.*, **37**, 546

55. Tung, K. S. K. (1976). Human sperm antigens and anti-sperm antibodies. III. Studies on acrosomal antigens. *Clin. Exp. Immunol.*, **24**, 292

56. Tung, K. S. K., Cook, W. D., Terestia, A., McCarty, T. A. and Robitaille, R. (1976). Human sperm antigens and antisperm antibodies. II. Age related incidence of antisperm antibodies. *Clin. Exp. Immunol.*, **25**, 73

57. Clarke, G. M., Boyd, R. L. and Muller, H. K. (1977). Actin-like protein in human sperm heads. In Boettcher, B. (ed.) *Immunological Influence on Human Fertility*, pp. 211–214. (Sydney: Academic Press)

58. Boettcher, B., Hjort, T., Rumke, P., Shulman, S. and Vyazov, O. (1977a). Auto- and isoantibodies to antigens of the human reproductive system. *Acta Path. Microbiol. Scand.*, Sect. C, Suppl. 258

59. Chen, C. and Simons, M. J. (1977a). Modified seminal plasma antigens and subfertility. In Boettcher, B. (ed.) *Immunological Influence on Human Fertility*, pp. 255–262. (Sydney: Academic Press)

60. Chen, C. and Simons, M. J. (1977b). Modified seminal plasma antigens: further characterisation of antigenic activity. In Boettcher, B. (ed.) *Immunological Influence on Human Fertility*, pp. 263–270. (Sydney: Academic Press)

61. Amos, D. B. (1974). HL-A, fertility and natural selection. In Diczfalusy, E. (ed.) *Immunological Approaches to Fertility Control*, p. 318. 7th Karolinska Symposium. (Stockholm: Karolinska Institute)

62. Edidin, M., Gooding, L. R. and Johnson, M. (1974). Surface antigens of normal early embryos and a tumour model system useful for their further study. In Diczfalusy, E. (ed.) *Immunological Approaches to Fertility Control*, p. 336. 7th Karolinska Symposium. (Stockholm: Karolinska Institute)

63. Edwards, R. G. (1976). Immunity and the control of human fertility. In Diczfalusy, E. (ed.) *Immunological Approaches to Fertility Control*, pp. 415–470. 7th Karolinska Symposium. (Stockholm: Karolinska Institute)

64. Johnson, M. H. (1976). Fertilisation and implantation. In Scott, J. S. and Jones, W. R. (eds.) *Immunology of Human Reproduction*, pp. 33–60. (London: Academic Press)

65. Rickson, R. P. (1977). Differentiation and other alloantigens of spermatozoa. In Edidin, M.

and Johnson, M. H. (eds.) *Immunobiology of Gametes*, pp. 85–114. (Cambridge: Cambridge University Press)

66. Landsteiner, K. and Levine, P. (1926). Polymorphism and intra-specific differences in human spermatozoa. *J. Immunol.*, **12**, 415

67. Kerek, G. (1974). Distribution of the blood group antigens A and B on human spermatozoa. *Int. J. Fertil.*, **19**, 181

68. Erickson, R. P. and Stites, D. P. (1975). Effect of murine spermatozoa on the mixed leukocyte reaction of mouse. *Transplantation*, **20**, 263

69. Halim, A. and Festenstein, H. (1975). HLA-D on sperm is haploid, enabling use of sperm for HLA-D typing. *Lancet*, **2**, 1255

70. Levis, W. R., Whalen, J. J. and Sherins, R. J. (1976). Mixed cultures of sperm and leukocytes as a measure of histocompatibility in man. *Science*, **191**, 302

71. Misko, I. S., Boettcher, B., Roberts, T. K. and Kay, D. J. (1978). Spermatozoal cells in human semen do not stimulate allogeneic leucocytes in culture. *Lancet*, **1**, 560

72. Koo, G. C., Boyse, E. A. and Wachtel, S. S. (1977). Immunogenetic techniques and approaches in the study of sperm and testicular cell surface antigens. In Edidin, M. and Johnson, M. H. (eds.) *Immunobiology of Gametes*, pp. 73–84. (Cambridge: Cambridge University Press)

73. Fellows, M., Colle, A. and Tonnelle, C. (1976). The expression of human beta-2 microglobulin on human spermatozoa. *Eur. J. Immunol.*, **6**, 21

74. El-Mahgoul, S. (1972). Anti-spermatozoal antibodies in infertile women with cervico-vaginal schistosomiasis. *Am. J. Obstet. Gynecol.*, **112**, 781

75. Friberg, J. and Gnarpe, H. (1973). Mycoplasma and human reproductive failure. III. Pregnancies in 'infertile' couples treated with doxycycline for T-Mycoplasmas. *Am. J. Obstet. Gynecol.*, **116**, 23

76. Lord, E. M., Sensabaugh, G. F. and Stites, D. P. (1977). Immunosuppressive activity of human seminal plasma. I. Inhibition of *in vitro* lymphocyte activation. *J. Immunol.*, **118**, 1704

77. Husted, S. and Hjort, T. (1975). Microtechniques for simultaneous determination of immobilising and cytotoxic sperm antibodies. *Clin. Exp. Immunol.*, **22**, 256

78. Kovary, P. M., Dykgers, A. and Nurmann, H. (1978). C_{1q} precipitins in human seminal plasma. *Arch. Androl.*, **1**, 99

79. Cinader, B. and de Weck, A. (1976). *Immunological Response of the Female Reproductive Tract*. (Copenhagen: Scriptor)

80. Jones, W. R. (1976b). Immunological factors in infertility. In Jordan, J. and Singer, A. (eds.) *The Cervix*, pp. 184–191. (London: W. B. Saunders)

81. Schumacher, G. F. B. and Yang, S.-L. (1977). Cyclic changes in immunoglobulins and specific antibodies in human and rhesus monkey cervical mucus. In Insler, V. and Bettendorf, G. (eds.) *The Uterine Cervix in Reproduction*, pp. 187–203. (Stuttgart: Geo. Thième)

82. Lippes, J., Ogra, S. S., Tomasi, T. B. and Tourville, D. R. (1970). Immunohistochemical localisation of IgG, IgA, IgM, secretory piece and lactoferrin in the human female genital tract. *Contraception*, **1**, 163

83. Lippes, J., Enders, R. G., Pragay, D. A. and Bartholomew, W. R. (1972). The collection and analysis of human fallopian tube fluid. *Contraception*, **5**, 85

84. Linnet, L. and Hjort, T. (1977). Sperm agglutinins in seminal plasma and serum after vasectomy. Correlation between immunological and clinical findings. *Clin. Exp. Immunol.*, **30**, 413

85. Lucas, P. L. and Rose, N. R. (1978). Immunological consequences of vasectomy: a review. *Ann. d'Immunol. (Instit. Pasteur)*, **129**, 301

86. Friberg, J. and Tilly-Friberg, I. (1977). Antibodies in human seminal fluid. In Hafez, E. S. E.

(ed.) *Human Semen and Fertility Regulation in Men*, pp. 258–264. (St Louis: C. V. Mosby Co.)

87. Rose, N. R., Hjort, T., Rumke, P., Harper, M. J. K. and Vyazov, O. (1976). Techniques for the detection of iso- and autoantibodies to human spermatozoa. *Clin. Exp. Immunol.*, **23**, 175

88. Boettcher, B., Hjort, T., Rumke, P., Schulman, S. and Vyazov, O. (1977b). Auto- and isoantibodies to antigens of the human reproductive system. *Clin. Exp. Immunol.*, **30**, 173

89. Hjort, T. and Hansen, K. B. (1971). Immunofluorescent studies on human spermatozoa. I. The detection of different spermatozoal antibodies and their occurrence in normal and infertile women. *Clin. Exp. Immunol.*, **8**, 9

90. Husted, S. (1975). Sperm antibodies in men from infertile couples. *Int. J. Fertil.*, **20**, 113

91. Marcus, Z. H., Soffer, Y., Ben-David, A., Peleg, S. and Nebel, L. (1973). Studies on sperm antigenicity. I. Delayed hypersensitivity to spermatozoa. *Eur. J. Immunol.*, **3**, 75

92. Soffer, Y., Marcus, Z. H., Bukovsky, J. and Caspi, E. (1975). Immunological factors and post coital test in unexplained infertility. *Int. J. Fertil.*, **21**, 89

93. Moghissi, K. (1977). Significance and prognostic value of post-coital test. In Insler, V. and Bettendorf, G. (eds.) *The Uterine Cervix in Reproduction*, pp. 231–238. (Stuttgart: Geo. Thieme)

94. Morgan, H., Stedronska, J., Hendry, W. F., Chamberlain, G. V. P. and Dewhurst, C. J. (1977). Sperm and cervical mucus crossed hostility testing and anti-sperm antibodies in the husband. *Lancet*, **1**, 1228

95. Kremer, J. and Jager, S. (1976). The sperm cervical mucus contact test: a preliminary report. *Fertil. Steril.*, **27**, 335

96. Sung, J. S., Shiyuya, H., Black, D. D. and Mumford, D. M. (1977). A radioimmunoassay for cytotoxic antibody to human spermatozoa. *Clin. Exp. Immunol.*, **27**, 469

97. Boettcher, B. and Boettcher, M. J. (1979). Spermatotoxic antibodies in sera from infertile couples determined with H[3]-actinomycin D. *Proc. Fourth Symp. Immunology of Reproduction*. (Sofia: Bulgarian Academy of Sciences Press) (In press)

98. Southam, A. L. (1960). What to do with the 'normal' infertile couple. *Fertil. Steril.*, **11**, 543

99. Rumke, P., van Amstel, N., Messer, E. N. and Bezemer, P. D. (1974). Prognosis of fertility of men with sperm agglutinins in serum. *Fertil. Steril.*, **25**, 393

100. Shivers, C. A. (1977). The zona pellucida as a possible target in immunocontraception. In Boettcher, B. (ed.) *Immunological Influence on Human Fertility*, p. 25. (Sydney: Academic Press)

101. Shivers, C. A. (1975). Immunological interference with fertilisation. In Diczfalusy, E. (ed.) 7th Karolinska Symposium on Immunological Approaches to Fertility Control. *Acta Endocrinol.* (Suppl. 194), **78**, 223

102. Sacco, A. G. (1977). Antigenic cross reactivity between human and pig zona pellucida. *Biol. Reprod.*, **16**, 164

Section II
Immunological
Aspects of
Fertility Control

6
Inhibition of Reproductive Function by Antibodies to Luteinizing Hormone Releasing Hormone

H. M. FRASER

INTRODUCTION

The hypothalamus regulates the pituitary secretion of luteinizing hormone (LH) and follicle-stimulating hormone (FSH) by the release of the deca-peptide luteinizing hormone releasing hormone (LHRH) into the hypo-physeal portal blood vessels. During the isolation of LHRH in the 1960s it was thought that a separate releasing hormone existed for FSH, but most of the chemical evidence is against this idea and LHRH is now considered the releasing hormone for both LH and FSH[1-3]. If the action of LHRH is inhibited one would anticipate that the secretion of LH and FSH would be prevented. Since LH and FSH control the processes of spermatogenesis and ovulation and the production of the sex steroid hormones it follows that the ultimate effect of inhibiting the action of LHRH is to inhibit fertility. This chapter describes the way in which this can be achieved by the use of antibodies to LHRH. We will see how this work has played an important part in elucidating the physiological role of the releasing hormone and examine some of the possibilities for practical application of the techniques developed in control of fertility in animals and man.

GENERATION OF ANTIBODIES TO LHRH

LHRH is a decapeptide (Figure 6.1) and it appears to be without species specificity among mammals[1]. As an immunogen it has the disadvantage that it

pGLU ——HIS–TRP——SER–TYR—GLY—LEU–ARG–PRO—GLY-NH$_2$

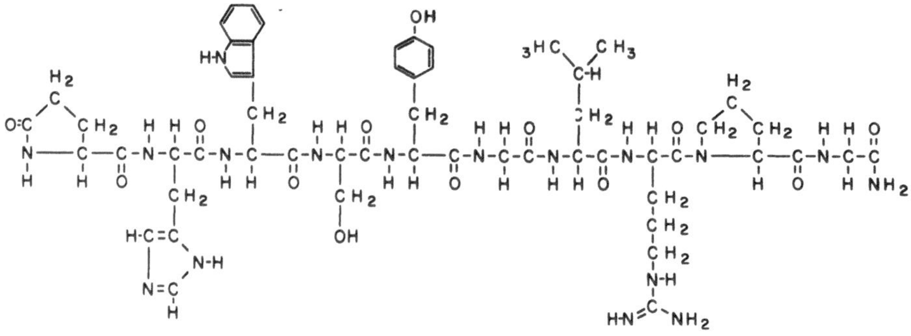

Figure 6.1 Structure of luteinizing hormone releasing hormone. From Guillemin[2]

is a naturally occurring peptide with a low molecular weight of 1183, but has the advantage that its structure is known and it can be easily synthesized by classical or solid phase methods for peptide synthesis[1] and is thus readily available in purified form.

Despite its apparent lack of immunogenicity, antibodies can be produced to LHRH given with Freund's complete adjuvant if it is first absorbed to alhydrogel[4,5], polyvinylpyrrolidone[6] or charcoal[7], and there has even been a unique instance of inadvertent production of antibodies in a male patient undergoing self-administered LHRH therapy[8,9]. However, there is no doubt that for the reliable production of good antibodies the conjugation of LHRH to a carrier protein molecule is obligatory. Bovine serum albumin (BSA) has been most widely employed as a carrier[5–7, 10–20] although human serum albumin[14,21], thyroglobulin[20,22], guinea-pig γ-globulins[23], keyhole limpet haemocyanin[24], tetanus toxoid[25], horse-radish peroxidase[26] and a synthetic copolymer of glutamic acid, lysine, alanine and tyrosine (MW 30 000)[27] have also been used successfully.

Several different methods of conjugating LHRH to the carrier molecule have been used. Conjugation using carbodi-imide is a simple and widely used technique[5, 7, 11, 13, 15, 17–20, 24] although only four to six molecules of LHRH are incorporated on to the carrier molecule[7, 28]. This may be because carbodi-imides primarily act by joining free amino or carboxyl groups on a peptide to respective groups on the carrier molecule[29]. Since neither of these groups exists in the LHRH molecule it seems that the reaction must take place through the hydroxyl groups on serine or tyrosine. Some workers have used LHRH with the N terminal pyroglutamine changed to glumatic acid or the C terminal glycine-amide changed to a free carboxyl group to make the conventional groups available sites for conjugation[11, 14]. Gluataraldehyde condensation has been used widely to polymerize LHRH with a carrier molecule[9, 15, 21, 23] and there is one report of the use of di-isocyanate toluene as a conjugating agent[21]. It is generally believed that the introduction of a chemical 'bridge' between peptide and carrier improves immunogenicity because the peptide can be more easily 'seen' by the antibody-producing cells. This type of link can be achieved using bis diazotized benzidine which introduces two aromatic rings between the tyrosine and histidine residues of LHRH and the conjugation sites on the carrier molecule. The resulting conjugate has been used successfully by several groups[7, 12, 13, 22] although the method has the disadvantage that benzidine is a known carcinogen.

A problem in these one-step conjugation methods is that one not only gets carrier–hapten conjugation but also hapten–hapten conjugation. The two step procedure described by Koch et al.[10] is an attempt to overcome this. LHRH itself is first reacted with p-diazomium phenylacetic acid to produce an azo-LHRH derivative at the histidine position and to a lesser extent at the tyrosine position. The derivative can then be coupled to a carrier using carbodi-imide. High incorporation rates of 27[10] and 20[16] molecules of LHRH per molecule of BSA have been reported and satisfactory antisera produced[7, 10, 16].

Specificity of resulting antisera is of crucial importance if they are being used for radioimmunoassay and also requires consideration when the antibodies are being used to inhibit endogenous LHRH in vivo. With the availability of an extensive range of fragments and analogues of LHRH a number of detailed studies on antibody specificity have been carried out[5, 7, 9, 10, 12, 14, 20, 30]. Copeland et al.[20] have divided LHRH antisera into three groups according to their specificity. The highly specific antisera are termed conformational. They do not bind any fragments of LHRH although they will cross-react with some analogues. It seems that the antigenic determinant is not localized to a sequence of amino acids but is a function of a three-dimensional feature of the molecule. Such antisera are exceptional and the most widely used currently in radioimmunoassay is that of Nett et al.[12] produced as early as 1973. The second group are termed sequential as they cross-react with certain fragments of the decapeptide molecule as well as with some analogues. Many sequential antisera have been produced; for example those which have specifically for a C-terminal portion of the molecule such as the 7–10 fragment[5, 7, 14, 18]. The third group of antisera recognize several fragments of LHRH but with no precise relation to sequence, suggesting that these individual antisera are composed of several subpopulations of antibodies.

There is a high possibility that a single conjugate will generate antibodies of varying specificity in different animals, but it would be desirable to establish some guidelines from all we know about the immunogenicity of LHRH to select a conjugate which would provide the best chance of producing a specific antiserum. Unfortunately, we are forced to conclude that no particular method of conjugation gives consistently highly specific antisera. Conformational antisera have been produced using bis diazotized benzidene and carbodi-imide[12, 20] but the use of these agents has most often produced sequential or subpopulation antisera[5, 20]. All the conjugates described above can produce antisera of high titre and affinity and no particular one is outstanding in this respect. It is important to note that antibodies to unconjugated LHRH do not lead to the production of highly specific antibodies[5, 9, 14] and no benefit is obtained by allowing conjugation to occur at only one particular end of the molecule, other than increasing the chances of producing an antiserum to the portion most distant from the site of conjugation[11, 14]. The use of the azo LHRH conjugate with its high degree of incorporation at a known site of conjugation[10] would seem to be the most promising approach for further development.

For the purpose of inhibition of LHRH *in vivo* it is not essential to have complete antibody specificity; in studies of active immunization uniform specificity would seem to be virtually impossible. The chief concern is that the antibodies should not also inhibit other endogenous hormones. The LHRH antisera studied in detail seem to be free of cross-reaction with other known peptides but it should be remembered that the existence of subpopulations of antibodies capable of binding other hormones is not sought after in general specificity studies. What we can say is that while animals immunized against LHRH show gross inhibition in function of the pituitary gonadotrophs and of the gonads and accessory sex organs no inhibitory effects have been observed in the function of the other anterior pituitary cells or endocrine glands.

Before leaving the subject of antibody production it is useful to look at the immunization techniques employed to produce antisera to LHRH. Freund's complete adjuvant has been used exclusively as the best stimulator of the immune response; although *Bordetella pertussis* has sometimes also been given[28] there is no firm evidence that this will improve the antibody response induced by Freund's complete adjuvant. It is astonishing how the vast majority of groups[5–7, 10–22] employed the multiple intradermal site technique for immunization. There are only two reports describing immunization by the subcutaneous route[26, 31] with one using intramuscular[27] and another lymph node injection[23]. Since an intradermal route would be unsatisfactory for practical use of LHRH immunization it is appropriate to point out that while we have also largely employed the intradermal site technique we have also been consistently successful in raising antisera in rats, sheep and monkeys by subcutaneous injection. The final dose of LHRH conjugate is rarely accurately documented but a starting amount of LHRH for conjugating of 500 μg for rats and 1 mg for rabbits is standard. Booster immunization at intervals of 1 month or longer will increase antibody levels but is not obligatory for the production of high titre antisera[13, 28, 30].

INHIBITION OF LHRH *IN VIVO* BY ANTIBODIES

Most reports on the production of antisera to LHRH concern individual antisera being characterized for use in radioimmunoassays or for immunohistochemical studies. These antisera have been raised almost exclusively in rabbits but the use of immunization against LHRH as a means of inhibiting the action of the hormone has been widely practised in the rat, sheep, marmoset monkey and stump-tailed monkey. Studies on passive transfer have been carried out in rats, chickens, hamsters, sheep and rhesus monkeys using homologous or heterologous antisera. For such work it is best to raise antisera in species with a large blood volume, such as the sheep, to obtain large quantities of antiserum and to avoid interference from rabbit immuno-globulin present in the serum from the recipient animal if the radioimmuno-assay for its gonadotrophin depends upon precipitation by anti-rabbit γ-globulin.

Site of action of LHRH antibodies

Inhibition of a hormone by antibodies is a classical technique in studying its physiological role, but the unique difficulty when extending this approach to the hypothalamic releasing hormones is that they travel only a few millimetres in the hypophyseal portal blood vessels to reach their target gland, making antibody–antigen contact particularly elusive.

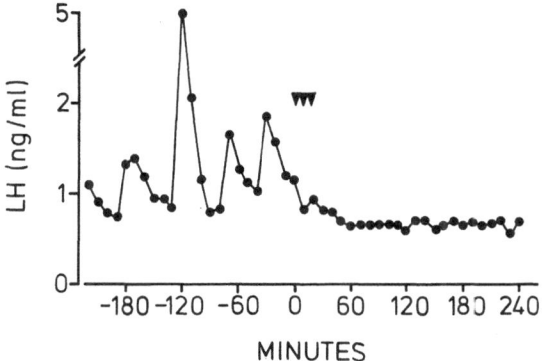

Figure 6.2 Cessation of pulsatile release of LH in the blood of a ewe after an intravenous injection of 100 ml anti-LHRH during a 20 min period (arrows). Blood samples were collected at 10 min intervals. H. M. Fraser and A. S. McNeilly (unpublished)

The most obvious site of action of antibodies to releasing hormones is in the hypophyseal portal blood itself. It is conceivable that they could also act at the level of the gonadotroph cell membrane or even gain entry into the median eminence where LHRH is stored in nerve terminals prior to release[32], although it seems safe to assume that they would be excluded from the brain itself. The action of the antibodies is essentially immediate. This can be seen from Figure 6.2 which shows the inhibitory effect of an intravenous injection of antibodies to LHRH on the pulsatile release of LH in the ewe. In this particular animal one pulse of LH was occurring every 60 min and the antibodies were administered within 10 min of the onset of the expected pulse.

To investigate the possibility of the antibodies to LHRH entering the median eminence we studied rats producing high-titre antibodies to LHRH 12 months after primary immunization. Using the technique normally employed in the immunohistochemical localization of LHRH in the rat[32] we added fluorescent-labelled rat γ-globulin to sections of the median eminence. If antibodies to LHRH had been present in the median eminence fluorescent labelling would have been expected, but negative reactions were observed in all six rats studied. To show that the animals' own serum contained antibodies capable of combining with LHRH in the nerve terminals, dilutions of the individual sera were added to the respective brain sections and a positive reaction was obtained for each rat. It is possible that this technique is not sufficiently sensitive to pick up small amounts of antibody, but the results clearly give no support to the idea that the antibodies actually can enter the median eminence.

We do not know if anti-LHRH has any action at the level of the anterior pituitary. LHRH is thought to act by attachment to the cell membrane[33] so it is conceivable that the antibody could combine with an exposed portion of the LHRH molecule. But the configuration of the decapeptide may change once it has combined with its receptor, rendering it immunochemically distinct, and in any case one would expect that the affinity of the membrane receptor for LHRH would be greater than that of the antibody. It should be noted, however, that using *in vitro* immunocytochemical techniques it has been reported that antiserum to LHRH appears to be able to bind to LHRH occupying receptors in the plasma membrane, and also to gonadotrophin secretion granules[26, 34].

INHIBITION OF LHRH IN THE MALE

An intravenous injection of a high-titre, high-affinity antibody to LHRH is probably the most effective and clearly defined way of inducing the immediate selective inhibition of LHRH. Injection of antibodies to LHRH in the Soay ram causes an immediate block in the pulsatile release of LH with a corresponding decrease in the secretion of testosterone from the testes (Figure 6.3), thus showing that the episodic secretion of LH is dependent on LHRH from the hypothalamus[35]. In contrast to LH there was no change in blood levels of FSH during the 24 h sampling period following antibody injection. One of the objects of the first experiments using antibodies to LHRH was to find if the inhibition of the releasing hormone affected FSH as well as LH, to help answer the controversy over whether LHRH controlled both pituitary hormones. We believe that this apparent absence of effect on FSH release in the ram can still be explained on the basis of LHRH controlling both hormones. When physiological amounts of LHRH are administered in a pulsatile manner to rams in the inactive phase of the breeding season it takes several days to raise the secretion of FSH, and when such treatment is stopped it takes several days for FSH secretion to decline[39]. A similar situation could occur after administration of LHRH antibodies. There is no doubt that the active immunization of rats[36,37] and rabbits (H. M. Fraser and A. S. McNeilly, unpublished observations) and the passive immunization of castrate rats[16,38] results in an unequivocal decrease in the levels of both gonadotrophins in the blood and supports the chemical evidence for the one releasing hormone for LH and FSH. Some FSH is detectable even after prolonged active immuniz- ation and although in the rat a proportion represents non-specific interference

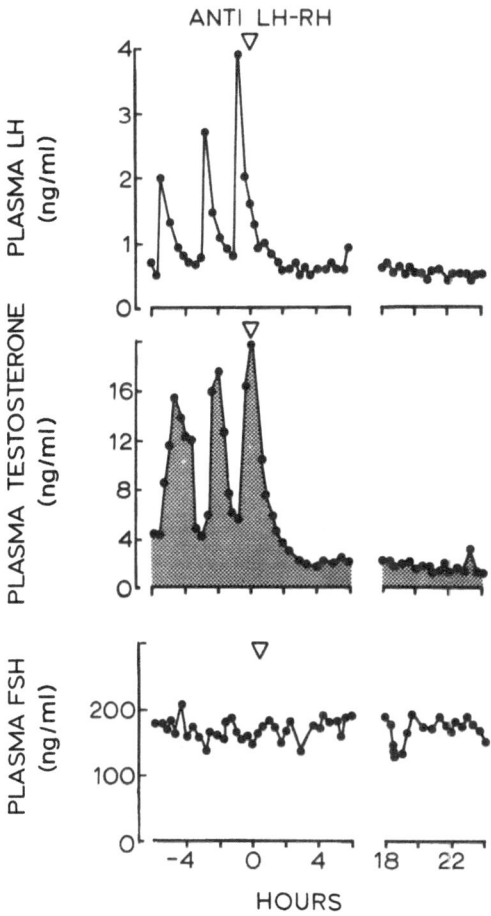

Figure 6.3   Changes in the plasma concentration of LH, FSH and testosterone in a Soay ram after an intravenous injection of 75 ml anti-LHRH (arrow). Blood samples were collected at 20 min intervals. From Lincoln and Fraser[35]

in the radioimmunoassay[36] it does seem that small amounts of this hormone are still released. This could be an autonomous secretion of FSH but it is more likely that it is released by a minute fraction of LHRH which reaches the pituitary despite the presence of the antibodies. There is evidence from work using hypophysectomized pituitary-grafted rats that when the pituitary is exposed to very small amounts of LHRH the release of low levels of FSH is favoured without release of LH[40, 41].

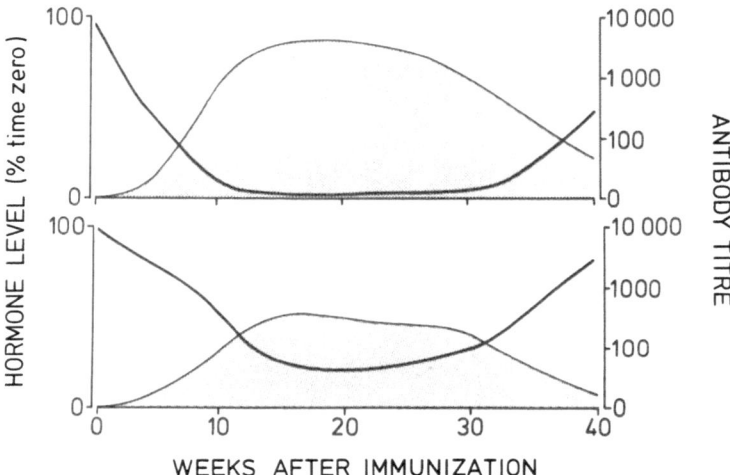

WEEKS AFTER IMMUNIZATION

Figure 6.4 Diagram illustrating how active immunization against LHRH can lead to production of high levels of antibody with a subsequent severe and prolonged reduction in hormone levels (LH and testosterone) (upper panel). Low levels of antibody result in an incomplete and short-lived reduction in hormone levels (lower panel). (Antibody titre represented by shaded area)

The process of inhibition of a hormone by active immunization has some important differences to passive immunization induced by injecting antiserum. Instead of an immediate response, the degree of inhibition of LHRH will be minimal for some time as antibody levels rise slowly, so that it takes several weeks for a significant effect on hormone levels to be obtained; but after 3–4 months a dramatic involution of the testes is evident. While the administration of a standard dose of antiserum will result in a relatively uniform response between animals, the active immunization of a group of animals with an immunogen under uniform conditions will produce a variable response because of individual variations in the immune system. Thus, by 2 or 3 months after immunization some animals will have antibodies of high titre which are sustained for several months, while others will have a short-lived period of low antibody production. Consequently, high antibody producers will have non-detectable or low gonadotrophin levels in the blood with a reduction of testosterone secretion and involution of the testes over this prolonged time-period, while the poor responders will show a less marked effect on hormone levels and testicular function (Figure 6.4). This variability can be reduced by booster immunizations, so that poor responders may reach the threshold levels of antibody to achieve successful inhibition of LHRH.

It is therefore important to be able to assess antibody production for individual animals so as to predict the success of the immunization. Our own studies have shown that measurement of LHRH antibody titre is a convenient way of achieving this, despite the fact that it does not give a complete assessment of the properties of the antiserum. We standardize the method as follows: To doubling dilutions of antiserum is added ^{125}I-labelled LHRH (10 000 cpm, approx. 10 pg) in a final volume of 300 μl in 0.1% BSA[42]. After overnight incubation free hormone is separated from bound by mixing with 1.5 ml of ice-cold ethanol and centrifugation for 15 min at 4 °C. Titre is

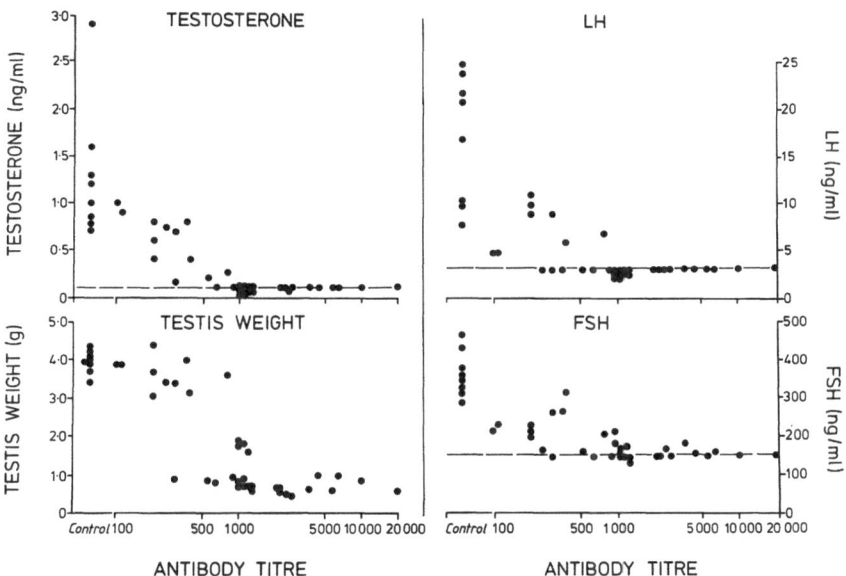

Figure 6.5 Effect of LHRH antibody titre (1:100 to 1:20 000) on levels of testosterone, LH and FSH in the blood and on testes weight in individual male rats immunized against LHRH for 40 weeks. Values for control rats are shown on the left-hand side of each panel. Broken line shows detection limit of assays. H. M. Fraser (unpublished)

expressed as the dilution of antiserum binding 33% of label. Usually, if an antibody titre of 1:1000 or more is maintained then the necessary inhibition of LH and FSH is achieved to reduce testosterone levels and testicular weight (e.g. Figure 6.5). It is of interest to note that in the experiments on passive immunization in the sheep shown in Figures 6.2 and 6.3 we obtained circulating antibody titres of between 1:1000 and 1:2000. The results in the rat

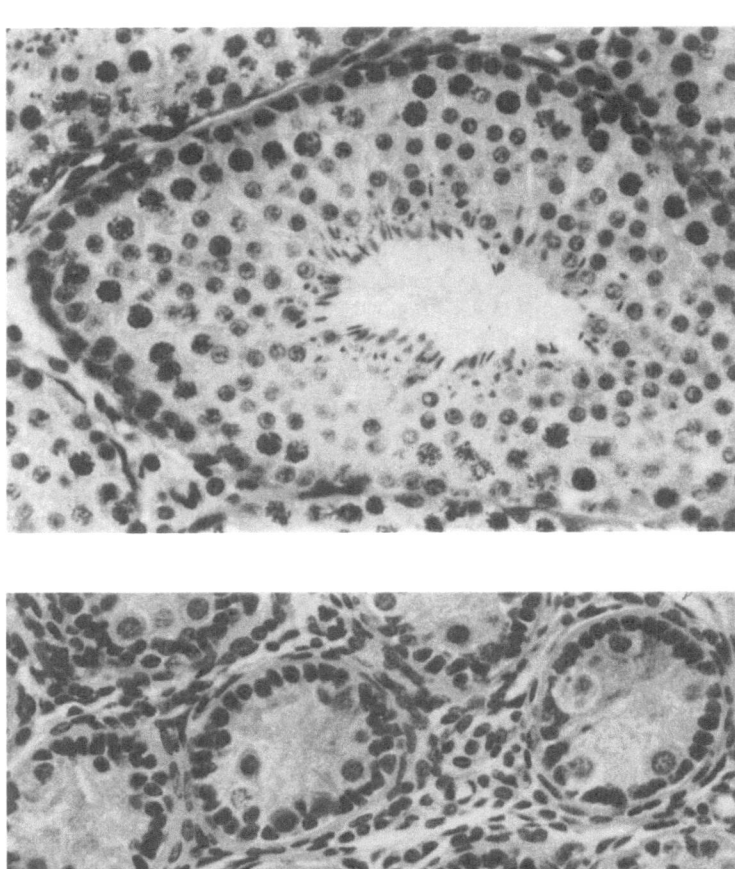

Figure 6.6   Testicular biopsy from a rabbit at time of primary immunization against LHRH (top) and 4 months after immunization (bottom). From Fraser[44]

(Figure 6.5) also show a preferential reduction of LH and testosterone in some animals, since these hormones were undetectable while some FSH was clearly being secreted and the testes were not as reduced in size as when complete inhibition was established.

From studies in rats[36] and rabbits[43–45] we know that successful active immunization against LHRH results in a reduction in the levels of pituitary gonadotrophins in the blood, and that this is associated with a reduction in secretion of testosterone[36, 45] and involution of the seminal vesicles and prostate[36]. The testes also involute, the tubules decrease in diameter and an arrest of spermatogenesis is observed in each species similar to that following hypophysectomy. The tubules are lined with Sertoli cells and in the rat and marmoset monkey primary spermatocytes are still present[36, 46] while in the rabbit the arrest of spermatogenesis is even more complete (Figure 6.6)[6, 44, 45]. Because of the outward sign of testicular involution the measurement of changing testicular size can be a good indication of the effectiveness of immunization[46].

The pituitary content of LH and FSH is also reduced after active immunization against LHRH, indicating that LHRH is required for the synthesis of the gonadotrophins[36]. Histological examination of pituitaries from rats immunized against LHRH has been carried out by histochemically identifying gonadotrophic cells by staining adjacent sections using (1) the Alcian blue–periodic acid Schiff–orange G procedure; and (2) the peroxidase–antiperoxidase (PAP) unlabelled antibody enzyme using antiserum to the β-subunit of rat LH[47]. The histochemical staining indicated that there is a decrease in the number of gonadotrophin cells in LHRH-immunized rats but this is probably because they do not stain, having only a low LH and FSH content. The more sensitive PAP method revealed that there was no real reduction in cell numbers. However, the gonadotroph cells in LHRH-immunized rats were smaller than those from control rats and were irregular in shape. No typical cytoplasmic features such as vacuoles or intensely stained areas were evident, and in some cells staining was sparse and most of the cytoplasm appeared unstained, indicating inactivity. There was no evidence of stromal abnormalities, inflammatory infiltrate or areas of necrosis.

The LHRH-immunized rat has provided a new model for studying the effects of long-term gonadotrophin deprivation on testicular function, being superior to the hypophysectomized rat since inhibition of hormone release is selective and the animals can be maintained for longer periods of time. In particular, detailed studies of Leydig cell function in these rats have been described[25, 48].

The Leydig cells appear reduced in size and the number of cells per cross-sectional area is greater than those of control rats; this is largely because of the reduction in tubule diameter so that when the differences in testicular weight are taken into account the number of Leydig cells is actually about 30% lower than in controls. However, the number of fibroblast-like cells is increased in LHRH-immunized rats and these may be inactive Leydig cells.

We have seen how testosterone levels in the blood are reduced considerably after inhibition of LHRH. In addition the capacity of the testes of LHRH-immunized rats to secrete testosterone basally or in response to human chorionic gonadotrophin (HCG) or cyclic AMP *in vitro* is reduced (Figure 6.7).

Presumably this is due to a change in the synthetic capacity of the Leydig cells following deprivation of LH.

However, the Leydig cells of the LHRH-immunized rat remain sensitive to HCG stimulation (Figure 6.8). This is despite the fact that they are unable to bind as much HCG as the controls, the number of LH/HCG receptors being severely reduced (Figure 6.9). Hypophysectomy also causes a reduction in the binding capacity of the Leydig cells, but short-term selective inhibition of LHRH by passive immunization is without effect on receptor numbers,

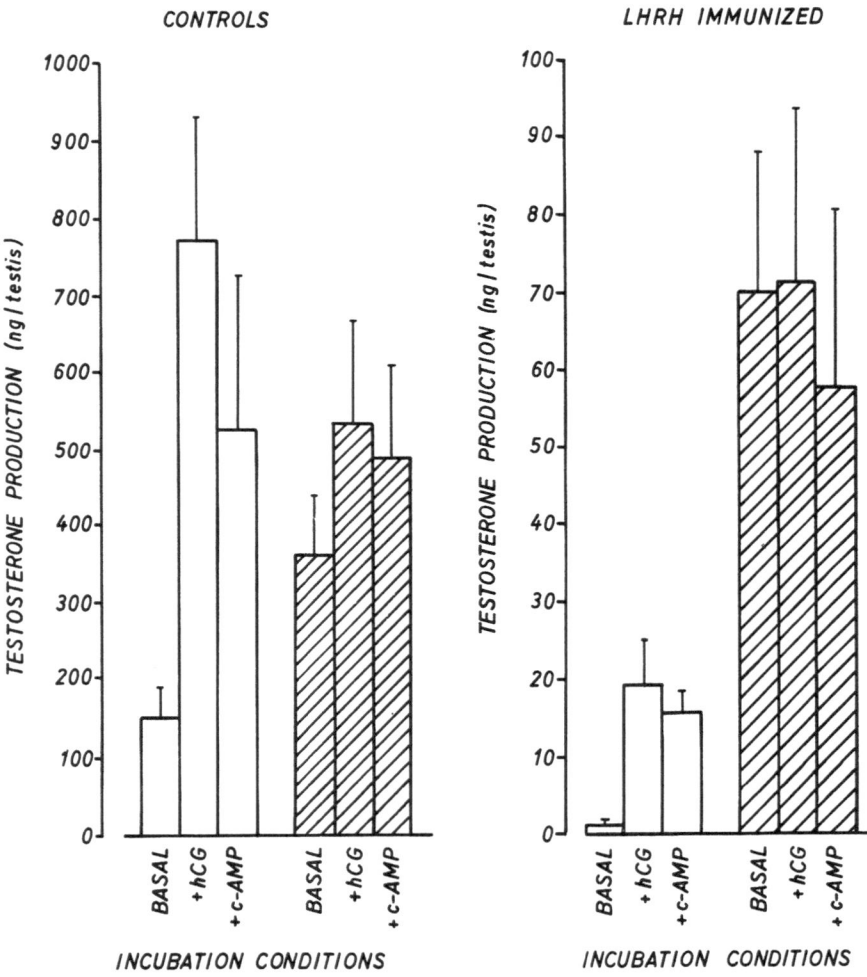

Figure 6.7 *In vitro* testosterone production from testes of control rats and rats immunized against LHRH in the absence (basal) or in the presence of either HCG or dibutyryl cAMP (open bars). Results from rats injected 48 h previously with HCG are shown by the hatched bars. From Sharpe and Fraser[48]

suggesting that other hormones such as prolactin and growth hormone may have a role in maintaining Leydig cell receptors[16]. The results using the actively immunized rat therefore confirm the importance of the gonadotrophins in maintaining LH/HCG receptors.

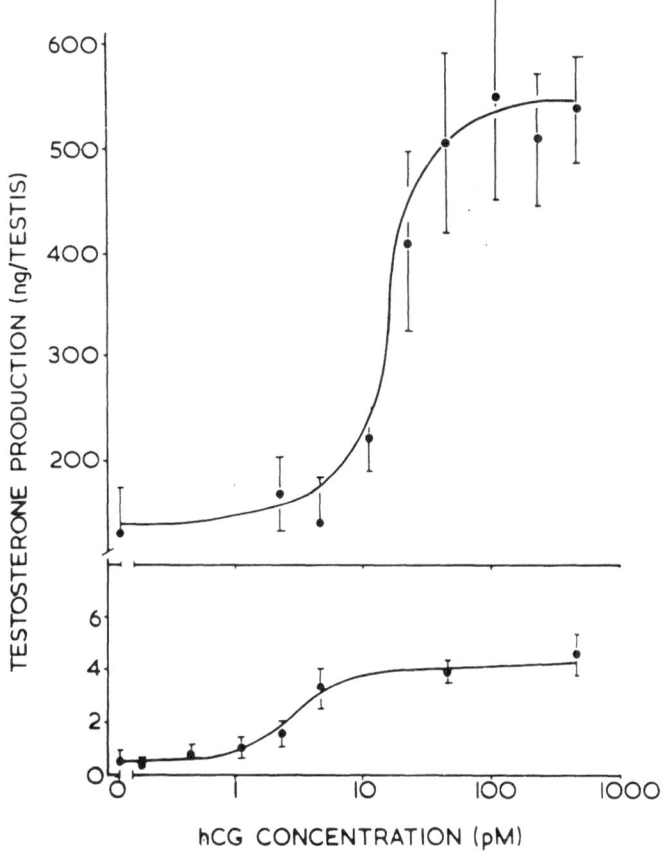

Figure 6.8   *In vitro* testosterone production from testes of control rats (upper panel) and rats immunized against LHRH (lower panel) in the presence of increasing amounts of HCG. From Sharpe and Fraser[25]

Injection of HCG or elevation of endogenous LH by injection of LHRH causes a reduction in the number of testicular LH/HCG receptors[48, 50] (Figure 6.9); the so-called 'down regulation' phenomenon. It is of interest that despite the lower number of receptors in LHRH-immunized rats injection of HCG also produces down-regulation (Figure 6.9). In the normal rat this treatment also reduces the capacity of Leydig cells to secrete testosterone in response to HCG *in vitro*[49, 50] (Figure 6.7). However, in the LHRH-immunized rat pretreatment with HCG *in vivo* has a strikingly different effect on the steroidogenic responsiveness of the testis, causing an increase in responsiveness of the Leydig cells to further stimulation by HCG *in vitro* (Figure 6.7). This suggests that doses of HCG which are inhibitory in the normal animal may be stimulatory when endogenous gonadotrophin levels have been low. In LHRH-immunized rats injected with HCG 48 h previously, the basal

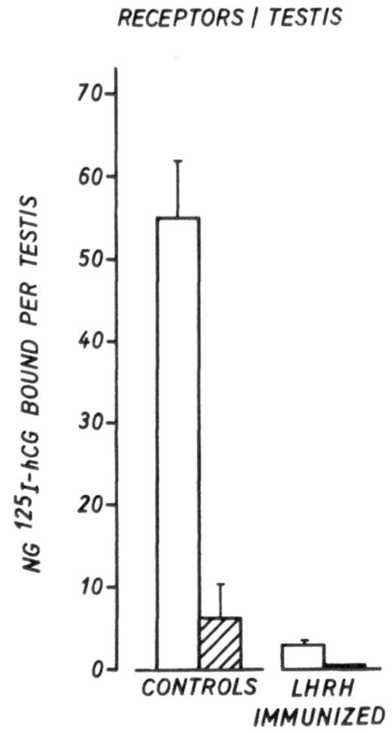

Figure 6.9 The *in vitro* binding of [^{125}I] HCG by testicular homogenates from control rats and rats immunized against LHRH (open bars) and for rats injected 48 h previously with HCG (hatched bars). From Sharpe and Fraser[48]

production of testosterone by the testis *in vitro* was equal to the maximal possible output (Figure 6.7); this suggests the interesting possibility that the Leydig cells in the gonadotrophin-deprived rat are in some way capable of perpetuating the stimulus resulting from the initial interaction of HCG with LH receptor.

INHIBITION OF LHRH IN THE FEMALE

Perhaps the most intriguing question in the reproductive cycle is how the negative feedback effect of oestrogen from the developing follicle on LH release can change to positive feedback and bring about the midcycle LH surge. It is still not clear whether: (1) there is a surge of LHRH, composed of an increase in the number and/or amplitude of LHRH pulses; or (2) whether the increased responsiveness of the pituitary which is induced by the rising oestrogen levels in the blood is the primary cause of the LH surge, with LHRH secretion remaining constant; or (3) whether both systems act together to cause the LH surge. The production of antibodies to LHRH provided two new methods of studying the role of LHRH in the female reproductive cycle. Radioimmunoassays were developed capable of measuring down to a few picograms of LHRH. Since LHRH is a locally-acting hormone, it is active in very small amounts and is virtually undetectable in peripheral blood, so that a true indication of the pattern of LHRH release from the hypothalamus can only be achieved by collecting hypophyseal portal blood. This obviously imposes limitations on the application of the technique. The few results available have shown a rise in LHRH output associated with the LH surge in the rat[51] and an indication that highest levels occur at mid-cycle in the rhesus monkey[52]. The problems of measuring the pattern of LHRH release have increased the importance of using inhibition by antibodies to study its physiological role. It is also important to use immunization to determine the long-term effects of inhibition of LHRH in the female because much effort has been put into the development of antagonists to LHRH as a potential means of fertility control in women. These antagonists can inhibit ovulation in rodents[53] but the high doses required preclude studies in non-human primates or women.

Role of LHRH throughout the ovulatory cycle

Let us first consider the effects of inhibiting LHRH on tonic secretion of LH and FSH in the female. We have seen previously (Figure 6.2) how injection of antibodies to LHRH brings about an immediate cessation of pulsatile release of LH in the ewe. As in the ram (Figure 6.3) this is not accompanied by a lowering of FSH levels. This apparent lack of effect of FSH secretion is even found in ewes actively immunized against LHRH in which LH levels are low and the animals stop cycling[31]. As discussed previously, FSH secretion may continue under low levels of LHRH. We can assume that antibodies to LHRH reduce tonic gonadotrophin secretion in the cycling rodent, as injection of anti-LHRH during dioestrus in the rat prevents the normal oestrogen-dependent enlargement of the uterus at pro-oestrus[43] and prevents the normal cyclic rise in oestradiol-17β in the hamster[54]. Active immunization of the rat leads to a lowering of both LH and FSH levels in the blood, and suppresses follicular development[55-57].

In all species studied, the inhibition of LHRH in the ovariectomized animal leads to a striking reduction in release of LH and FSH. This occurs in LHRH-immunized ewes and rats following ovariectomy[19,31,56] as well as after passive[58] or active[59] immunization of ovariectomized rats. The same effect occurs after injection of anti-LHRH in the ovariectomized rhesus monkey[60] (Figure 6.10) and it is of interest to note how LH levels decline within hours while it takes several days for maximal inhibition to occur for FSH.

The most dramatic effect of the administration of antibodies to LHRH in the female is their ability to prevent ovulation. Thus in cycling rats and hamsters injection of antibodies to LHRH a few hours before the critical period on the afternoon of pro-oestrus prevents the pre-ovulatory surge of LH and FSH and subsequently abolishes the expected ovulation[54, 58, 61, 62]. In these species it is a simple matter to pinpoint the time of expected

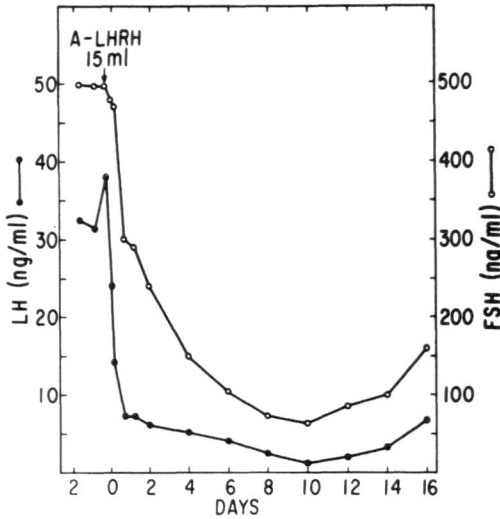

Figure 6.10   Lowering of the levels of LH and FSH in the blood of an ovariectomized rhesus monkey after an intravenous injection of antiserum to LHRH. From McCormack *et al.*[60]

hypothalamic involvement in the LH surge, as it always occurs on the afternoon on the day of pro-oestrus. It is much more difficult to extend this approach to species in which the timing of the surge is not influenced by the time of day. The problem is that injection of antibodies before levels of oestradiol-17β have reached a critical level might cause a reduction in oestrogen secretion, which in itself could abolish positive feedback since it is required to increase pituitary responsiveness to LHRH[33]. To overcome this, exogenous oestrogen can be given during the early follicular phase of the cycle or in the ovariectomized animal. Positive feedback in response to oestradiol benzoate is clearly abolished in ovariectomized ewes immunized against LHRH[63] (Figure 6.11). The actively immunized animal has the disadvantage that the pituitary will be deficient in LH and we have repeated the experiment by injecting antibodies to LHRH into normal ovariectomized ewes after giving oestradiol benzoate and again the positive response was absent or reduced (H. M. Fraser and A. S. McNeilly, unpublished). In the bird it is progesterone, not oestrogen, which induces the LH surge, and treatment of laying hens with anti-LHRH 30 min prior to administration of progesterone prevents the surge, and the hens stop laying for several days[64]. In marked

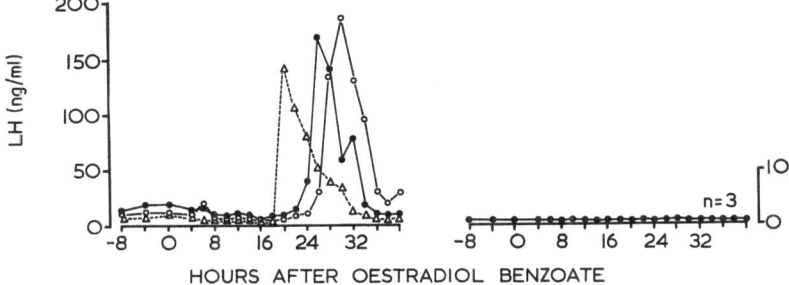

Figure 6.11 Plasma levels of LH after intramuscular injection of 50 μg oestradiol benzoate (time 0) in three ovariectomized control ewes (left-hand side) and in three ovariectomized ewes actively immunized against LHRH (right-hand side). Data from Fraser *et al.*[63]

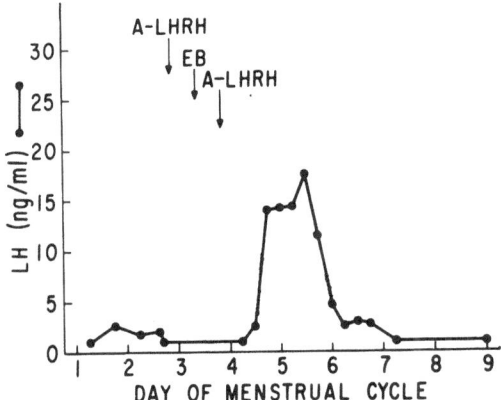

Figure 6.12 Occurrence of an LH surge in response to injection of oestradiol benzoate in an intact cycling female Rhesus monkey despite passive immunization to LHRH. From McCormack *et al.*[60]

contrast to other species, it appears that injection of antibodies to LHRH in the ovariectomized or intact Rhesus monkey in the follicular phase has no effect on oestrogen-induced positive feedback[60] (Figure 6.12), yet this same antiserum reduced tonic gonadotrophin secretion in these animals (Figure 6.10) and inhibited ovulation in the rat[58].

These results suggest that while in the rodent, bird and sheep LHRH is actively involved in inducing the LH surge, in the primate the sensitizing effect of oestrogen acting directly on the pituitary gonadotrophs may be sufficient to cause the surge. The situation is more clearly defined by using the alternative technique of inhibiting LHRH release by placing lesions in the arcuate nucleus of Rhesus monkeys. This causes a cessation of LH and FSH release, and the animals fail to respond to an oestrogen provocation test. When the animals are given exogenous LHRH in a pulsatile manner of one pulse per hour at a uniform dose this not only restores LH and FSH levels in the blood, it also restores normal negative and positive feedback responses to oestrogen[65]. Perhaps after the injections of antibodies to LHRH a small amount of biologically active LHRH remained and the results of both experiments in the monkey would suggest that, unlike the other species, only a small constant level of LHRH is required during the LH surge.

Antibodies to LHRH have also been used very effectively to determine whether the pituitary or the hypothalamus is the important site of action of prostaglandin E in inducing LH release in the rat[66, 67]. While injection of PGE into control rats induces a rapid release of LH, treatment of rats 1 h previously with antibodies to LHRH blocks the response, indicating that its action is directly on the hypothalamus, inducing LHRH release, rather than at the level of the pituitary.

Long-term inhibition of LHRH

From studies on active immunization against LHRH there is no doubt that the continual secretion of LHRH is required for normal follicular growth and ovulation in the marmoset monkey[46] and stump-tailed macaque (this chapter) as well as in the rat[55–57] and sheep[31]. The slow increase in antibody levels reduces output of gonadotrophins more gradually than passive administration of antibody, thus follicular stimulation is reduced with a subsequent decline in oestrogen levels in the blood so that the normal hypothalamic–pituitary–ovarian relationship is disrupted and cycles stop.

Active immunization against LHRH in the rat causes a gradual increase in the length of the oestrous cycles[57] before persistent dioestrous vaginal smears, with complete cessation of cycles and sterility[56, 57]. These rats have low levels of LH and FSH in the blood and pituitary[55, 56], although FSH appears less reduced than LH[56]. The ovaries are small and have no active luteal tissue, but small developing and atretic follicles. These are unlikely to secrete much oestrogen, as shown by the small uteri of these rats even when compared to dioestrous controls[56]. Interestingly, in low antibody producers in which the inhibition of LHRH is presumably less effective, LH and FSH levels in the blood are in the normal range for dioestrous rats and the ovaries are of almost normal weight[56]. While active luteal tissue still is absent, these rats have large antral or cystic follicles suggesting that gonadotrophins are stimulating follicles to develop, but that the LH surge does not occur and they fail to ovulate. The presence of oestrous vaginal smears and normal uterine weights in these rats indicates that some of the follicles are secreting oestrogen[56].

Attempts have been made to induce ovulation in rats and in ewes immunized against LHRH. LHRH can induce gonadotrophin release in immunized rats[57], ewes[19] and marmoset monkeys[46] while a more pronounced release is obtained using an LHRH agonist immunochemically different from LHRH[19, 31, 37]. However, this was unable to produce LH levels comparable to the pre-ovulatory LH surge, probably because of the low levels of gonadotrophins in the pituitary. However, injection of pregnant mares' serum into LHRH-immunized rats induced follicular development, as shown by the occurrence of pro-oestrous vaginal smears, and ovulation can then be induced by injecting LH[57].

Long-term inhibition of LHRH has also been studied in two primate species, the marmoset monkey and the stump-tailed macaque (*Macaca arctoides*). In adult marmosets kept in stable male–female pairs, immunization against LHRH was successful in preventing ovulation for about 1 year[46]. Luteal tissue was absent in all immunized animals and in high antibody producers only the early stages of follicular maturation were observed, while in marmosets with low antibody titres all stages of follicular development were taking place.

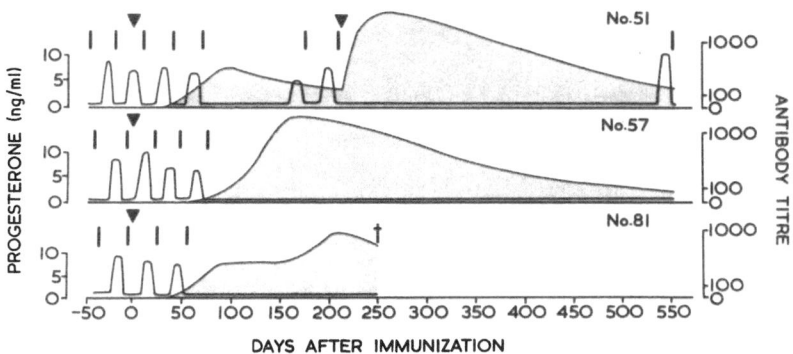

Figure 6.13   Effect of immunization against LHRH (arrows) in three cycling female stump-tailed monkeys showing development of LHRH antibody titre (shaded area), the plasma levels of progesterone and menstruation (bars). H. M. Fraser (unpublished)

The stump-tailed macaque has a menstrual cycle similar to that of women. After a single immunization of three monkeys with LHRH conjugated to tetanus toxoid, ovulation and menstruation stopped once antibody levels had become established at levels $\geqslant 1:800$ (Figure 6.13). In monkey No. 51 cycles started again once antibody levels declined, but a booster immunization during the late follicular phase of the third cycle produced a rapid rise in antibody levels and prevented the expected ovulation. An anovulatory state was maintained until antibody levels fell again. In monkey No. 57, an anovulatory state has continued despite a fall in antibody levels, and a similar inhibition of ovulation occurred in the remaining monkey but unfortunately it died from an unknown cause during the course of the study. The ovaries of this animal were devoid of corpora lutea but there was extensive hyperplasia of the interstitial tissue which superficially resembled a mass of granulosa lutein cells. The primordial and 'growing' (non-antral) follicles appeared normal, as did some medium-sized antral follicles; however, most of the Graffian follicles showed extensive degenerative changes. The ovaries of the immunized animals were probably secreting little oestrogen, as very low levels of oestradiol-17β were found in the blood (Figure 6.14).

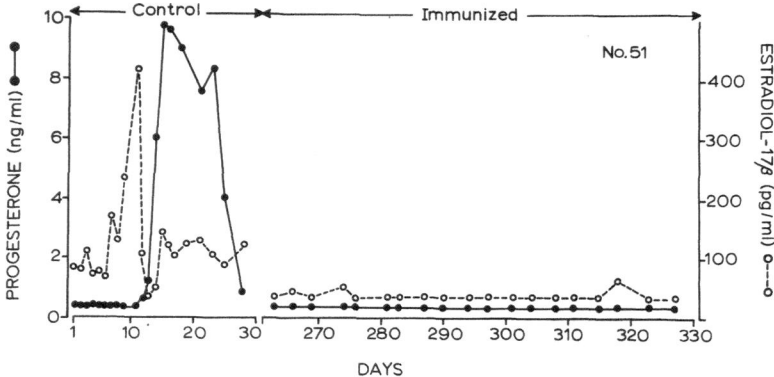

Figure 6.14   Plasma levels of oestradiol 17β and progesterone in a stump-tailed monkey during a control cycle and during a typical 70-day period after immunization against LHRH. H. M. Fraser (unpublished)

These results, showing conclusively that inhibition of LHRH by active immunization prevents ovulation in the primate, are not necessarily at variance with the results of McCormack et al.[60] in which rhesus monkeys passively immunized against LHRH could still produce an LH surge in response to oestrogen. In the latter study the monkeys received a dose of oestrogen which would trigger an LH surge at a time when their pituitaries contain a normal amount of gonadotrophin; after active immunization to LHRH the pituitary content of gonadotrophins is likely to be reduced and oestrogen levels are low.

How does the LHRH-immunized monkey compare with the monkey with lesions in the arcuate nucleus as a model for studying the relative roles of the hypothalamus and pituitary in causing the LH surge? Immunization, which can achieve specific inhibition of LHRH, has the advantage over a neuro-surgical technique in that it is a relatively simple chemical procedure. The injection of antibodies to LHRH is the best method of short-term inhibition of LHRH, but would not be suitable for the type of experiment in which LHRH replacement over a long time-period was being attempted. The exogenous LHRH would reduce the effectiveness of the antibodies to inhibit endogenous LHRH making active immunization the better method of guaranteeing efficient elimination of endogenous LHRH. The difficulty then is that exogenous LHRH would have to be given in very high doses in order to act on the pituitary, as the circulating antibodies would be highly effective in blocking its action[37]. An alternative approach is to use an LHRH agonist which does not cross-react with the antibody but is effective in small doses in immunized animals[37, 68]. An example of the effect of injecting 1 µg of the agonist into ovariectomized LHRH-immunized ewes is shown in Figure 6.15.

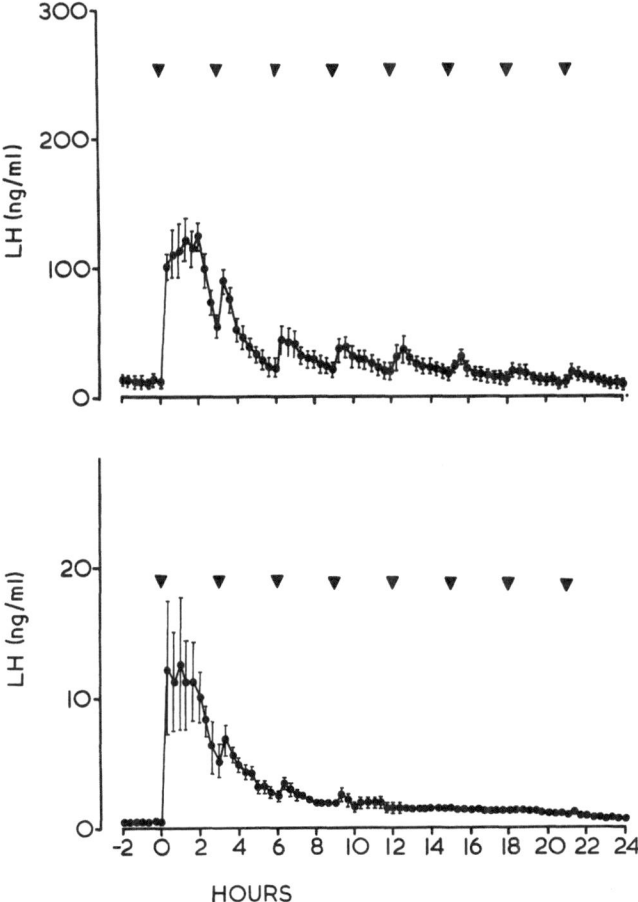

Figure 6.15 Effect of eight consecutive intravenous injections of 1 µg LHRH agonist on plasma levels of LH in three control ovariectomized ewes (top panel) and in three ovariectomized ewes immunized against LHRH (note 10-fold difference in scales). H. M. Fraser (unpublished)

Although LH release is induced the response is 10-fold lower than in control ewes; this probably reflects the lower amount of stored gonadotrophin, lower activity within the cell for the release of hormone and transfer of stored hormone to the releasable form, and it is also possible that the number of LHRH receptors on the gonadotroph cell is reduced following immunization. It is, therefore, necessary to try and stimulate synthesis of gonadotrophins by giving repeated injections of agonist but, as shown in Figure 6.15, when the injections were given 3 h apart the release of hormone was not sustained. This decreasing responsiveness also occurs in controls, and it is now becoming clear that the administration of LHRH agonist must be spaced out at intervals of a number of days to avoid this. However, a more encouraging result might have been expected in the animals deprived of a native trophic hormone since, as we have seen, the testis deprived of gonadotrophins shows a sustained response to HCG.

Although correct spacing and dose of agonist might be successful in stimulating sustained gonadotrophin release in LHRH-immunized animals, this would not mimic the normal pattern of LHRH secretion, since LHRH is thought to have a one-to-one relationship with LH pulses which occur several times per day[35]. The property of an LHRH agonist which enables it to stimulate LH release for long periods of time is its resistance to enzymic breakdown in the pituitary[68] and concomitantly it is this property which renders the pituitary unresponsive to repeated short-term stimulation. Therefore, to use this as an experimental model to superimpose possible normal patterns of LHRH stimulation a peptide immunologically different from LHRH, but with the same biological half-life, would have to be synthesized.

Inhibition of LHRH during implantation and pregnancy

We would expect implantation to be delayed or prevented, or a pregnancy to be aborted, if LHRH is inhibited during the time the corpus luteum is dependent on stimulation by LH for survival, a period which varies considerably between species. Studies have been confined to the rat, in which injection of antibodies to LHRH between days 1 and 7 of pregnancy prevents or delays implantation[69], while injections of antibodies on single days show that day 4 is crucial in requiring LHRH for implantation to occur on day 8. This inhibition can be overcome by injections of LHRH or a single dose of oestradiol[69]. Although LH levels in the rat are very low during pregnancy and no decrease could actually be detected after treatment, it is likely that LHRH is required on day 4 to maintain low levels of LH for secretion of oestradiol. Since oestradiol is not required in higher species for implantation, it is unlikely that antibodies to LHRH could prevent implantation in this way, but they could have a luteolytic action and thus lower progesterone levels. In women this would only be effective if given prior to day 7 of pregnancy, because after this time chorionic gonadotrophin is secreted. In the rat antibodies to LHRH are effective in lowering progesterone levels and causing resorption of fetuses if injected on days 9 or 10, an effect which could be reversed by administration of LHRH twice daily or by an injection of progesterone[70]. The treatment was without effect on prolactin levels after fertilization. One other report[71] described no effect of antibodies on LHRH on pregnancy in rats, but this may have been the result of insufficient lowering of basal gonadotrophin levels by the antibodies.

PRACTICAL APPLICATIONS

We have seen how inhibition of LHRH by antibodies has been used to study the physiological role of the releasing hormone in male and female reproduction. Passive administration of antibodies is a selective method of immediately stopping the action of LHRH; it blocks the secretion of testosterone in the male and inhibits ovulation in the female. Although an elegant experimental tool, it could not be used in any form of fertility control because of its short-term action, the large amounts of antiserum required and the dangers associated with injecting antibodies, particularly those from another species.

Active immunization also causes these inhibitory effects on reproduction. Inhibition is gradual, taking several weeks, but the effect is long-lasting and in the male results in involution of testicular size, cessation of spermatogenesis and severe reduction in testosterone secretion. In the female ovulation ceases and oestrogen secretion is considerably lower than normal. This long-lasting effectiveness of active immunization suggests the possibility of practical application in control of fertility. As far as controlling fertility in the human is concerned prospects seem rather remote. Testicular involution and decline in testosterone levels would be unacceptable to men. Women are probably less dependent on their sex hormones for the maintenance of normal libido; some might welcome amenorrhea as a byproduct of contraception[72]. Low oestrogen levels could produce a protection from the increased risk of breast cancer thought to be associated with recurring menstrual cycles[73]. However, we do not know if sufficient oestrogen would be produced to support the oestrogen-dependent tissues. As with other immunological approaches to fertility control dependent on inhibiting the action of naturally occurring protein, an efficacy of less than 100% would have to be acceptable. Also, there is always the possibility that a population of antibodies could be induced which could interfere with the action of circulating proteins; an unacceptable risk in the application to normal healthy women. The technique might have an application in patients with cancer of the breast or prostate gland who would currently be subjected to gonadectomy, some without deriving benefit.

Prospects for practical application of LHRH immunization in veterinary practice seem much more encouraging. It has been suggested that the technique could be used as a method for spaying cats and dogs[74], but it might be difficult to keep up antibody levels to abolish behavioural effects and fertility over the long lifetime of these animals while, on the other hand, the possibility of reversing the procedure by allowing antibody levels to decline might appeal to many pet-owners. The most appropriate area seems to be in meat production where the short-term manipulation of sex hormones can have considerable effects on the body composition of an animal being kept for 1–2 years for slaughter. For example, in several countries, including the UK and the USA, it is common practice to castrate bull calves not required for breeding purposes. Thus, the animal is made sterile, his aggressive behaviour decreased and by encouraging fat disposition the carcase quality is considered to be improved. The castration is carried out when the animal is only about 3 months old so that it can be done without anaesthetic. This imposes a considerable potential loss in meat production since the male depends on testicular androgens for increased muscular development, so that the male castrate will be lighter in body weight than his intact male counterpart. A better prospect might be to delay castration until the time of puberty, i.e. 9 months of age, so that some benefit can be attained from the testicular androgens. Now, surgical castration at this time is not practised because the animal requires an anaesthetic for what at this time is major surgery; it would suffer considerable trauma, run a risk of infection and would undoubtedly suffer a check in growth. It has been suggested that this late castration could be feasible if it were carried out by immunization against LHRH[75]. Bull calves could be immunized at about 6 months of age to allow antibody titre to reach effective levels at about 9 months, at which time a booster immunization could be administered. In a recent pilot study we have been able to establish that antibodies to LHRH can be produced in the bull calf using Freund's complete adjuvant and that they are capable of preventing the normal pubertal changes in testicular growth[76]. It has yet to be established whether this approach would achieve a sufficiently higher weight gain over the prepubertal castrate to make the treatment economically viable, and it also remains to be seen how effectively aggression and mounting behaviour would be eliminated.

As in the application of any immunization technique there is a challenging array of immunological problems. An adjuvant is required which has minimal side-effects but can stimulate the immune response sufficiently to cause successful inhibition of the hormone, and the effect must be long-lasting. For practical purposes the number of booster immunizations must be limited to one or two per year. The immunogen, with its carrier protein, must be acceptable and not lead to the production of antibodies which might be injurious to the recipient.

The techniques employed successfully in the laboratory to induce active immunization need considerable refinement for practical application. Freund's complete adjuvant cannot be used because of the risk of reaction at the site of injection and other side-effects. It consists of an emulsifier – Aracel A, and a mineral oil – Bayol F and *Mycobacterium butyricum*. Omission of the *Mycobacterium* reduces its side-effects and the incomplete adjuvant maintains much of the stimulatory activity. Changing the mineral oil component to marcol still gives a good immune response but results have been poor when adjuvants with low side-effects, such as adjuvant 65 – which contains a metabolizable vegetable oil – and alhydrogel, have been used[45]. It should also be noted that immunizations in the laboratory have mostly employed multiple-site immunization to disperse the immunogen to increase immunogenicity. For practical application one would be restricted to one or two subcutaneous injections.

Individual variation in the immune response is an inherent problem and can only be reduced by giving booster immunizations to raise antibody levels in all recipients to a threshold level which will cause sufficient neutralization of LHRH to inhibit reproductive function. Boosters would have to be limited to 3–6 months after immunization and yearly intervals thereafter. If antibody titres were left to decline then a return to full fertility would be expected to occur eventually.

There is considerable scope for improvement in attempts to develop an inexpensive highly immunogenic LHRH conjugate. Since the cost of purification of a peptide is considerably more than the cost of producing it, it is important that the 3–10-octapeptide of LHRH, which is a precursor of its synthesis, has been shown to induce antibodies which cross-react with an inhibit endogenous LHRH[44]. The choice of carrier molecule should be determined by the species being immunized. Thus, tetanus toxoid, which women can be safely immunized against, acts as a suitable carrier for HCG (Chapter 9) and can also be used successfully as a carrier for LHRH in the monkey (this chapter). If LHRH immunization were to be used in veterinary practice it may be possible to extend this principle by using a carrier protein against which the animals were normally immunized.

Fortunately, the major challenges in developing a vaccine for LHRH are universal. We need to know more about the immune response, how to make more immunogenic conjugates and to produce acceptable adjuvants. The fact that the antibody response will vary between individuals will always have to be considered, but, as our knowledge increases, the production of an LHRH vaccine giving considerable benefit, particularly in the veterinary field, can be envisaged.

References

1. Schally, A. V., Arimura, A. and Kastin, A. J. (1973). Hypothalamic regulating hormones. *Science*, **179**, 341
2. Guillemin, R. (1972). Physiology and chemistry of the hypothalamic releasing factors for gonadotropins: a new approach to fertility control. *Contraception*, **5**, 1

3. Lincoln, G. A. and Short, R. V. (1980). Seasonal breeding: nature's contraceptive. *Recent Prog. Horm. Res.*, **36** (In press)

4. Kerdelhue, B., Jutisz, M., Gillesen, D. and Studer, R. O. (1973). Obtention of antisera against a hypothalamic decapeptide (luteinizing hormone/follicle-stimulating hormone releasing hormone) which stimulates release of pituitary gonadotrophins and development of its radioimmunoassay. *Biochem. Biophys. Acta*, **297**, 540

5. Jeffcoate, S. L., Holland, D. T. and Fraser, H. M. (1976). Anti-LH-RH sera in the investigation of reproduction. In Edwards, R. G. and Johnston, M. H. (eds.) *Physiological Effects of Immunity Against Hormones*, pp. 121–136. (Cambridge: Cambridge University Press)

6. Arimura, A., Sato, H., Kumasaka, T., Worobec, R. B., Debeljuk, L., Dunn, J. and Schally, A. V. (1973). Production of antiserum to LH-releasing hormone (LH-RH) associated with gonadal atrophy in rabbits: development of radioimmunoassays for LH-RH. *Endocrinology*, **93**, 1092

7. Pique, L., Cesselin, F., Strauch, G., Valcke, J. C. and Bicaire, H. (1978). Specificity of anti-LH-RH antisera induced by different immunogens. *Immunochemistry*, **15**, 55

8. van Loon, G. R. and Brown, G. M. (1975). Secondary drug failure occurring during chronic treatment with LHRH: appearance of an antibody. *J. Clin. Endocrinol. Metab.*, **41**, 640

9. Brown, G. M., van Loon, G. R., Hummel, B. C. W., Grota, L. J., Arimura, A. and Schally, A. V. (1977). Characteristics of antibody produced during chronic treatment with LHRH. *J. Clin. Endocrinol. Metab.*, **44**, 784

10. Koch, Y., Wilchek, M., Fridkin, M., Chobsieng, P., Zor, U. and Lindner, H. R. (1973). Production and characterisation of an antiserum to synthetic gonadotrophin-releasing hormone. *Biochem. Biophys. Res. Commun.*, **55**, 616

11. Makino, T., Takahashi, M., Yoshinaga, K. and Greep, R. O. (1973). Ovulation blockade in rats by rabbit anti-luteinizing hormone releasing factor serum. *Contraception*, **8**, 133

12. Nett, T. M., Akbar, A. M., Niswender, G. D., Hedlund, M. T. and White, W. F. (1973). A radioimmunoassay for gonadotrophin-releasing hormone (Gn-RH) in serum. *J. Clin. Endocrinol. Metab.*, **36**, 880

13. Fraser, H. M., Gunn, A., Jeffcoate, S. L. and Holland, D. T. (1974). Preparation of antisera to luteinizing hormone releasing factor. *J. Endocrinol.*, **61**, ix

14. Arimura, A., Sato, H., Coy, D. H., Worobec, R. B., Schally, A. V., Yanaihara, N., Hashimoto, T., Yanaihara, C. and Sukura, N. (1975). The antigenic determinant of the LH-releasing hormone for the three different antisera. *Acta Endocrinol.*, **78**, 222

15. Sorrentino, S. and Sundberg, D. K. (1975). Measurement of plasma and hypothalamic luteinizing-hormone releasing hormone in pregnant mare serum induced ovulating immature rats. *Neuroendocrinology*, **17**, 274

16. Hauger, R. L., Kelch, R. P., Chen, Y. D. I. and Payne, A. H. (1977). Testicular receptors for luteinizing hormone after immunoneutralization of gonadotrophin releasing hormone in the male rat. *J. Endocrinol.*, **75**, 23

17. Eskay, R. L., Mical, R. S. and Porter, J. C. (1977). Relationship between luteinizing hormone releasing hormone concentration in hypophysial portal blood and luteinizing hormone release in intact, castrated, and electrochemically stimulated rats. *Endocrinology*, **100**, 263

18. Root, A. W., Reiter, E. O. and Duckett, G. E. (1977). Urinary excretion of immunoreactive gonadotrophin-releasing hormone-like material in prepubertal and pubertal children. *J. Clin. Endocrinol. Metab.*, **44**, 909

19. Jeffcoate, J. A., Foster, J. P. and Crighton, D. B. (1978). Effect of active immunization of ewes against synthetic luteinizing hormone releasing hormone. *Theriogenology*, **10**, 323

20. Copeland, K. C., Aubert, M. L., Rivier, J. and Sizonenko, P. C. (1979). Luteinizing hormone-releasing hormone: sequential versus conformational specificity of anti-luteinizing hormone-releasing hormone sera. *Endocrinology*, **104**, 1504

21. Barry, J., Dubois, M. P. and Poulain, P. (1973). LRF producing cells of the mammalian hypothalamus. *Z. Zellforsch.*, **146**, 351

22. Bercu, B. B., Jackson, I. M. D., Sawin, C. T., Safaii, H. and Reichlin, S. (1977). Permanent impairment of testicular development after transient immunological blockade of endogenous luteinizing hormone releasing hormone in the neonatal rat. *Endocrinology*, **101**, 1871

23. Kerdelhue, B., Catin, S., Kordon, C. and Jutisz, M. (1976). Delayed effects of *in vivo* LH-RH immunoneutralization on gonadotrophins and prolactin secretion in the female rat. *Endocrinology*, **98**, 1539

24. Hendricks, S., Millar, R. and Pimstone, B. (1975). A specific radio-immunoassay for gonadotrophin-releasing hormone. *S. Afr. Med. J.*, **49**, 1559

25. Sharpe, R. M. and Fraser, H. M. (1978). The influence of sexual maturation and immunization against LH-RH on testicular sensitivity to gonadotrophin stimulation *in vitro*. *Int. J. Androl.*, **1**, 501

26. Sternberger, L. A., Petrali, J. P., Joseph, S. A., Meyer, H. G. and Mills, K. R. (1978). Specificity of the immunocytochemical luteinizing hormone-releasing hormone receptor reaction. *Endocrinology*, **102**, 63

27. Rosenblum, N. G. and Schlaff, S. (1976). Gonadotrophin-releasing hormone radioimmunoassay and its measurement in normal human plasma, secondary amenorrhoea, and postmenopausal syndrome. *Am. J. Obstet. Gynecol.*, **124**, 340

28. Fraser, H. M. (1975). Effects of antibodies to luteinizing hormone releasing hormone on reproductive functions in rodents. In Nieschlag, E. (ed.) *Immunization with Hormones in Reproduction Research*, pp. 107–116. (Amsterdam: North-Holland)

29. Goodfriend, T. L., Levine, L. and Fasman, G. D. (1964). Antibodies to bradykinin and angiotensin: a use of carbodiimides in immunology. *Science*, **144**, 1334

30. Jeffcoate, S. L., Holland, D. T., Fraser, H. M. and Gunn, A. (1974). Preparation and specificity of antibodies to luteinizing hormone releasing hormone. *Immunochemistry*, **11**, 75

31. Clarke, I. J., Fraser, H. M. and McNeilly, A. S. (1978). Active immunization of ewes against luteinizing hormone releasing hormone, and its effects on ovulation and gonadotrophin, prolactin and ovarian steroid secretion. *J. Endocrinol.*, **78**, 39

32. Hokfelt, T., Johansson, O., Fuxe, K., Goldstein, M., Park, D., Ebstein, R., Fraser, H. M., Jeffcoate, S. L., Efendic, S., Luft, R. and Arimura, A. (1976). Mapping and relationship of hypothalamic neurotransmitters and hypothalamic hormones. *Proceedings of the Sixth International Congress of Pharmacology*, **3**, 93

33. Labrie, F., Drouin, J., Ferland, L., Lagace, L., Beaulieu, M., deLean, A., Kelly, P. A., Caron, M. G. and Raymond, V. (1978). Mechanism of action of hypothalamic hormones in the anterior pituitary gland and specific modulation of their activity by sex steroids and thyroid hormones. *Recent Prog. Horm. Res.*, **34**, 25

34. Sternberger, L. A. and Petrali, J. P. (1975). Quantitative immunocytochemistry of pituitary receptors for luteinizing hormone-releasing hormone. *Cell. Tissue Res.*, **162**, 141

35. Lincoln, G. A. and Fraser, H. M. (1979). Blockade of episodic secretion of luteinizing hormone in the ram by the administration of antibodies to luteinizing hormone-releasing hormone. *Biol. Reprod.*, **21**, 1239

36. Fraser, H. M., Gunn, A., Jeffcoate, S. L. and Holland, D. T. (1974). Effect of active immunization to luteinizing hormone releasing hormone on serum and pituitary gonadotrophins, testes and accessory sex organs in the male rat. *J. Endocrinol.*, **63**, 399

37. Fraser, H. M. and Sandow, J. (1977). Gonadotrophin release by a highly active analogue of luteinizing hormone releasing hormone in rats immunized against luteinizing hormone releasing hormone. *J. Endocrinol.*, **74**, 291

38. Arimura, A., Shino, M., de la Cruz, K. G., Rennels, E. G. and Schally, A. V. (1976). Effect of active and passive immunization with luteinizing hormone-releasing hormone on serum luteinizing hormone and follicle-stimulating hormone levels and the ultrastructure of the pituitary gonadotrophs in castrated male rats. *Endocrinology*, **99**, 291

39. Lincoln, G. A. (1979). Differential control of luteinizing hormone and follicle-stimulating hormone by luteinizing hormone releasing hormone in the ram. *J. Endocrinol.*, **80**, 133

40. Debeljuk, L., Arimura, A., Shiino, M., Rennels, E. G. and Schally, A. V. (1973). Effects of chronic treatment with LH/FSH-RH in hypophysectomized pituitary-grafted male rats. *Endocrinology*, **92**, 921

41. McNeilly, A. S., de Kretser, D. M. and Sharpe, R. M. (1979). Modulation of prolactin, LH and FSH secretion by LHRH and bromocriptine (CB154) in the hypophysectomized pituitary-grafted male rat and its effect on testicular LH receptors and testosterone output. *Biol. Reprod.*, **21**, 141

42. Jeffcoate, S. L., Fraser, H. M., Holland, D. T. and Gunn, A. (1974). Radioimmunoassay of luteinizing hormone releasing hormone in serum from man, sheep and rat. *Acta Endocrinol.*, **75**, 625

43. Fraser, H. M. and Gunn, A. (1973). Effects of antibodies to luteinizing hormone-releasing hormone in the male rabbit and on the rat oestrous cycle. *Nature (London)*, **244**, 160

44. Fraser, H. M. (1976). Physiological effects of antibodies to LH-RH. In Edwards, R. G. and Johnston, M. H. (eds.) *Physiological Effects of Immunity Against Hormones*, pp. 137–165. (Cambridge: Cambridge University Press)

45. Fraser, H. M. (1976). Immunization against hypothalamic hormones. In Peters, D. K. (ed.) *Advanced Medicine*, Vol. 12, pp. 425–434. (Tunbridge Wells: Pitman Medical)

46. Hodges, J. K. and Hearn, J. P. (1977). Effect of immunisation against luteinizing hormone releasing hormone on reproduction of the marmoset monkey. *Callithrix jacchus. Nature (London)*, **265**, 746

47. Turner, G. E. (1978). The histology and ultrastructure of the anterior pituitary glands of male rats actively immunized against luteinizing hormone-releasing hormone. *B.Sc. Med. Sci.* Thesis. Dept. of Pathology, University of Edinburgh

48. Sharpe, R. M. and Fraser, H. M. (1979). Leydig cell function in rats chronically deprived of normal gonadotrophic stimulation: the effect of treatment with hCG. *Int. J. Androl.*, **2**, 395

49. Sharpe, R. M. (1976). hCG-induced decrease in availability of rat testis receptors. *Nature (London)*, **264**, 644

50. Sharpe, R. M., Fraser, H. M. and Sandow, J. (1979). Effect of treatment with an agonist of luteinizing hormone releasing hormone on early maturational changes in pituitary and testicular function in the rat. *J. Endocrinol.*, **80**, 249

51. Sarkar, D. K., Chiappa, S. A., Fink, G. and Sherwood, N. M. (1976). Gonadotrophin-releasing hormone in pro-oestrous rats. *Nature (London)*, **264**, 461

52. Neill, J. D., Patton, J. M., Dailey, R. A., Tsou, R. C. and Tindall, G. T. (1977). Luteinizing hormone releasing hormone (LHRH) in pituitary stalk blood of rhesus monkeys: relationship to level of LH release. *Endocrinology*, **101**, 430

53. Nishi, N., Coy, D. H., Coy, E. J., Arimura, A. and Schally, A. V. (1976). Suppression of LH-RH induced ovulation in hamsters and rats by synthetic analogues of LH-RH. *J. Reprod. Fertil.*, **48**, 119

54. de la Cruz, A., Arimura, A., de la Cruz, K. G. and Schally, A. V. (1976). Effect of administration of antiserum to luteinizing hormone-releasing hormone on gonadal function during the estrous cycle in the hamster. *Endocrinology*, **98**, 490

55. Koch, Y. (1977). Effects of antibodies against luteinizing hormone-releasing hormone on reproduction. In James, V. H. T. (ed.) *Proceedings of the V International Congress of Endocrinology*, Hamburg, July 18–24, 1976, Vol. 1, pp. 374–378. (Amsterdam: Excerpta Medica)

56. Fraser, H. M. and Baker, T. G. (1978). Changes in the ovaries of rats after immunization against luteinizing hormone releasing hormone. *J. Endocrinol.*, **77**, 85

57. Takahashi, M., Ford, J. J., Yoshinaga, K. and Greep, R. O. (1978). Active immunization of female rats with luteinizing hormone releasing hormone (LHRH). *Biol. Reprod.*, **17**, 754

58. Koch, Y., Chobsieng, P., Zor, U., Fridkin, M. and Lindner, H. R. (1973). Suppression of

gonadotrophin secretion and prevention of ovulation in the rat by antiserum to synthetic gonadotrophin-releasing hormone. *Biochemical and Biophysical Research Communications*, **55**, 623

59. Fraser, H. M., Jeffcoate, S. L., Gunn, A. and Holland, D. T. (1975). Effect of active immunization to luteinizing hormone-releasing hormone on gonadotrophin levels in ovariectomized rats. *J. Endocrinol.*, **64**, 191

60. McCormack, J. T., Plant, T. M., Hess, D. L. and Knobil, E. (1977). The effect of luteinizing hormone releasing hormone (LHRH) antiserum administration on gonadotrophin secretion in the rhesus monkey. *Endocrinology*, **100**, 663

61. Arimura, A., Debeljuk, L. and Schally, A. V. (1974). Blockade of the preovulatory surge of LH and FSH and of ovulation by anti-LH-RH serum in rats. *Endocrinology*, **95**, 323

62. Fraser, H. M. (1977). Reversal of the inhibitory action of an antiserum of luteinizing hormone releasing hormone (LH-RH) by an inactive fragment of LH-RH. *J. Endocrinol.*, **73**, 393

63. Fraser, H. M., Clarke, I. J. and McNeilly, A. S. (1977). Inhibition of ovulation and absence of positive feedback in ewes immunized against luteinizing hormone releasing hormone. *J. Endocrinol.*, **75**, 45P

64. Fraser, H. M. and Sharp, P. J. (1978). Prevention of positive feedback in the hen (*Gallus domesticus*) by antibodies to luteinizing hormone releasing hormone. *J. Endocrinol.*, **76**, 181

65. Nakai, Y., Plant, T. M., Hess, D. L., Keogh, E. J. and Knobil, E. (1978). On the sites of negative and positive feedback actions of estradiol in control of gonadotrophin secretion in the rhesus monkey. *Endocrinology*, **102**, 1008

66. Chobsieng, P., Naor, Z., Koch, Y., Zor, U. and Lindner, H. R. (1975). Stimulatory effect of prostaglandin E$_2$ on LH release in the rat: evidence of hypothalamic site of action. *Neuroendocrinology*, **17**, 12

67. Drouin, J., Ferland, L., Bernard, J. and Labrie, F. (1976). Site of the *in vivo* stimulatory effect of prostaglandin on LH release. *Prostaglandins*, **11**, 367

68. Sandow, J., von Rechenberg, W., Koenig, W., Hahn, M., Jerzabek, G. and Fraser, H. M. (1978). Physiological studies with highly active analogues of LH-RH. In Gupta, D. and Voelter, W. (eds.) *Hypothalamic Hormones – Chemistry, Physiology and Clinical Applications*, pp. 307–326. (Weinheim: Verlag, Chemie)

69. Arimura, A., Nishi, N. and Schally, A. V. (1976). Delayed implantation caused by administration of sheep immunogammaglobulin against LHRH in the rat. *Proc. Soc. Exp. Biol. Med.*, **152**, 71

70. Nishi, N., Arimura, A., de la Cruz, K. G. and Schally, A. V. (1976). Termination of pregnancy by sheep anti-LH-RH gammaglobulin in rats. *Endocrinology*, **98**, 1024

71. Makino, T., Shiina, M., Nakashima, S., Ilzuka, R., Tamaoki, B. and Greep, R. O. (1977). Role of luteinizing hormone-releasing factor (LH-RF) and LH on maintenance of early gestation in rats. *Endocrinol. Jpn.*, **24**, 83

72. Louden, N. B., Foxwell, M., Potts, D. M., Guild, A. L. and Short, R. V. (1977). Acceptibility of an oral contraceptive that reduces the frequency of menstruation: the tri-cycle pill regimen. *Br. Med. J.*, **2**, 487

73. Short, R. V. (1975). Man, the changing animal. In Coutinho, E. M. and Fuchs, F. (eds.) *Physiology and Genetics of Reproduction*, Part A, pp. 3–15. (New York: Plenum)

74. Fraser, H. M., Gunn, A., Borthwick, R. and Fraser, A. F. (1975). Sterilising by immunization. *Vet. Rec.*, **96**, 323

75. Short, R. V. (1980). The hormonal control of growth at puberty. In Lawrence, T. L. J. (ed.) *Growth in Animals*. (London: Butterworths) (In press)

76. Robertson, I. S., Wilson, J. C. and Fraser, H. M. (1979). Immunological castration in male cattle. *Vet. Rec.*, **105**, 556

7
Immunization against Zona Pellucida Antigens

R. J. AITKEN and D. W. RICHARDSON

INTRODUCTION

Whatever new forms of contraception the twenty-first century brings it is likely that some kind of vaccine against pregnancy will be amongst them. The advantages associated with this form of fertility control include the speed and ease with which it can be administered by paramedical personnel, a long duration of action and potential reversibility. An additional attraction is the possibility of producing dual-purpose vaccines by linking highly immunogenic antigens such as tetanus toxoid to a contraceptive immunogen[1,2]. Work has already reached an advanced stage with the development of a vaccine incorporating tetanus toxoid and the beta-subunit of human chorionic gonadotrophin (see Chapter 8) or analogues of this moiety (see Chapter 9). Even though certain aspects of this research programme have now reached the stage of clinical trials there are still a number of potentially serious problems associated with this approach. In particular, the development of a specific immunogen which will not induce the formation of antibodies cross-reacting with LH[3], the risk of late abortion in the face of falling antibody titres[4], and finally the ethical dilemma which confronts any abortifacient method. In an attempt to side-step some of these issues, research has been initiated on the development of a vaccine which would inhibit fertilization. The target for this vaccine is the zona pellucida, a glycoprotein shell which surrounds the oocyte and serves to bind spermatozoa during the early stages of fertilization (Figure 7.1). In the following discussion we shall consider the anti-fertility effect of passive and active immunization against the zona pellucida in different species, the specificity of zona antigens and the realistic prospects for this approach to contraception. To begin with, however, let us

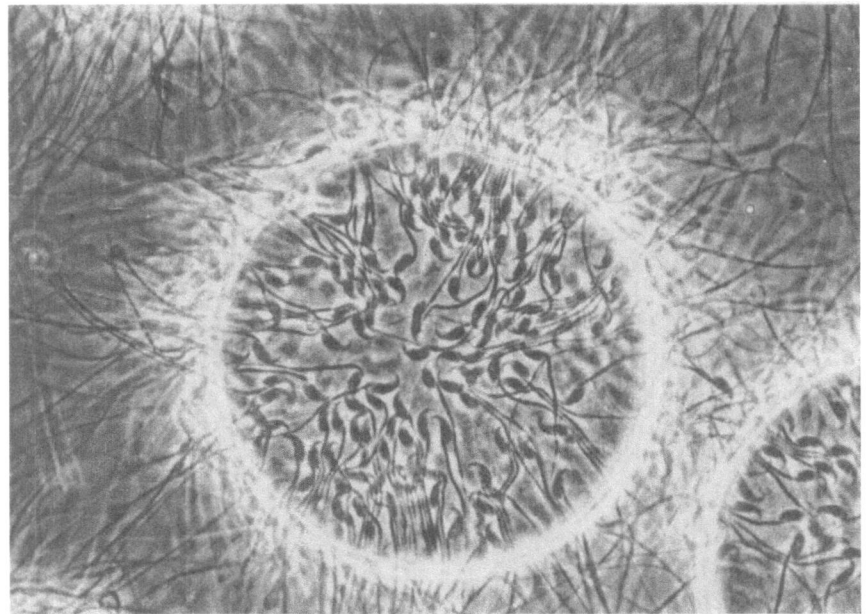

Figure 7.1   Binding of spermatozoa to a cumulus-free mouse egg

remind ourselves of the composition and function of the zona pellucida and recall why it is such a potentially important target for the inhibition of fertility.

STRUCTURE AND FUNCTION OF THE ZONA PELLUCIDA

Zona structure

The zona pellucida is rich in both protein and carbohydrate and is synthesized during folliculogenesis by the joint action of the oocyte and the surrounding granulosa cells[5-15]. The ground substance of the zona is mucopolysaccharide in nature judging by its affinity for stains such as Alcian blue and Schiffs reagent[16]. The carbohydrate fraction includes glycosaminoglycans such as heparan sulphate and chondroitin sulphate[16] which are probably covalently bound to a protein core to form a proteoglycan subunit. The solubility of the zona pellucida in 2-mercaptoethanol indicates that disulphide bonds play a major role in stabilizing the structure of the zona[17]. The zona pellucida does not appear to be a homogeneous structure but shows distinct regional specialization[16, 18]. Of particular importance is the presence of a layer in the outermost region of the zona which, judging by its ability to bind ferritin-conjugated plant lectins, is rich in terminal saccharide residues[19]. The lectin-binding sites on the surface of rat, mouse and hamster zonae exhibit a marked affinity for *Ricinus communis* and wheat-germ agglutinins indicating the presence of D-galactose and *N*-acetyl-D-glucosamine (or *N*-acetylneuraminic acid) residues in this region. In addition receptors for concanavalin A have been observed throughout the zonae of these species suggesting the presence of α-D-mannose or α-D-glucose residues in the structural matrix of the zona[19,20]. Although little is known about the protein composition of the zona pellucida it is clear that there are pronounced species differences in this respect, the hamster zona pellucida being much more soluble in trypsin than that of the mouse[21,22]. Polyacrylamide gel electophoresis of SDS (sodium dodecyl sulphate) denatured proteins obtained from isolated porcine zonae solubilized in 2-mercaptoethanol has revealed the presence of at least five protein bands[23]. Four of these bands did not appear to be specific to the zona because proteins of similar mobility were observed in follicular fluid or extracts of porcine oocytes. The remaining protein band appeared to be confined to the zona pellucida and exhibited a molecular weight of 120 000–150 000; this band was also PAS-positive, suggesting the presence of carbohydrate residues[23].

Zona function

The first function the zona pellucida has to perform is to bind spermatozoa during the initial stages of fertilization (Figure 7.1). The nature of the binding process is poorly understood[24] and there is even disagreement as to which portion of the sperm head is involved – the plasma membrane overlying the acrosome[25] or the inner acrosomal membrane[26]. *In vitro* there can be no doubt that both membranes possess the ability to bind to the zona pellucida of

Table 7.1 Comparison of the binding affinities of uncapacitated[27] and capacitated acrosome-reacted[26] sperm

Spermatozoa	Zona pellucida		
	Mouse	*Hamster*	*Guinea-pig*
Uncapacitated			
Hamster	+	+	+
Guinea-pig	±	−	+
Capacitated, acrosome-reacted			
Hamster	+	+	+
Guinea-pig	−	−	+

homologous and even heterologous eggs[26,27]. This is revealed in a comparison of the results obtained in two independent studies on the binding affinities of spermatozoa *in vitro* (Table 7.1). In one study[27] uncapacitated sperm were used (and so the binding observed was due to the interaction between the sperm plasma membrane and the zona pellucida) while in the other[26], acrosome-reacted sperm were employed (hence the binding involved the inner acrosomal membrane and the zona pellucida). The results obtained in the two experiments are virtually identical. *In vivo*, the first contact between male and female gametes appears to involve the plasma membrane overlying the acrosomal cap and the zona pellucida. Investigation of the sequence of sperm–egg interactions during the early stages of fertilization *in vivo* indicate that the acrosome reaction is initiated as the spermatozoa are passing between the granulosa cells which surround the egg[14, 28–31]. At this stage multiple fusions between the outer acrosomal membrane and sperm plasma membrane lead to perforation of the acrosomal cap and the release of soluble enzymes, such as hyaluronidase[25, 29, 30, 32–36]. The hyaluronidase subsequently attacks the intercellular matrix holding the cumulus mass together and clears a path through to the surface of the zona[25, 26, 28, 29, 33]. In most species the vesiculated acrosomal cap still appears to be intact when the spermatozoa first bind to the surface of the zona pellucida[37]. This initial contact probably corresponds to the tenuous 'attachment' phase of sperm–egg association described by Hartmann, Gwatkin and Hutchison[38]. The vigorous tail movements exhibited by capacitated, 'activated' spermatozoa[26, 35, 39–42], then serve to drive the head of the sperm down into the zona pellucida, forcing off the acrosomal cap, which is left at the zona surface[25]. Loss of the acrosomal cap exposes the inner acrosomal membrane and in so doing brings into play a membrane-bound proteolytic enzyme, acrosin[43–45], which is thought to digest a path through the zona in advance of the penetrating sperm. The interaction between the inner acrosomal membrane of the sperm head and the zona pellucida results in the formation of a tenacious bond which probably corresponds to the 'binding' stage of sperm–egg interaction described by Hartmann *et al.*[38]. The tenacious binding of hamster sperm to the zona pellucida takes about 30–40 min; the process is temperature-dependent but not as species-specific as was once thought (Table 7.1)[26, 38].

It has been postulated that the binding of sperm to the zona pellucida involves specific recognition sites on the sperm and the zona. The sperm receptor sites on the zona pellucida of the hamster egg are sensitive to trypsin, chymotrypsin and trypsin-like acrosin preparations from hamster, ram, and boar spermatozoa[37, 46, 48]. Species differences are apparent here, however, because the receptor-for-sperm in rabbit[49] and mouse[50] zonae is not destroyed by trypsin treatment (Figure 7.2). If the sperm receptor is a protein it must be a small one because Gwatkin and Williams[47] have demonstrated that the hamster sperm receptor retains its binding capacity after freezing and thawing and even boiling. The abundance of terminal saccharide residues in the outer regions of the zona has also been equated with the presence of sperm-binding sites[26]. While it is true that saturation of the N-acetyl-D-glucosamine-like or N-acetylneuraminic acid-like residues on the surface of hamster zonae with lectins will block sperm binding, this does not necessarily mean that these groups are an integral part of the binding site[20]. Indeed it is extremely unlikely that these saccharide groups do contribute in any direct way to the sperm-binding properties of the zona pellucida because spermatozoa will bind to the inner as well as the outer surface of the zona[47]. The fact that the sperm receptor of the hamster egg is resistant to glycosidases[51] also suggests that terminal sugars are not of critical importance in the process of sperm binding.

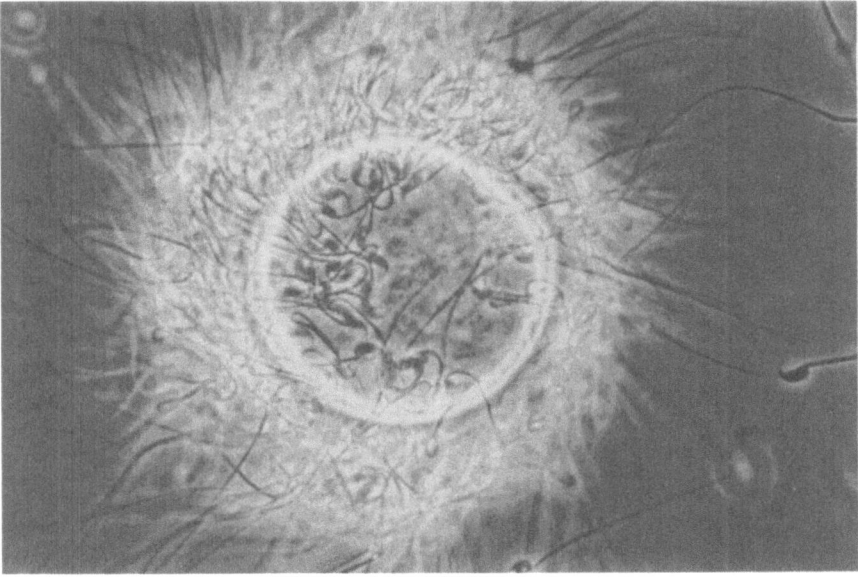

Figure 7.2 Binding of spermatozoa to a cumulus-free mouse egg following a 30 min pre-incubation in medium containing 1 mg trypsin/ml

A second function of the zona pellucida is to participate in the block to polyspermy. The role played by the zona in preventing the entry of excess sperm into the perivitelline space has been particularly well documented for such species as the hamster, rat and mouse[52]; however in other species, such as the rabbit, the responsibility for implementing the block to polyspermy rests entirely with the vitelline membrane[53]. The post-fertilization change in the zona pellucida which leads to a sudden increase in its resistance to sperm penetration, and a decrease in its capacity for sperm binding, has been termed the 'zona reaction'. The zona reaction appears to be induced by the contents of the cortical granules which are discharged into the perivitelline space as soon as fusion has occurred between the post-acrosomal membrane of the sperm head and the oolemma[26,54,55]. It has been suggested by Gwatkin[37,46] that the cortical granules of the hamster egg contain a heat-labile trypsin-like serine protease which destroys or inactivates the receptor-for-sperm in the zona pellucida. It has also been observed that the cortical granule exudate from hamster oocytes is capable of inducing a loss of sperm-binding activity in the mouse zona pellucida[37]. However, since the sperm-binding activity of mouse zonae is not reduced by trypsin treatment[49] (Figure 7.2) it follows that the active component of hamster cortical granules may be something other than, or additional to, a trypsin-like protease. A similar conclusion has also been drawn by Oikawa, Nicolson and Yanagimachi[56] who observed that trypsin treatment so modifies the structure of the hamster zona that it is no longer capable of binding plant lectins. Since this change is not observed following normal fertilization it is possible that the influence of trypsin on sperm-binding activity is not strictly physiological and does not reflect the normal mechanism by which polyspermy is prevented *in vivo*. An alternative possibility is that the glycoproteins or mucopolysaccharides present in the cortical granules are capable of masking or altering the configuration of sperm-binding sites[15,57]. In addition to a loss of sperm-binding activity the product of the cortical granules is also responsible for rendering the zona more resistant to sperm penetration. In the rat and mouse, but not the hamster[58], this increased resistance to sperm penetration is associated with a reduction in the zona's susceptibility to digestion by lytic agents such as 2-mercaptoethanol, heat, sodium periodate, trypsin, pronase and presumably, acrosin[59-62]. This increased resistance to solubilization is thought to involve a rise in the degree of cross-linking between peptide chains in the zona pellucida. For this reason it is possible to artificially render the zona pellucida both less susceptible to solubilization and less penetrable by sperm using either plant lectins[20] or anti-zona antibodies[63-65] as the cross-linking agents. *In vivo* increased cross-linking of the zona structure after fertilization is presumably achieved by proteins or glycoproteins released from the cortical granules.

After fertilization has taken place the zona pellucida continues to surround the developing egg during its journey through the Fallopian tube and into the uterus. During this time its functions are those of protection and physical isolation from the glandular mucosae of the oviduct and uterus. Isolation is particularly important during a process known as compaction[66], which occurs during the formation of the morula and involves a sudden increase in the adhesiveness of the blastomeres. If it were not for the isolating properties of the zona pellucida the embryo would adhere to the lining of the oviduct during this stage of development. The zona pellucida is finally disposed of just before the initiation of implantation. The precise mechanism of zona removal shows considerable variation between species involving, to varying degrees, proteases of trophoblastic or endometrial origin and the physical expansion of the blastocyst[67-70].

The zona pellucida therefore performs at least three major functions: sperm binding during the initial stages of fertilization; loss of sperm-binding capacity and susceptibility to penetration during the post-fertilization block to polyspermy; and finally the physical isolation of the developing embryo up to the time of implantation. In the following sections we shall consider the ways in which these functions are modified by the presence of anti-zona antibodies.

ACTIVITY OF ANTI-ZONA ANTIBODIES *IN VITRO*

The ability of antibodies raised against ovarian antigens to inhibit fertilization *in vitro* was first demonstrated by Shivers *et al.*[71] in the hamster. Subsequently parallel studies in the rat[72] and mouse have[73, 74] confirmed the effectiveness of heteroimmune anti-ovary antisera in this respect. The mouse ovary appears to be a particularly potent source of the effective antigen since isoimmunization with homologous ovarian antigens induces infertility in this species and, furthermore, ova recovered from isoimmunized animals are extremely difficult to fertilize *in vitro*[75]. The inhibitory activity displayed by anti-ovary antisera *in vitro* can be negated by absorption with ovarian extracts in hamster[64], mouse[76], and rat[72]. In contrast absorption with somatic tissues does not reduce the effectiveness of these antisera *in vitro* in the mouse[74] and hamster[64], indicating that in these species at least specific ovarian antigens are involved.

Studies in the rabbit[77], hamster[64], guinea-pig[78, 79], mouse[80], rat[72], cow[81], pig[82], and human[83], indicate that the major source of ovary-specific antigens is the zona pellucida. As a consequence, experiments have been designed to investigate the anti-fertility activity of more specific antisera. To this end antibodies raised against cumulus-free mouse ova[84] and isolated murine zonae pellucidae[85] have been assessed for their anti-fertility activity *in vitro* and shown to be extremely effective[84, 85].

The mechanism by which anti-zona antibodies block fertilization is not clear, although the process appears to involve, like the natural block to polyspermy, the inhibition of both sperm binding and penetration. In the mouse[63, 73], hamster[71], and to a lesser extent the rat[72], the interaction between anti-zona antibodies and the zona pellucida results in the formation of a precipitate on the outer surface of the zona (Figure 7.3); never on the inner surface. The location of this immune precipitate corresponds to the region which, because of its ability to bind plant lectins, is known to be rich in terminal saccharide residues and is therefore extremely antigenic. The ability of an antiserum to inhibit sperm binding *in vitro* correlates extremely well with its ability to form an immune precipitate on the zona surface (Figure 7.4)[63, 72, 86]. However, since the receptors-for-sperm are not located exclusively at the zona surface[37] the interaction between anti-zona antibodies and the outer region of the zona must presumably limit sperm binding indirectly by cross-linking glycoprotein chains at the zona surface and preventing access to the binding sites. The cross-linking activity of anti-zona antibodies also serves to stabilize the structure of the zona so that it becomes resistant to digestion by proteolytic

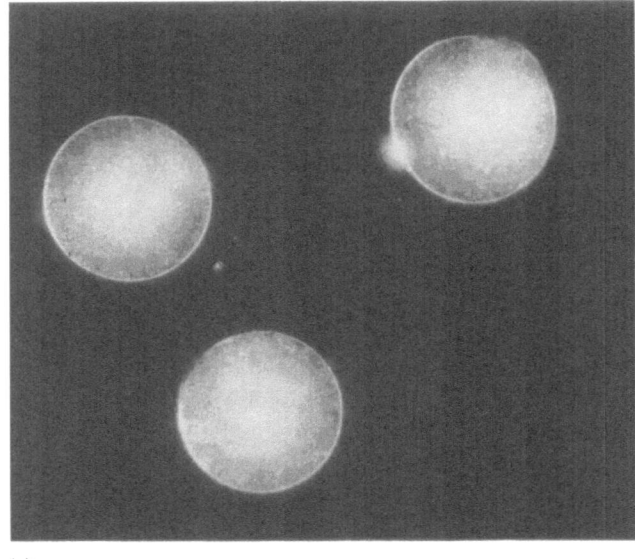

(a)

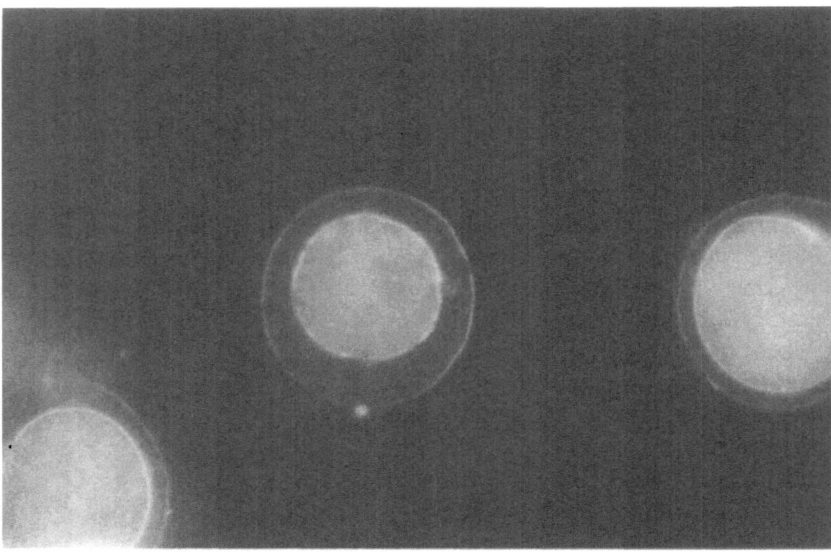

(b)

Figure 7.3   Precipitation of anti-zona antibodies on the surface of the zona pellucida. (a) Mouse eggs treated with an antiserum against mouse serum proteins which has been absorbed with liver, kidney and serum, and heat-inactivated. No zona precipitate is observed. (b) Mouse eggs treated with an antiserum against mouse ovarian antigens which has been absorbed with liver, kidney and serum, and heat-inactivated. A pronounced precipitate is visible on the surface of the zona

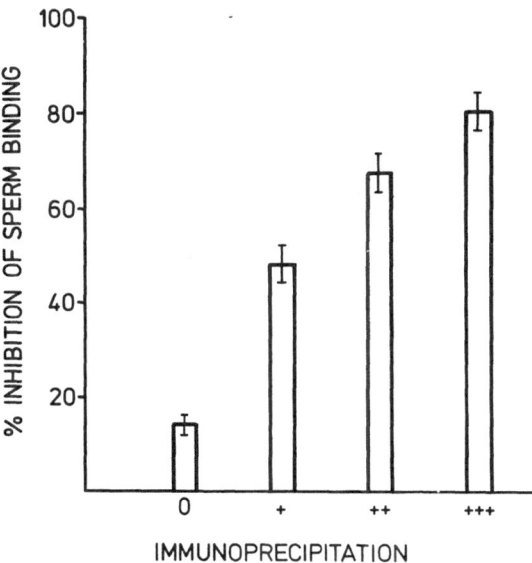

Figure 7.4 Relationship between the amount of precipitate observed on the zona surface and sperm binding in the mouse. The antisera were raised against mouse ovarian extracts heat-inactivated and absorbed with liver, kidney and serum before use. 0 = antisera in which anti-zona antibodies were detected by immunofluorescence but which failed to induce the formation of an immunoprecipitate on the zona surface; +, ++, +++ = intensity of precipitate in positive samples

enzymes or reducing agents[63, 64, 84, 85] (Table 7.2). Similarly the ability of sperm acrosin to digest a path through the zona pellucida must presumably be inhibited as a consequence of this cross-linking activity. The ability of anti-zona antibodies to block fertilization *in vitro* therefore appears to depend

Table 7.2 Influence of fertilization and anti-zona antibodies on the sperm-binding capacity and solubility of mouse zonae

Ova	Inhibition of sperm-binding capacity (%)	Percentage increase in solubilization time in 0.1% pronase
Unfertilized	0	0
Fertilized	100*	12
Antisera		
1	58	266
2	44	266
3	37	187
4	0	0

* Reference 99

upon their ability to cross-link glycoprotein chains in the highly antigenic, outer regions of the zona with its complement of terminal saccharide residues. The ability of plant lectins to block fertilization[87] probably depends upon a similar mechanism. In contrast the natural block to polyspermy, in a species such as the mouse, manages to achieve a dramatic decrease in sperm binding and penetrability by a mechanism which does not appear to rely entirely on cross-linking effects (Table 7.2).

ACTIVITY OF ANTI-ZONA ANTIBODIES *IN VIVO*

Passive immunization

As a consequence of the *in vitro* studies described above passive immunization experiments were initiated to determine the anti-fertility activity of anti-zona antibodies *in vivo*. Passive immunization of hamsters[64, 86], mice[73], and rats[72] with antisera raised against ovarian antigens has been found to be extremely effective in blocking fertilization. Absorption of non-specific antibodies with somatic tissues does not reduce the effectiveness of these antisera in the hamster[76] and mouse[74, 76], but does apparently negate the anti-fertility activity of antisera raised against extracts of rat ovary[72, 76]. Crude γ-globulin preparations of heteroimmune anti-ovary serum have also been shown to block fertilization on passive administration[64]. In addition immunoglobulin preparations of antisera raised against cumulus-free mouse eggs, or mechanically isolated mouse zonae, inhibit fertilization when given as an intra-peritoneal injection[85]. One remarkable feature of such passive immunization procedures is the prolonged protection against pregnancy afforded by a single injection. This was first demonstrated by Oikawa and Yanagimachi[64] using a γ-globulin preparation of an anti-hamster ovary antiserum. A single injection of this material gave complete protection against fertilization for 12 days and partial protection for a further 16 days. Using more specific antisera raised against mechanically isolated mouse zonae a single injection has been found to prevent conception for 24–30 days[88, 89]. The prolonged period of infertility observed following the passive administration of anti-zona antisera is due to the ability of these antibodies to bind to the zonae pellucidae surrounding follicular oocytes as well as ovulated eggs[64]. The effectiveness of these antisera *in vivo*, as *in vitro*, appears to lie primarily in their ability to block sperm binding and penetration by cross-linking glycoprotein chains on the zona surface. Ova recovered from passively-immunized animals exhibit an immune precipitate on the outer region of the zona pellucida and an increased resistance to digestion by lytic agents[64, 72, 76, 85]. In addition to the inhibition of fertilization, passive immunization with antisera directed against the zona pellucida may also block pregnancy by inhibiting the 'hatching' of the blastocyst just before implantation[90]. The antigenic determinants in the zona pellucida do not show any detectable alteration after fertilization, and even at the blastocyst stage of development appropriate antisera will produce an immunoprecipitate on the outer surface of the zona[90]. In order to determine whether cross-linking of the zona structure at this stage of development would impair the blastocysts' ability to gain access to the endometrial surface, hamster embryos have been incubated in antisera and then transferred to synchronized pseudopregnant hosts. In this experiment only five out of 110 (4.5%) blastocysts implanted after treatment with an anti-ovary antiserum compared with 15 out of 111 (13.5%) following treatment with pre-immune serum[90]. Tsunoda and Chang[91] also observed that treatment of eight-cell mouse embryos with antisera raised against either denuded mouse eggs or isolated zonae pellucidae significantly inhibited blastocyst hatching in vitro. However they observed no inhibition of fertility when mice were passively immunized with anti-egg serum after fertilization, during the pre-implantation period. Whether the ability of anti-zona antisera to inhibit blastocyst hatching will contribute significantly to the contraceptive efficacy of this approach remains to be determined.

Active immunization

The data from passive immunization studies indicate that antibodies directed against the zona pellucida are capable of inhibiting fertilization in vivo. In order to investigate such questions as the duration of infertility following immunization, the correlation between antibody titre and infertility, the establishment of normal fertility after antibody titres have waned, the effectiveness of booster injections and the possible existence of harmful side-effects it is necessary to utilize active immunization procedures. Active immunization might be achieved by using homologous zona antigens, or analogues thereof, coupled to immunogenic molecules such as bovine serum albumin or tetanus toxoid, or cross-reacting zona antigens obtained from another species. In view of our poor state of knowledge concerning the composition of the zona pellucida, the use of heterologous zona antigen is the only approach which is feasible at the present time. Initial studies on the rabbit ovary indicated that antisera prepared against this tissue did not cross-react in agar-gel diffusion tests with mouse, guinea-pig or hamster ovarian antigens[92]. However evidence was soon forthcoming to suggest a substantial degree of cross-reactivity between the zona antigens of other species. Of potential importance to the future of the zona pellucida as a target for contraception has been the demonstration that antibodies raised against human ovarian antigens cross-react with pig zona pellucida[82,93]. Furthermore, in the converse experiment, antibodies raised against pig ovarian antigens induced the formation of a precipitate on the surface of the human zona and inhibited the fertilization of human ova in vitro[83,94]. The cross-reactivity observed between human and porcine zona antigens does not appear to extend to the sperm-binding sites because human spermatozoa will not attach to porcine zonae in *vitro*[82]. Immunofluorescence and immunoprecipitation techniques have also been used to demonstrate cross-reactivity between human and marmoset zona antigens[95] and antisera raised against human ovarian antigens have been found to block sperm binding to marmoset zonae *in vitro*. However, since human sperm will not bind to the zonae of sub-hominoid primates[27] it is also doubtful whether the cross-reactivity observed in this case involves the receptors-for-sperm. Immunofluorescent techniques have similarly succeeded in demonstrating cross-reactivity between an antiserum raised against heat-solubilized hamster zonae and the zonae pellucidae of rhesus and squirrel monkeys[96]. Since the spermatozoa of both these primates will bind to hamster eggs[27] the cross-reactivity, in this instance, does appear to include the sperm-binding sites. For this reason active immunization of rhesus or squirrel monkeys with hamster zona antigens would appear to be both feasible and desirable. Of equal importance would be the construction of an active immunization model involving laboratory rodents as both the donor and the recipient of the zona antigen. In our own studies we have selected the rat as a suitable model because of the ease with which frequent blood samples can be taken from the tail vein, their high fertility and the short duration of the oestrous cycle. Active immunization has been achieved using cross-reacting zona antigens obtained from the mouse. Cross-reactivity between the zona antigens of the rat and the mouse has been established using an antiserum

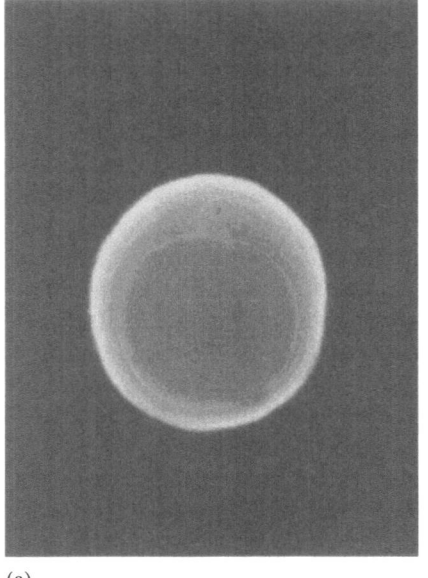
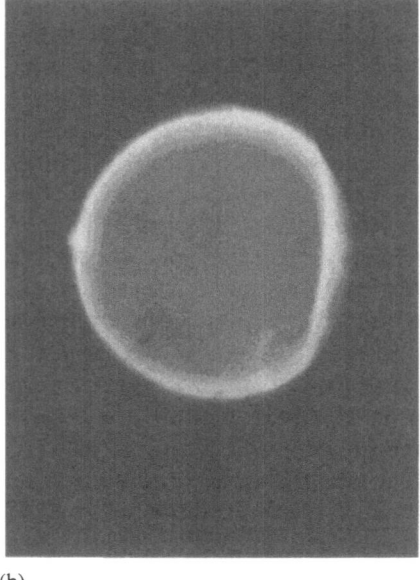

(a)   (b)

Figure 7.5 Labelling of: (a) mouse zona; and (b) rat zona, by indirect immunofluorescence using a fluorescein-conjugated antibody against rabbit IgG and a rabbit antiserum (heat-inactivated and absorbed with liver, kidney and serum) against cumulus-free mouse eggs

raised in rabbits against cumulus-free mouse eggs and made specific for the zona by repeated absorptions with mouse kidney, liver and serum[84]. An indirect immunofluorescence technique, employing fluorescein-labelled anti-rabbit IgG, was then used to demonstrate cross-reactivity between the antigenic determinants on rat and mouse zonae (Figure 7.5)[97]. A fluorescein-labelled antibody against the C3 component of human complement was also used to demonstrate complement fixation on rat and mouse zonae in the presence of a rabbit antiserum against mouse zona pellucida[97]. In addition absorbed antisera raised in rats against saline extracts of mouse ovary or cumulus-free mouse eggs have been shown to form an immune precipitate on

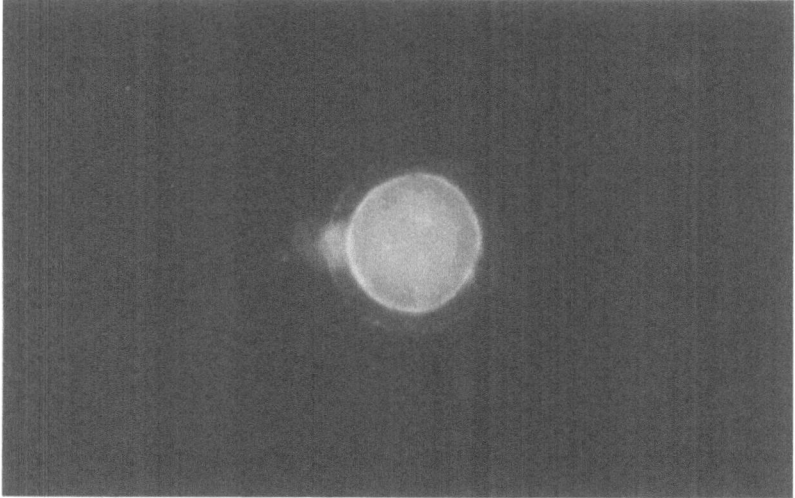

Figure 7.6   Immunoprecipitate on the zona surface of an egg recovered from a rat which had been immunized with cumulus-free mouse ova 6 months previously

the surface of both rat and mouse eggs[97]. Similarly ova recovered from rats exhibiting a high antibody titre against mouse zona antigens exhibit a precipitate on the surface of the zona pellucida (Figure 7.6)[97]. Although the above data suggest that mouse and rat zonae share common antigenic determinants they do not indicate whether this cross-reactivity extends to the sperm-binding sites. That this probably is the case was demonstrated when mouse sperm were shown to bind with equal avidity to both rat and mouse eggs[97] (Table 7.3). It has also been demonstrated that antisera raised against isolated mouse zonae pellucidae will inhibit the fertilization of both rat and mouse eggs *in vitro*[85]. In the light of this information it was decided to immunize rats against mouse zona determinants in an attempt to establish an active immunization model. Before this study could proceed, however, it was necessary to devise a procedure for estimating antibody titres in the

Table 7.3 Binding of mouse spermatozoa to the surface of rat and mouse zonae

Species	Number of eggs examined	Concentration of sperm/mm² zona surface ± SE
Rat ova	8	2947 ± 151
Mouse ova	8	2954 ± 174

immunized animals. For this purpose a sperm-binding assay was developed[98]. This procedure involves incubating cumulus-free mouse ova in HEPES buffered medium 199 for 1 h in the presence of capacitated mouse sperm at a concentration of 2 million/ml. At the end of the culture period the eggs are washed to remove loosely adhering sperm, compressed under coverslips and photographed (Figure 7.7). The photographs are subsequently used to

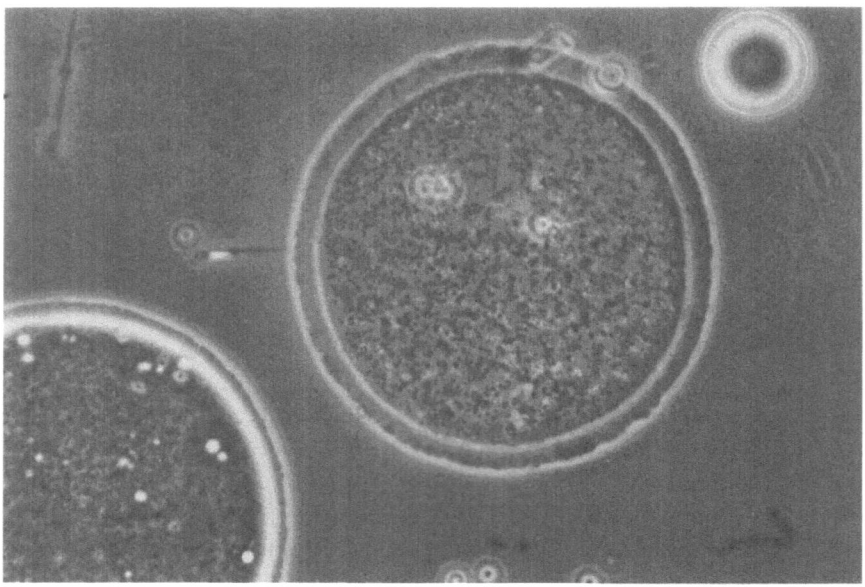

Figure 7.7 Complete suppression of sperm binding in the mouse with a high-titre antibody raised against mouse ovarian antigens

calculate the concentration of sperm per unit area of zona surface. If the eggs are pre-incubated in the presence of serum containing anti-zona antibodies sperm binding during the subsequent incubation period is suppressed (Figure 7.7) and the degree of inhibition is proportional to the antibody titre (Figure 7.8). Both complement and the presence of antibodies against serum interfere with the assay, and for this reason all antisera are heat-inactivated

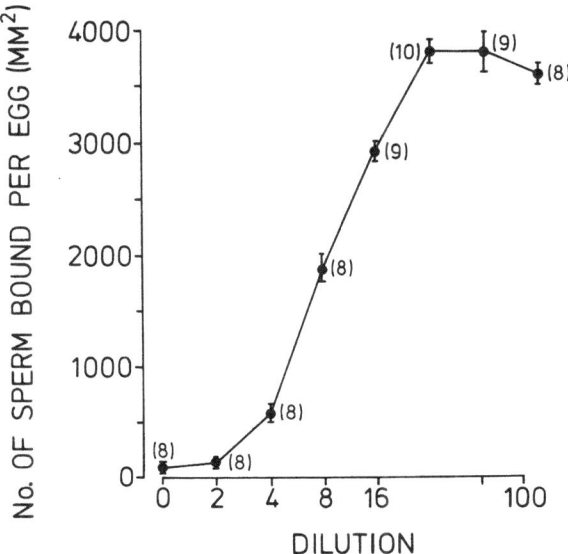

Figure 7.8 Correlation between the concentration of sperm bound per mm² zona surface and dilution of an absorbed antiserum raised against cumulus-free mouse eggs

and repeatedly absorbed before analysis. Examples of control values (sperm binding in the absence of antibody) for a number of separate experiments is given in Table 7.4. It will be noted that although the standard error observed within each experimental run is small there are noticeable differences between experiments, because of minor variations in the assay conditions and the fact that each determination is carried out using sperm from a different male. For

Table 7.4 Concentration of sperm bound to control ova – not treated with antiserum – in separate experiments

Date	Number of eggs scored	Sperm concentration per mm² of zona surface ± SE
16.1.79	8	5001 ± 140
30.1.79	10	4104 ± 134
8.2.79	9	4822 ± 129
23.2.79	8	4695 ± 194
27.2.79	9	5286 ± 141
6.3.79	9	4379 ± 89
6.3.79	8	2750 ± 95
3.4.79	8	5109 ± 158
3.4.79	8	4257 ± 168
4.4.79	9	4102 ± 174
4.4.79	9	2936 ± 98
11.5.79	8	2936 ± 99
24.5.79	8	3691 ± 91

this reason the degree of inhibition due to any given antiserum is always expressed as a percentage of the binding observed in the absence of antibody in a parallel culture using the same population of sperm.

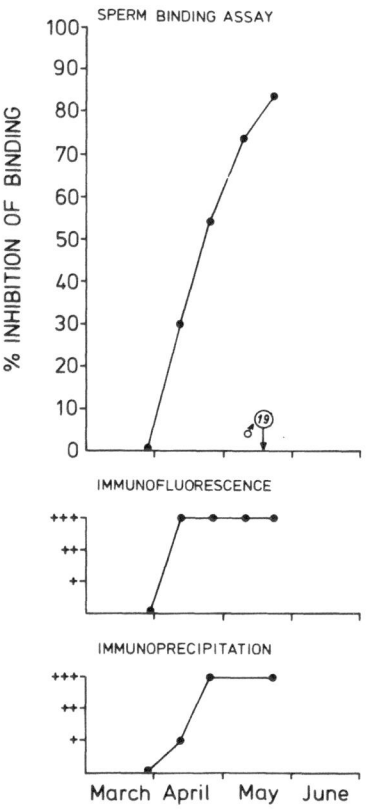

Figure 7.9 Antibody titres in a female rat immunized with mouse ovarian antigens as determined by sperm binding, immunofluorescence, and immunoprecipitation. All serum samples were heat-inactivated and absorbed with liver, kidney and serum before analysis. ♂ = Introduction of male; ↓ = sperm observed in vaginal smear; number = date

Since previous studies had shown[73, 74] that saline extracts of homogenized mouse ovaries were a rich source of zona antigen, one of the initial experiments to be carried out involved the immunization of female rats with the 600 g supernatant of homogenized mouse ovaries. The immunization schedule involved three injections of 6 mg protein separated by 14-day intervals; the primary injection incorporated Freund's complete adjuvant while incomplete adjuvant was used for the subsequent boosters. The antibody response was followed using the sperm-binding assay as well as immunofluorescence and immunoprecipitation techniques. The results indicate a close correlation between the values obtained with each method (Figure 7.9), the antibody titre showing a progressive rise following immunization. Fourteen days after the final booster injection the animal was mated and subsequently autopsied 9 days later. Close inspection of the reproductive tract revealed that although ovulation has occurred there was no sign of conception having taken place. A similar experiment was then carried out employing cumulus-free mouse eggs (about 750 per injection) as the source of zona antigen. As a consequence of immunization the antibody titre rose rapidly and

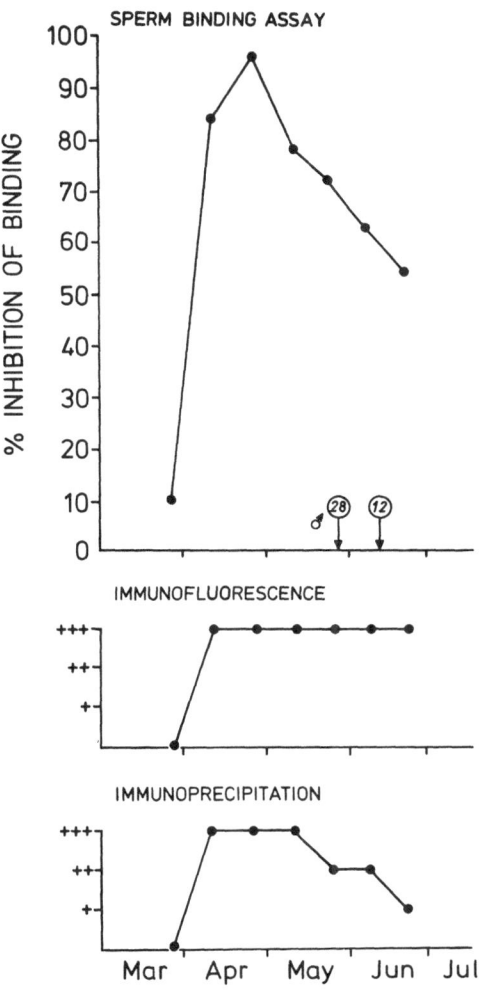

Figure 7.10 Antibody titres in a female rat immunized with cumulus-free mouse eggs as determined by sperm binding, immunofluorescence and immunoprecipitation. All serum samples were heat-inactivated and absorbed with liver, kidney and serum before analysis. ♂ = Introduction of male; ↓ = sperm observed in vaginal smear; number = date

then showed a gradual fall over the next 50 days. Once again there was a close correlation between the results obtained with the sperm-binding assay, immunofluorescence and immunoprecipitation (Figure 7.10). Immunofluorescence was found to be the most sensitive indicator of antibody presence since this procedure continued to register a maximum titre when the sperm-binding and immunoprecipitation techniques indicated a fall in antibody concentration (Figure 7.10). As in the previous experiment this female was exposed to a male of proven fertility 14 days after the completion of the

Table 7.5 Fertility of rats immunized with mouse serum proteins, mouse ovarian antigens and cumulus-free mouse ova

Immunization procedure	Number of animals	Number of matings	Number of pregnancies	Percentage of matings successful
Mouse serum	7	8	7	87.5
Mouse ovarian extract	6	46	2	4.3
Cumulus-free mouse eggs	6	46	2	4.3

Table 7.6

Immunization procedure	Animal Number	Duration of infertility (months)	Number of infertile matings	Pregnancy	Litter size
Serum	1	0	0	+	7
	2	0.5*	1	+	10
	3	0	0	+	6
	4	0	0	+	2
	5	0	0	+	5
	6	·0	0	+	16
	7	0	0	+	11
Ovary	1	0	0	+	4
	2	1	1	Died prematurely	—
	3	2	8	+	5
	4	>6	12	—	—
	5	>6	13	—	—
	6	>6	10	—	—
Denuded ova	1	1	2	+	10
	2	2	2	Died prematurely	—
	3	1	2	+	2
	4	>6	17	—	—
	5	>6	12	—	—
	6	>6	9	—	—

* One pseudopregnancy preceded the establishment of pregnancy

immunization schedule. Pregnancy was not established after the first mating and a 15-day pseudopregnancy ensued. This animal was subsequently autopsied 14 days after a second mating and once again, no sign of pregnancy was observed (Figure 7.10). As a result of these experiments a larger series of animals were immunized against mouse ovarian antigens or denuded mouse ova in order to obtain data on the duration of infertility, the correlation between antibody titre and infertility and the possible existence of adverse side-effects. A control series of animals were immunized against mouse serum proteins using identical immunization schedules. The results of these experiments are summarized in Table 7.5. It is evident that active immunization of rats against mouse zona antigens has a profound effect upon their fertility. Only one mating in the serum-immunized series failed to established pregnancy; in contrast, 96% of matings in rats immunized against zona antigens proved infertile. Information on the duration of infertility in individual animals is presented in Table 7.6. All of the serum-immunized

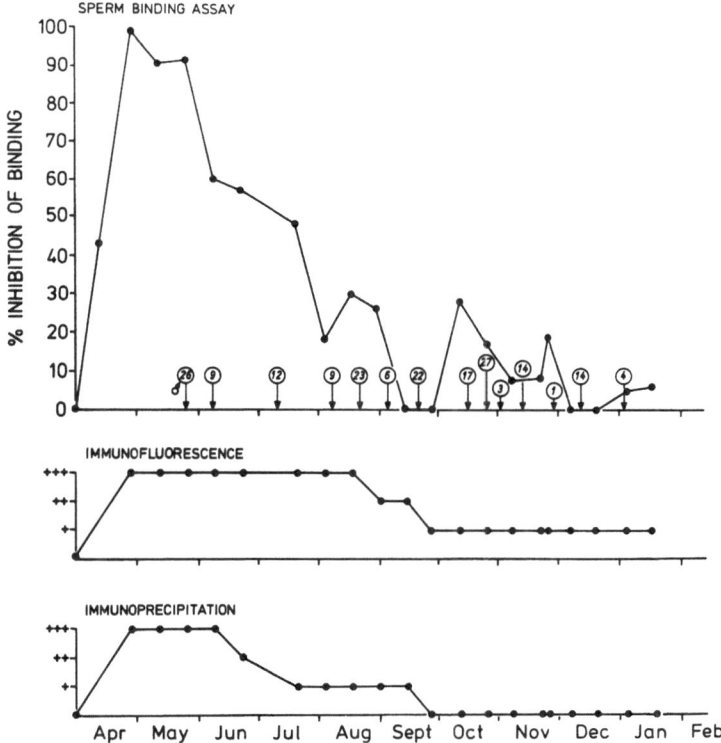

Figure 7.11 Antibody titres in a female rat immunized against cumulus-free mouse eggs as determined by a sperm-binding test, immunofluorescence and immunoprecipitation. All serum samples were heat-inactivated and absorbed with liver, kidney and serum before analysis. ♂ = Introduction of male; ↓ = sperm observed in vaginal smear; Number = date

animals eventually became pregnant and the mean litter size was about eight. In contrast, five out of six animals immunized against mouse ovarian extracts experienced some degree of infertility, and in half the animals pregnancies were never established despite repeated matings. In the two animals which did ultimately become pregnant the litters were small but the young were normal and were subsequently shown to be fertile. All of the animals immunized against denuded mouse ova experienced some degree of infertility and, once again, half the animals never became pregnant despite repeated matings. Those which did give birth produced normal healthy fertile young.

The relationship between antibody concentration and the duration of infertility is shown in Figures 7.11–7.14. Figures 7.11 and 7.12 illustrate the

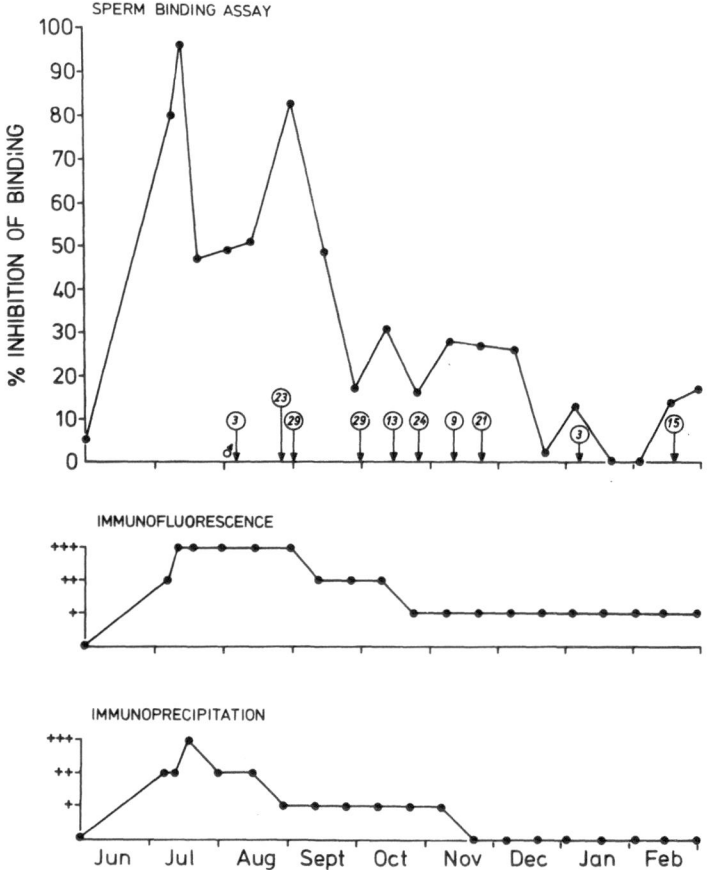

Figure 7.12 Antibody titres in a female rat immunized against mouse ovarian antigens as determined by a sperm-binding test, immunofluorescence and immunoprecipitation. All serum samples were heat-inactivated and absorbed with liver, kidney and serum before analysis. ♂ = Introduction of male; ↓ = sperm observed in vaginal smear; number = date

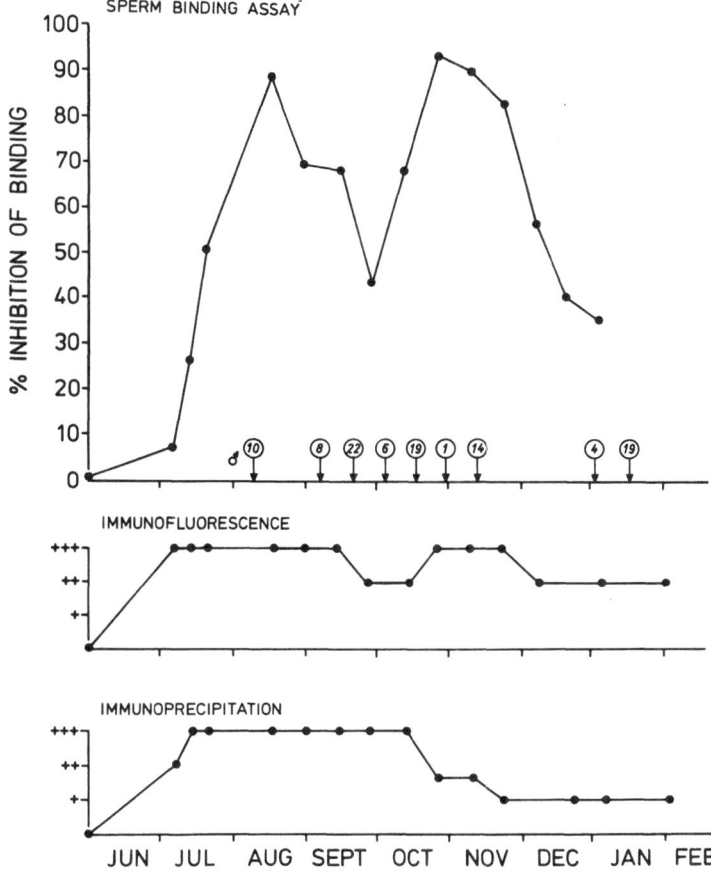

Figure 7.13 Antibody titres in a female rat immunized against cumulus-free mouse eggs as determined by a sperm-binding test, immunofluorescence and immunoprecipitation. All serum samples were heat-inactivated and absorbed with liver, kidney and serum before analysis. ♂ = Introduction to male; ↓ = sperm observed in vaginal smear; number = date

changes observed in two animals, one immunized against ovarian antigens and the other against denuded ova, which never became pregnant. The rat immunized with cumulus-free mouse eggs (Figure 7.11) showed a rapid rise in antibody titre during the immunization procedure which remained maximal for about 1 month. The titre then declined over the next 4 months so that serum samples collected 5 or more months after immunization could not induce the formation of an immune precipitate on the zona surface or inhibit sperm-binding by more than 25%. Nevertheless a low level of antibody could still be detected at this time by indirect immunofluorescence and was still present as long as 10 months after the completion of the immunization schedule. A similar pattern was observed in the rat immunized against mouse ovarian antigens. In this animal the antibody titre rose rapidly after the first two injections and then fell just before the final booster was given. The final injection subsequently stimulated a second rise in antibody titre which gradually declined during the next 4–5 months. Samples collected after this time did not produce a precipitate on the zona surface or inhibit sperm binding by more than 25%.

A similar sequence of antibody rise and fall was observed in all but one (see

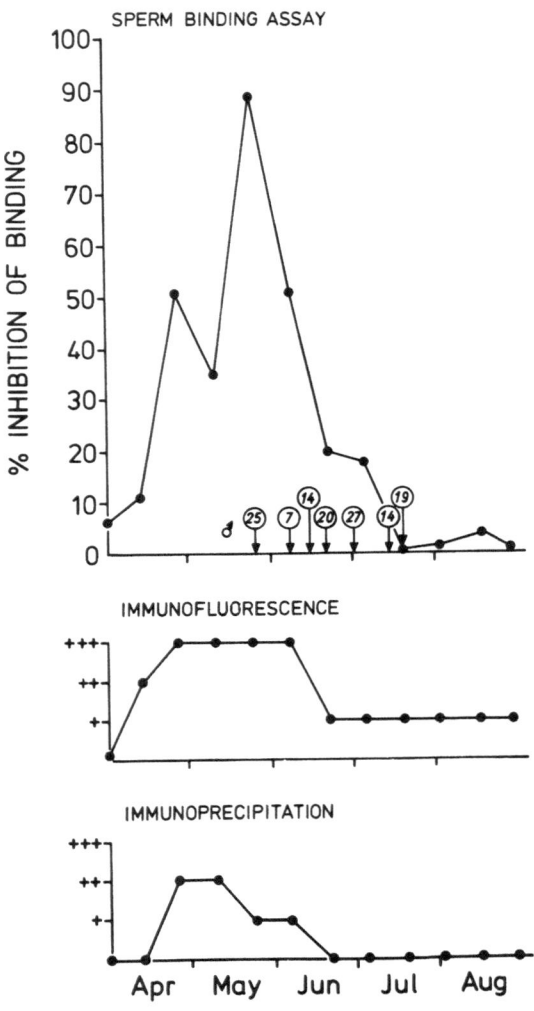

Figure 7.14 Antibody titres in a female rat immunized against mouse ovarian antigens as determined by a sperm-binding assay, immunofluorescence and immunoprecipitation. All serum samples were heat-inactivated and absorbed with liver, kidney and serum before analysis. ♂ = Introduction of the male; ↓ = sperm observed in vaginal smear; number = date

below) of the remaining animals which failed to conceive. It is evident from these analyses that the immunization procedures employed in these studies result in the formation of anti-zona antibodies which persist for at least 10 months. After 4 or 5 months, however, the titres have reached such a low level that they fail to form a precipitate on the surface of mouse zonae and, consequently (Figure 7.8), fail to exert a marked effect on sperm binding. When the antibody titres are high the lack of conception in the immunized animals is presumably due to the inhibition of fertilization, as observed *in vitro* or following passive immunization[85]. However, when antibody titres are low and sperm binding is obviously not being inhibited to a significant degree how

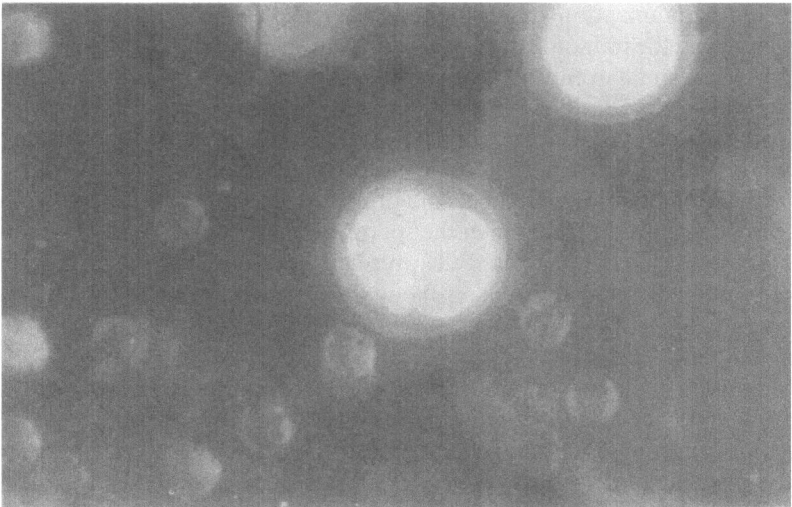

Figure 7.15 A two-cell egg recovered from a rat 6 months after being immunized against mouse ova. Note the precipitation layer on the outer surface of the zona

is the anti-fertility effect maintained? Tsunoda and Chang[72] observed that the fertilization of rat eggs often failed in the presence of an antiserum against rat ovarian antigens without the formation of a visible precipitate on the zona surface. It is therefore possible that fertilization in the rat is particularly sensitive to low levels of antibody. However, analysis of an animal which showed an exceptional pattern of antibody production (Figure 7.13) suggests that at least part of the anti-fertility effect operating in this active immuniz-ation model is achieved after fertilization. In this animal the antibody titre rose and fell in the normal manner but then showed a secondary rise which was sustained for a further 2 months. As the antibody levels were falling for a second time this animal was autopsied 24 h after spermatozoa were found in the vaginal smear. Eleven eggs were recovered from the Fallopian tubes and all possessed a distinct precipitate around the periphery of the zona, even though the last injection of antigen had been given 6 months previously. Nine of the 11 eggs recovered from this animal were degenerating but the remaining two were apparently normal two-cell eggs (Figure 7.15). At the time of autopsy the serum from this animal inhibited sperm binding by about 35% (Figure 7.13). In a parallel experiment one out of four eggs were found to be at the two-cell stage in an animal immunized against cumulus-free mouse eggs and exhibiting a sperm-binding inhibition titre of 35%. It is possible that the few eggs which are fertilized when antibody titres are low fail to implant because of an inhibitory effect on the ability of blastocyst 'to hatch' from the zona pellucida just before implantation[90].

Figure 7.14 illustrates the antibody profile of a rat which did conceive following immunization against zona antigens. The antibody titres rose rapidly during the immunization procedure but then fell rapidly over a 50-day period. The animal eventually conceived when the sperm-binding inhibition and immunoprecipitation scores had reached zero. A second animal which conceived after immunization against denuded mouse ova exhibited a similar decline in antibody titre just before conception. Preliminary results from the two remaining animals which became pregnant after immunization indicate that fertilization took place when the sperm-binding inhibition and immuno-precipitation tests still registered the presence of a significant antibody titre. Determination of the minimum antibody titre needed to ensure the complete suppression of fertility is obviously an extremely important fact to establish in future studies.

In summary, active immunization of rats against zona antigens has established for the first time that long-term suppression of fertility is possible using this procedure. The zona pellucida, particularly the terminal saccharide-rich outer region, is obviously extremely antigenic and antibodies against this structure were detected, by immunofluorescence, throughout the study period in all the immunized animals. None of the treated animals suffered any overt adverse side-effects following immunization and those which did give birth produced normal healthy young. Encouraging results of a similar nature have also been obtained using an active immunization system in which mice were immunized with heat-solubilized hamster zonae[95]. The variable degree of infertility observed in our own experiments probably reflects variations in the total amount of zona antigen administered to individual animals. Because of the possible influence of antigen dose on the duration of infertility, experiments are currently under way employing carefully graded doses of immunogen.

FUTURE PROSPECTS

The prospects for this approach to contraception are difficult to assess at the present time owing to a lack of information in certain critical areas. In particular, a great deal of research needs to be carried out on the composition of the zona pellucida, especially the sperm-binding sites. Progress in this direction will facilitate the use of purer antigens for immunization purposes and also help evaluate the feasibility of preparing synthetic analogues of critical zona components. In addition the availability of antibodies against purified zona constituents will be of value in determining the specificity of these antigens. Preliminary analyses indicate that antisera prepared against mechanically isolated zonae are not specific to this structure but also contain antibodies directed against follicular fluid and/or oocyte proteins[23]. Whether such non-specific antigens are normally present within the zona or are contaminants acquired during the isolation process is not known at the present time. The fact that absorption of antisera prepared against hamster ovary with somatic tissues removes all but one of the precipitin bands formed against ovarian homogenates is encouraging[65]. However, it has also been reported that absorption of antisera raised against rat ovary with liver and kidney removes all cross-reactivity with ovarian tissue and destroys the ability of the antiserum to inhibit fertilization[72]. The observation that certain women appear to exhibit a state of autoimmunity against the antigenic determinants on the human zona without any obvious side-effects[82] suggests that the use of this structure as a target for contraception is feasible.

References

1. Talwar, G. P., Sharma, N. C., Dubey, S. K., Salahuddin, M., Das, Ç., Ramakrishna, S., Kumar, S. and Hingorani, V. (1976). Isoimmunization against human chorionic gonadotrophin with conjugates of processed β-subunit of the hormone and tetanus toxoid. *Proc. Natl. Acad. Sci. USA*, **73**, 218

2. Talwar, G. P., Dubey, S. K., Salahuddin, M. and Shastri, N. (1976). Kinetics of antibody response in animals injected with processed beta-HCG conjugated to tetanus toxoid (Pr-β-HCG-TT). *Contraception*, **13**, 153

3. Stevens, V. (1973). Antifertility effects from immunization with intact, subunits and fragments of HCG. In Edwards, R. G. and Johnson, M. H. (eds.) *Physiological Effects of Immunity Against Reproductive Hormones*, pp. 249–274. (Cambridge: Cambridge University Press)

4. Hearn, J. (1976). Immunization against pregnancy. In Short, R. V. and Baird, D. T. (eds.) *Contraceptives of the Future*, pp. 149–160. (London: The Royal Society)

5. Braden, A. W. H. (1952). Properties of the membranes of rat and rabbit eggs. *Austr. J. Sci. Res. (B)*, **5**, 460

6. Odor, D. L. (1960). Electron microscopic studies on ovarian oocytes and unfertilized tubal ova in the rat. *J. Biophys. Biochem. Cytol.*, **7**, 567

7. Stegner, H. E. and Wartenberg, H. (1961). Electronen-mikroskopische and histotopochemische untersuchangen über Struktur and bildung der zona pellucida menschlicher eizellen. *Z. Zellforsch.*, **53**, 702

8. Jacoby, F. (1962). Ovarian histochemistry. In Zuckerman, S. (ed.) *The Ovary*, pp. 189–245. (New York: Academic Press)

9. Seshachar, B. R. and Bagga, S. (1963). Cytochemistry of the oocyte of *Loris tardigradus lydekkerianus* and *Macaca mulatta*. *J. Morphol.*, **113**, 119

10. Loewenstein, J. E. and Cohen, A. I. (1964). Dry mass, lipid content and protein content of the intact and zona-free mouse ova. *J. Embryol. Exp. Morphol.*, **12**, 113

11. Norrevang, A. (1968). Electron microscopic morphology of oogenesis. *Int. Rev. Cytol.*, **23**, 113

12. Hope, J. (1965). The fine structure of the developing follicle of the rhesus ovary. *J. Ultrastruct. Res.*, **12**, 592

13. Austin, C. R. (1968). *Ultrastructure of Fertilization.* (New York: Holt, Rinehart & Winston)

14. Piko, L. (1969). Gamete structure and sperm entry in mammals. In Metz, C. and Monroy, A. (eds.) *Fertilization.* Vol. 2, pp. 325–403. (New York: Academic Press)

15. Flechon, J. E. (1970). Nature glycoprotéique des granules corticaux de l'oeuf de lapin. Mise en évidence par l'utilisation comparée de techniques cytochimiques ultra-structurales. *J. Microsc.*, **9**, 221

16. Newport, A. and Carrol, J. (1976). Structure and composition of the zona pellucida of the mouse oocyte. *Biochem. Soc. Trans.*, **4**, 896

17. Inoue, M. and Wolf, D. P. (1974). Comparative solubility properties of the zonae pellucidae of unfertilized and fertilized mouse ova. *Biol. Reprod.*, **11**, 558

18. Potts, D. M. and Wilson, I. B. (1967). The preimplantation conceptus of the mouse at 90 hours post coitum. *J. Anat.*, **102**, 1

19. Nicolson, G. L., Yanagimachi, R. and Yanagimachi, H. (1975). Ultrastructural localization of lectin binding sites on the zona pellucida and plasma membranes of mammalian eggs. *J. Cell. Biol.*, **66**, 263

20. Oikawa, T., Nicolson, G. L. and Yanagimachi, R. (1974). Inhibition of hamster fertilization by phytoagglutinins. *Exp. Cell. Res.*, **83**, 239

21. Bowman, P. and McLaren, A. (1970). The reaction of the mouse blastocyst and its zona pellucida to enzymes *in vitro. J. Embryol. Exp. Morphol.*, **24**, 331

22. Chang, M. C. and Hunt, D. M. (1956). Effects of proteolytic enzymes on the zona pellucida of fertilized and unfertilized mammalian eggs. *Exp. Cell. Res.*, **11**, 497

23. Sacco, A. G. and Palm, V. S. (1977). Heteroimmunization with isolated pig zonae pellucidae. *J. Reprod. Fertil.*, **51**, 165

24. Aitken, R. J. and Richardson, D. W. R. (1980). Active immunization of rats with mouse zona antigens; duration of infertility and antibody titres. (In preparation)

25. Franklin, L. E., Barros, C. and Fussell, E. N. (1970). The acrosomal region and the acrosome reaction in sperm of the golden hamster. *Biol. Reprod.*, **3**, 180

26. Yanagimachi, R. (1978). Specificity of sperm–egg interaction. In Edidin, M. and Johnson, M. H. (eds.) *Immunobiology of Gametes*, pp. 255–289. (Oxford: Alden Press)

27. Bedford, M. (1977). Sperm/egg interaction: the specificity of human spermatozoa. *Anat. Rec.*, **188**, 477

28. Austin, C. R. (1961). *The Mammalian Egg.* (Springfield: Charles C. Thomas)

29. Bedford, J. M. (1968). Ultrastructural changes in the sperm head during fertilization in the rabbit. *Am. J. Anat.*, **123**, 329

30. Bedford, J. M. (1972). Sperm transport, capacitation and fertilization. In Balin, H. and Glasser, S. (eds.) *Reproductive Biology*, pp. 338–392. (Amsterdam: Excerpta Medica)

31. Yanagimachi, R. and Mahi, C. A. (1976). Sperm acrosome reaction and fertilization in the guinea-pig: a study *in vivo. J. Reprod. Fertil.*, **46**, 49

32. Piko, L. and Tyler, A. (1964). Fine structural studies of sperm penetration in the rat. *Proceedings of the 5th International Congress on Animal Reproduction*, **2**, 372

33. Barros, C., Bedford, J. M., Franklin, L. E. and Austin, C. R. (1967). Membrane vesiculation as a feature of the mammalian acrosome reaction. *J. Cell. Biol.*, **34**, C1

34. Yanagimachi, R. and Noda, Y. D. (1970). Ultrastructural changes in the hamster sperm head during fertilization. *J. Ultrastruct. Res.*, **31**, 465

35. Yanagimachi, R. and Usui, N. (1974). Calcium dependence of the acrosome reaction and activation of guinea-pig spermatozoa. *Exp. Cell. Res.*, **89**, 161

36. Soupart, P. and Strong, P. A. (1974). Ultrastructural observations on human oocytes fertilized *in vitro*. *Fertil. Steril.*, **25**, 11

37. Gwatkin, R. B. L. (1977). *Fertilization Mechanisms in Man and Mammals*. (New York: Plenum Press)

38. Hartmann, J. F., Gwatkin, R. B. L. and Hutchinson, C. F. (1972). Early contact interactions between mammalian gametes *in vitro*: evidence that the vitellus influences adherence between sperm and zona pellucida. *Proc. Natl. Acad. Sci. USA*, **69**, 2767

39. Yanagimachi, R. (1969). *In vitro* capacitation of hamster spermatozoa by follicular fluid. *J. Reprod. Fertil.*, **18**, 275

40. Yanagimachi, R. (1969). *In vitro* acrosome reaction and capacitation of golden hamster spermatozoa by bovine follicular fluid and its fractions. *J. Exp. Zool.*, **170**, 269

41. Mali, C. A. and Yanagimachi, R. (1973). Effects of temperature osmolality and hydrogen ion concentration on the activation and acrosome of golden hamster spermatozoa. *J. Reprod. Fertil.*, **35**, 55

42. Yanagimachi, R. (1972). Fertilization of guinea-pig eggs *in vitro*. *Anat. Rec.*, **174**, 9

43. Zaneveld, L. J. D., Polakoski, K. L. and Williams, W. L. (1972). Properties of proteolytic enzyme from rabbit sperm acrosomes. *Biol. Reprod.*, **6**, 30

44. Barros, C. (1974). Capacitation of mammalian spermatozoa. In Coutinho, E. M. and Fuchs, F. (eds.) *Physiology and Genetics of Reproduction: Part B*, pp. 3–24. (New York: Plenum Press)

45. Stambaugh, R. and Buckley, J. (1969). Identification and subcellular localisation of the enzymes effecting penetration of the zona pellucida by rabbit spermatozoa. *J. Reprod. Fertil.*, **19**, 423

46. Hartmann, J. F. and Gwatkin, R. B. L. (1971). Alteration of sites on the mammalian sperm surface following capacitation. *Nature (London)*, **234**, 479

47. Gwatkin, R. B. L. and Williams, D. T. (1976). Receptor activity of the solubilized hamster and mouse zona pellucida before and after the zona reaction. *J. Reprod. Fertil.*, **49**, 55

48. Gwatkin, R. B. L., Wudi, L., Hartree, E. F. and Fink, E. (1977). Prevention of fertilization by exposure of hamster eggs to soluble acrosin. *J. Reprod. Fertil.*, **50**, 359

49. Overstreet, J. W. and Bedford, J. M. (1975). The penetrability of rabbit ova treated with enzymes or anti-progesterone antibody: a probe into the nature of a mammalian fertilizin. *J. Reprod. Fertil.*, **44**, 273

50. Aitken, R. J. and Richardson, D. W. R. (1980). Influence of trypsin on sperm binding in the mouse and hamster. (In preparation)

51. Gwatkin, R. B. L., Williams, D. T. and Anderson, O. F. (1973). Zona reaction of mammalian eggs: properties of the cortical granule protease (Cortin) and its receptor substrate in hamster eggs. *J. Cell. Biol.*, **59**, 128a

52. Austin, C. R. and Braden, A. W. H. (1956). Early reactions of the rodent egg to spermatozoon penetration. *J. Exp. Biol.*, **33**, 358

53. Braden, A. W. H., Austin, C. R. and David, H. A. (1954). The reaction of the zona pellucida to sperm penetration. *Austr. J. Biol. Sci.*, **7**, 391

54. Austin, C. R. (1956). Cortical granules in hamster eggs. *Exp. Cell Res.*, **10**, 533

55. Gwatkin, R. B. L., Rasmusson, G. H. and Williams, D. T. (1976). Induction of the cortical reaction in hamster eggs by membrane-active agents. *J. Reprod. Fertil.*, **47**, 299

56. Oikawa, T., Nicolson, G. L. and Yanagimachi, R. (1975). Trypsin-mediated modification of the zona pellucida glycopeptide structure of hamster eggs. *J. Reprod. Fertil.*, **43**, 133

57. Szollosi, D. (1967). Development of cortical granules and the cortical reaction in rat and hamster eggs. *Anat. Rec.*, **159**, 431

58. Inoue, M. and Wolf, D. P. (1975). Comparative solubility properties of rat and hamster zonae pellucidae. *Biol. Reprod.*, **12**, 535

59. Smithberg, M. (1953). The effect of different proteolytic enzymes on the zona pellucida of mouse ova. *Anat. Rec.*, **117**, 554

60. Cholewa-Stewart, J. and Massaro, E. J. (1972). Thermally induced dissolution of the murine zona pellucida. *Biol. Reprod.*, **7**, 166
61. Inoue, M. and Wolf, D. P. (1974). Comparative solubility properties of the zonae pellucidae of unfertilized and fertilized mouse ova. *Biol. Reprod.*, **11**, 558
62. Krzanowska, H. (1972). Rapidity of removal *in vitro* of the cumulus and zona pellucida in different strains of mice. *J. Reprod. Fertil.*, **31**, 7
63. Aitken, R. J. and Richardson, D. W. R. (1980). Active immunization of rats with cumulus free mouse eggs; induction of infertility and antibody titres. (In preparation)
64. Oikawa, T. and Yanagimachi, R. (1975). Block of hamster fertilization by anti-ovary antibody. *J. Reprod. Fertil.*, **45**, 487
65. Ownby, C. L. and Shivers, C. A. (1972). Antigens of the hamster ovary and effects of anti-ovary serum on eggs. *Biol. Reprod.*, **6**, 310
66. Ducibella, T. (1977). Surface changes of the developing trophoblast cell. In Johnson, M. H. (ed.) *Development in Mammals*, Vol. 1, pp. 5–30. (Oxford: North Holland)
67. Denker, H.-W. (1974). Trophoblastic factors involved in lysis of the blastocyst coverings and in implantation in the rabbit: observations on inversely orientated blastocysts. *J. Embryol. Exp. Morphol.*, **32**, 739
68. Denker, H.-W. and Hafez, E. S. E. (1975). Proteases and implantation in the rabbit: role of trophoblast vs. uterine secretion. *Cytobiologie*, **11**, 101
69. Pinsker, M. C., Sacco, A. G. and Mintz, B. (1974). Implantation-associated proteinase in mouse uterine fluid. *Devel. Biol.*, **38**, 285
70. McLaren, A. (1970). The fate of the zona pellucida in mice. *J. Embryol. Exp. Morphol.*, **23**, 1
71. Shivers, C. A., Dudkiewicz, A. B., Franklin, L. E. and Fussel, E. N. (1972). Inhibition of sperm–egg interaction by specific antibody. *Science*, **178**, 1211
72. Tsunoda, Y. and Chang, M. C. (1976). Effect of anti-rat ovary antiserum on the fertilization of rat, mouse and hamster eggs *in vivo* and *in vitro*. *Biol. Reprod.*, **14**, 354
73. Jilek, F. and Pavlok, A. (1975). Antibodies against mouse ovaries and their effect on fertilization *in vitro* and *in vivo* in the mouse. *J. Reprod. Fertil.*, **42**, 377
74. Tsunoda, Y. and Chang, M. C. (1977). Further studies on antisera on the fertilization of mouse, rat and hamster eggs *in vivo* and *in vitro*. *Int. J. Fertil.*, **22**, 129
75. Tsunoda, Y. and Chang, M. C. (1976). Reproduction in rats and mice isoimmunized with homogenates of ovary, testis with epididymis or sperm suspension. *J. Reprod. Fertil.*, **46**, 379
76. Tsunoda, Y. and Chang, M. C. (1976). The effect of passive immunization with hetero and iso immune anti-ovary antiserum on the fertilization of mouse, rat and hamster eggs. *Biol. Reprod.*, **15**, 361
77. Sacco, A. G. and Shivers, C. A. (1973). Localization of tissue specific antigens in the rabbit ovary, oviduct and uterus by the fluorescent antibody technique. *J. Reprod. Fertil.*, **32**, 415
78. Porter, C. W., Highfill, D. and Winovich, R. (1970). Guinea-pig ovary and testis: localization of common gonad specific antigens. *Int. J. Fertil.*, **15**, 177
79. Garavagno, A., Posado, J., Barros, C. and Shivers, C. A. (1974). Some characteristics of the zona pellucida antigen in the hamster. *J. Exp. Zool.*, **189**, 37
80. Glass, L. E. and Hanson, J. E. (1974). An immunologic approach to contraception: localization of anti-embryo and antizona pellucida serum during mouse pre-implantation development. *Fertil. Steril.*, **25**, 484
81. Shivers, C. A. (1974). Immunological interference with fertilization. In Diczfalusy, E. (ed.) *Immunological Approaches to Fertility Control*, pp. 223–244. (Karolinska Institute)
82. Shivers, C. A. and Dunbar, B. S. (1977). Auto antibodies to zona pellucida: a possible cause for infertility in women. *Science*, **197**, 1082
83. Sacco, A. G. (1977). Antigenicity of the human zona pellucida. *Biol. Reprod.*, **16**, 158
84. Tsunoda, Y. (1977). Inhibitory effect of anti-mouse egg serum on fertilization *in vitro* and *in vivo* in the mouse. *J. Reprod. Fertil.*, **50**, 353

85. Tsunoda, Y. and Chang, M. C. (1978). Effects of antisera on fertilization of mouse, rat and hamster egg. *Biol. Reprod.*, **18**, 468

86. Tsunoda, Y. and Chang, M. C. (1976). *In vivo* and *in vitro* fertilization of hamster, rat and mouse eggs after treatment with anti-hamster ovary antiserum. *J. Exp. Zool.*, **195**, 409

87. Oikawa, T., Yanagimachi, R. and Nicolson, G. L. (1973). Wheat germ agglutinin blocks mammalian fertilization. *Nature (London)*, **241**, 256

88. Sacco, A. G. (1979). Inhibition of fertility in mice by passive immunization with antibodies to isolated zonae pellucidae. *J. Reprod. Fertil.*, **56**, 533

89. Tsunoda, Y. and Sugrie, T. (1977). Inhibition of fertilization in mice by anti-zona pellucida antiserum. *Jpn. H. Zootech. Sci.*, **48**, 784

90. Dudkiewicz, A. B., Noske, I. G. and Shivers, C. A. (1975). Inhibition of implantation in the golden hamster by zona-precipitating antibody. *Fertil. Steril.*, **26**, 686

91. Tsunoda, Y. and Chang, M. C. (1978). Effect of antisera against eggs and zonae pellucidae on fertilization and development of mouse eggs *in vivo* and in culture. *J. Reprod. Fertil.*, **54**, 233

92. Sacco, A. G. and Shivers, C. A. (1973). Comparison of antigens in the ovary, oviduct and uterus of the rabbit and other mammalian species. *J. Reprod. Fertil.*, **32**, 421

93. Sacco, A. G. (1977). Antigenic cross reactivity between human and pig zona pellucida. *Biol. Reprod.*, **16**, 164

94. Trounson, A. O., Shivers, C. A., McMaster, K. and Lopata, A. (1979). Inhibition of sperm binding and fertilization of human ova by antibody to porcine zona pellucida and human sera. *Fertil. Steril.* (In press)

95. Shivers, C. A., Gengozian, N., Franklin, S. and McLaughlin, C. (1978). Antigenic cross-reactivity between human and marmoset zonae pellucidae, a potential target for immuno-contraception. *J. Med. Primatol.*, **7**, 242

96. Gwatkin, R. B. L., Williams, D. T. and Carlo, D. J. (1977). Immunization of mice with heat-solubilized hamster zonae: production of anti-zona antibody and inhibition of fertility. *Fertil. Steril.*, **28**, 871

97. Aitken, R. J. and Richardson, D. W. (1980). Cross-reactivity between the zonae pellucidae of the rat and mouse. (In preparation)

98. Aitken, R. J. and Richardson, D. W. (1980). A sperm-binding assay in the mouse: influence of anti-zona antibodies. (In preparation)

99. Inove, M. and Wolf, D. P. (1975). Fertilization-associated changes in the murine zona pellucida: a time sequence study. *Biol. Reprod.*, **13**, 546

8
The Current Status of Anti-pregnancy Vaccines Based on Synthetic Fractions of HCG

V. C. STEVENS

RATIONALE

Studies conducted during the past decade suggest that immunizations resulting in the inactivation of endogenous HCG in women would be an effective means of fertility regulation[1-3]. The relative advantages of this approach to fertility regulation have been previously presented[4] and other discussions of this subject can be found elsewhere in this volume. While this approach is very attractive, it should be emphasized that many problems must be overcome before a safe and effective method is available.

Although HCG is not a maternal antigen, women are immunologically tolerant to the hormone and an immune response is not normally elicited from parenteral administration of HCG for treatment of infertility. Therefore, antigens proposed for use in an anti-HCG vaccine must be modified or altered to cause macrophage and/or lymphocyte recognition in the recipient women. Also appropriate immune responses must be induced without use of unacceptable immunostimulants such as Freund's adjuvant. Probably the most critical requirement of an HCG vaccine is the necessity of the response to antigen to be specific towards the conceptus with no significant reactivity of antibodies or sensitized lymphocytes to maternal components.

Hapten-coupling of intact HCG has been shown to be adequate modification of the hormone to break immunological tolerance to it in women[5]; however, antibodies produced reacted extensively with the pituitary hormone

HLH. While these findings suggest HCG antigens can be made antigenic in humans, alternative antigens besides the intact hormone must be sought to obtain a more specific immune response. The first alternate antigen to be evaluated for producing specific HCG responses was the beta subunit of HCG. This subunit was chosen for testing since the alpha subunit of HCG is chemically identical with those of other maternal glycoprotein hormones, FSH, LH, and TSH. Despite the extensive similarities in the primary structures of the beta subunits of HCG and HLH, Vaitukaitus et al.[6] reported that antibodies raised to the beta subunit of HCG (β-HCG) could partially discriminate between HCG and HLH.

Immunization of female baboons with highly purified.β-HCG resulted in the production of high levels of antibodies to HCG and significant levels reacting to baboon CG[1]. No detectable cross-reaction with baboon LH was found in the sera from these animals, and they continued to exhibit normal ovulatory cycles. Repeated matings of 10 females with males of proven fertility, however, did not result in any sustained pregnancy. While menses occurred in the mated females at or before the expected time for a non-gravid cycle, fertility rates of non-immunized baboons in the same colony suggested that 80–90% of the females did conceive. The stage of gestation disrupted by the immunizations was not apparent, although a pre-implantation effect was suggested. Should CG be present on the cell surface of the pre-implantation blastocyst, antibodies in the uterine fluids could have reacted with the early conceptus and prevented implantation or destroyed the blastocyst by cytotoxic action. Also, lymphocyte populations sensitized to the CG antigen could have evoked cellular damage to the trophoblast. In any event, these data clearly indicated that CG immunization in primates was effective in disrupting fertility.

The antisera generated in baboons by β-HCG immunizations reacted not only with HCG and baboon CG but significantly with HLH also[7]. This observation caused concern that immunizations of human females with β-HCG may result in autoimmune damage to the pituitary gland or ovarian cells with receptors for LH or nephritis following accumulation of LH-antibody complexes in the glomerulus of the kidney. These concerns may represent only theoretical problems since studies in humans immunized with β-HCG conjugated to tetanus toxoid have not revealed any evidence of altered function of the pituitary, ovary, or kidney[8]. Since the immune response was weak in these reported studies, insufficient levels of antibody or numbers of sensitized lymphocytes may have been stimulated to reveal potential problems. Further study with more immunogenic antigens (prepared by other chemical alteration or conjugation or by using more effective adjuvants) will be necessary before definite conclusions on the safety of human immunizations with β-HCG can be made. However, in the absence of appropriate animal studies, continued experiments in humans with potentially hazardous consequences may not be possible.

Cross-reactivity of antibodies raised to β-HCG subunit with HLH is not surprising when one considers the extensive chemical similarities in the beta subunits of the two hormones. A comparison of the first 110 amino acid residues of HCG and HLH beta subunits reveal that 94 are identical (85%)[9]. However, HLH has only 115 amino acid residues in the subunit where β-HCG has 145. Excepting for one residue between 111 and 115 with the same amino acid, the 35 amino acids of the carboxyl terminal end of β-HCG is not represented in HLH (Figure 8.1). Therefore, peptides from the carboxy-terminal region of β-HCG provide an alternative source of antigens for eliciting a specific immune response to HCG. Several peptides representing this region of the molecule have been evaluated as potential antigens in an anti-fertility vaccine.

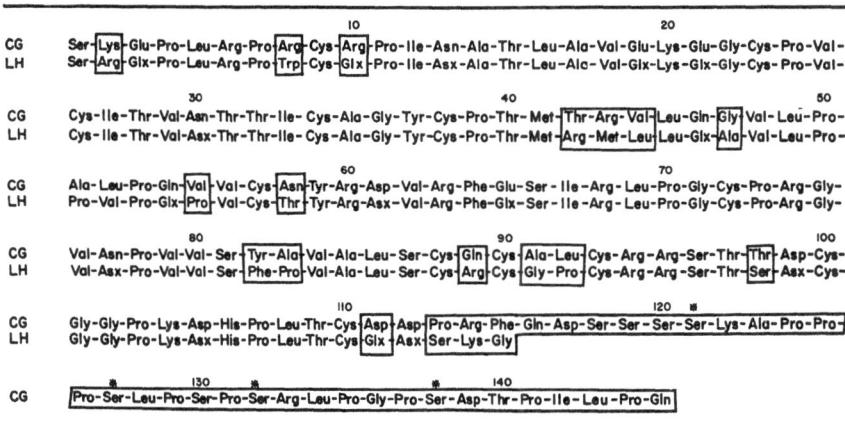

Figure 8.1 Amino acid sequences of the beta subunits of HCG and HLH. Residues in boxes represent areas of difference in the two hormones. Sites marked with an asterisk indicate points of carbohydrate attachment in the native molecule

SELECTION OF PEPTIDES FOR VACCINE DEVELOPMENT

Peptide chains of the COOH-terminal portion of β-HCG have been prepared by digesting the subunit with a variety of proteolytic enzymes and subsequently purifying the cleaved fragments. The number and length of peptide chains depends upon the enzyme used, concentrations and other factors present during digestion. Some of these peptides have been evaluated as antigens for producing antibodies to HCG.

A peptide representing β-HCG sequence 109–145 has been studied as a potential antigen for vaccine development. This structure, isolated after chymotryptic digestion of β-HCG, contains four serine-linked carbohydrate chains. Antibodies generated to this peptide are highly cross-reactive with intact HCG *in vitro* and will neutralize the biological activity of the hormone *in vivo*. Shorter peptides representing 116–145, 123–145, or 126–145 β-HCG elicit antibodies capable of reacting with HCG but have little ability to neutralize biological activity[10, 11, 7]. The reason for these differences has not been revealed, although data are available to suggest that the longer peptides possess an additional determinant on their N-terminal segment, and this facilitates production of multi-determinant antibodies following immunizations. Such antisera may then react with intact HCG at more than one site resulting in a larger immune complex than complexes found from antibodies to shorter peptides and HCG. It is well known that large immune complexes are removed from circulation rapidly whereas smaller ones persist commensurate with the half-life of the immune globulins.

For the above reasons, peptides with a length of at least 35 amino acid residues were selected for vaccine development. However, yields of natural peptides from digestion of β-HCG are low and the costs of production of these peptides for vaccine use are prohibitive. Therefore, the feasibility of producing a useful peptide antigen synthetically was investigated. Several peptides of various lengths have been prepared by solid-phase synthesis method, and the immunological characteristics of them studied. These peptides, of course, do not contain any carbohydrate moiety.

IMMUNOGENICITY OF PEPTIDES

Synthetic peptides containing 30–45 amino acid residues are weakly immunogenic even when injected into animals in Freund's complete adjuvant. Therefore, efforts have been made to enhance the immunogenicity of these molecules by conjugating them to various macromolecules using classical coupling methods. These efforts were only partially successful and a wide variation in immune responsiveness was observed in mice, rabbits, and baboons. Recently, new chemical procedures have been devised for preparing peptide-carrier conjugates and higher antibody responses have been obtained. Unfortunately, wide variation in response to immunization still remains.

Studies of cell-mediated immune responses to peptides have revealed that these molecules are capable of sensitizing T lymphocytes to some degree. Obviously, some B lymphocytes are capable of binding peptides as evidenced by antibody production. Conjugation of peptides to carrier molecules was performed to provide higher macrophage and/or lymphocyte recognition of antigens. It was believed, based on other experiments reported in the literature, that conjugation of peptides with a thymus-independent carrier would provide the optimal conjugate for antibody production. Therefore, polymerized flagellin and tetanus toxoid were used in the bulk of experiments in recent years. While there is some doubt that tetanus toxoid is truly a thymus-independent antigen, conjugates utilizing bovine γ-globulin as a carrier have elicited higher antibody levels in rabbits than similar conjugates of either tetanus toxoid or flagellin. Further studies are in progress currently to identify suitable carriers for providing greater helper function to peptide antibody production since most known effective proteins (such as bovine γ-globulin) are not acceptable for use in humans.

SPECIFICITY OF ANTIBODIES TO HCG PEPTIDES

The primary purpose of immunizations with COOH-terminal peptides of β-HCG is to produce antibodies reactive to intact HCG. Since isolated peptides, particularly synthetically prepared ones, cannot possess the identical structure as the same sequences in the native hormone, antibodies to peptides were assessed for their ability to react with HCG.

Antisera generated to a large number of peptides have been assessed for reactivity both to peptide and intact HCG. The results can be summarized by stating that antibodies to peptides of 35 amino acids or longer react to HCG on a molar basis nearly equivalent to the peptides used for immunization; antibodies to peptides of fewer than 20 amino acids react somewhat less to HCG than to peptides; and peptides 20–30 amino acids in length generate antisera with an intermediate cross-reactivity. The reasons for these differences in cross-reactivity are believed to be two-fold:

(1) Short peptides may present only part of a determinant existing on the native hormone and antibodies to them may have been a 'poor fit' to the intact determinant on HCG.

(2) Longer peptides have been shown to form confirmational determinants whereas short ones have only sequence specific determinants.

It is possible that cross-reactivity of anti-peptide antibodies with native HCG is high only when the peptides possess a similar structure to their analogous sequences existing in the whole hormone. While current data are not adequate to prove this hypothesis, suffice it to say that the use of longer peptides (35 residues or longer) for vaccine development appears to be most promising at this point in time.

None of the antisera to COOH-β-HCG peptides have shown significant reactivity with HLH or any other purified pituitary hormone; neither have any reactions of antisera with cells of human pituitary glands *in vitro* been found. Extensive testing for cross-reactivity of antisera with other organs and tissues has not yet been done.

Despite the hormone specificity displayed by these peptide antisera, radioimmunoassays employing them as ligands have demonstrated the presence of an HCG-like substance in extracts of human pituitary glands and in extracts of urine from post-menopausal women[12,13]. Figure 8.2 shows the reactivity of an antiserum to a synthetic peptide to human pituitary and urinary extracts. Reactive materials in these extracts have been partially characterized and shown to have a molecular size and isoelectric point similar to HCG. Extracts of pituitary glands from sheep, rats, and cows and sera from numerous species contain a small quantity of immunoreactive material in these COOH–peptide assay systems. Whether these observations are indicative of small amounts of HCG produced in the pituitaries of normal individuals, or whether they are a reflection of weak cross-reactivity of antisera with other components with a similar determinant is not clear at this

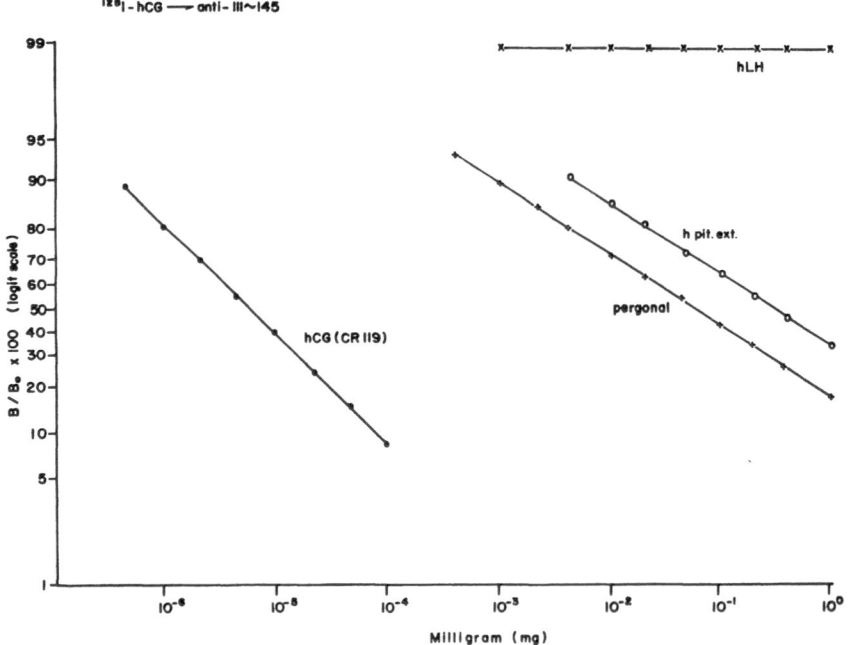

Figure 8.2   Responses of HCG, a crude pituitary extract, a urinary extract of post-menopausal urine (Pergonal) and HLH in a radioimmunoassay employing an antiserum to HCG-β peptide 111–145 and [125I]HCG

time. In any event, these data raise some questions about the absolute specificity of HCG peptide antibodies, and clearly point to the need to assess carefully the effects of immunizations upon the function of the endocrine organs in appropriate animal species prior to clinical trials.

Antibodies to HCG peptides are not species-specific. Fortunately, antisera raised to COOH-peptides will react with CG from baboons and chimpanzees; albeit at a lower level than to HCG. While highly purified preparations of these primate CGs are not available for testing, assays employing partially purified preparations suggest a 5–20% cross-reactivity of anti-HCG peptide antisera with CG preparations of non-human origin. Without this cross-reactivity it would not be possible to evaluate the efficacy and safety of a vaccine based on HCG peptides in animals. These evaluations are critical to the development of any method for human application.

CLASS AND AFFINITY OF ANTIBODIES TO COOH-β-HCG PEPTIDES

As with most antigens, the antibodies generated to HCG peptides during the first few weeks of immunizations in rabbits, mice, and baboons are a mixture of IgG and IgM. However, fractionalization of immune globulins collected at 70 days after the primary immunization with HCG peptide conjugates revealed greater than 95% of all antibodies produced were of the IgG class. No evidence, either from *in vitro* or *in vivo* studies, has been found that immunizations with peptides elicit any significant quantity of IgE antibody production.

The affinity of antibodies to peptides is relatively low both to HCG and to the peptides used as immunogen. Antibody affinity constants to HCG are in the order of 10^9 L/M. Antibodies to intact HCG and to its beta subunit usually have affinity constants of 10^{10} or 10^{11} L/M. The reason(s) for low affinity antibody production to peptide is not apparent; however, it may be related to the few determinants on the peptide molecule or to a higher disassociation rate of antibodies raised to the smaller peptide molecules. Another possibility is that these antigens have similar determinants as some other molecule(s) in the species immunized, and a state of partial tolerance exists to them.

ACTIONS OF PEPTIDE ANTISERA *IN VIVO*

Antibodies generated to peptides have been tested in various bioassay systems for their ability to neutralize the hormonal action of HCG. Some discrepancies have been found between *in vitro* and *in vivo* assay systems and caution must be applied to the interpretation of data obtained in systems where normal serum components can interfere with assay results. Most studies of anti-peptide sera have been performed by pre-incubating *in vitro* a quantity of HCG with a quantity of antisera capable of binding twice the amount of HCG. The incubates are injected into immature assay animals (usually rodents) for several days and the effects of antisera to inhibit the stimulatory action of HCG on the animal gonads assessed. Data obtained can be summarized by stating that antisera to peptides of less than 35 amino acids have only partial or no ability to neutralize the biological action of HCG, whereas those 35 residues or longer can effectively inhibit HCG activity (Figure 8.3). However, it should be noted that the quantity of HCG which an antisera will neutralize *in vivo* is less than the quantity which the same sera will bind *in vitro*. This finding supports the suggestion that more than one globulin molecule must bind to each HCG molecule for neutralization of biological activity to occur.

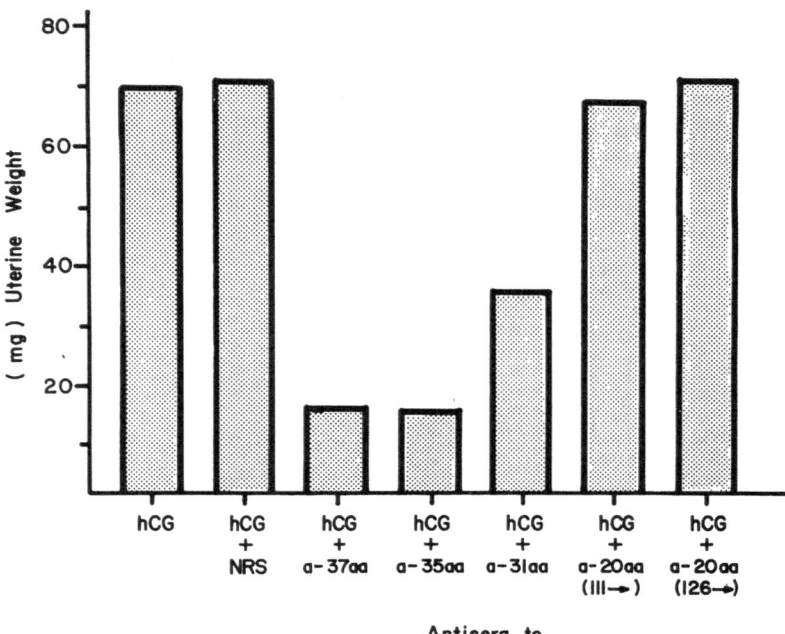

Figure 8.3 Uterine weights of immature mice receiving injections of HCG, HCG plus normal rabbit serum, and HCG plus various rabbit antisera to synthetic HCG peptides of differing chain lengths (aa = no. of amino acids). The two antisera raised to 20 aa peptides represent responses to peptides of the 111–130 and 126–145 sequence of β-HCG

Antiserum to β-HCG peptides do not appear to react with any available antigens in non-pregnant female baboons in the limited studies performed to date. Simultaneous injection of baboon anti-peptide globulin and baboon anti-rabbit serum albumin (RSA) intravenously into a non-pregnant female baboon showed the same clearance rate for both immunoglobulins (Figure 8.4). If it can be assumed that there was no unmasked determinant in the animal reactive to RSA, it can be concluded that no unmasked determinant in the non-pregnant baboon is reactive with antibodies to β-HCG COOH-peptides.

Antisera raised to these peptides, however, do have significant actions when administered to pregnant baboons. The intravenous instillation of

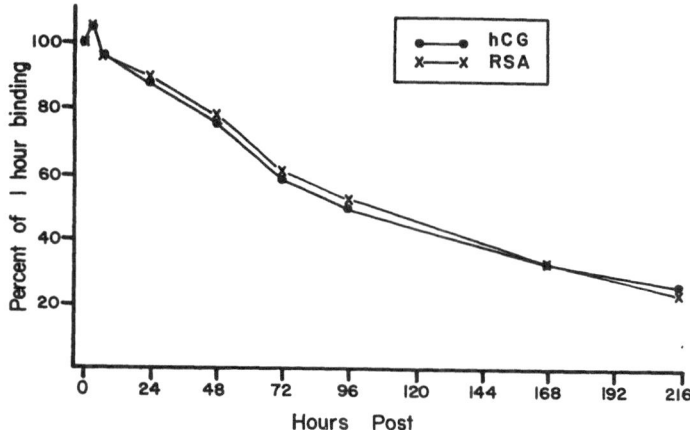

Figure 8.4 The simultaneous clearance of baboon IgG raised separately to a β-HCG peptide (HCG) and to rabbit serum albumin (RSA) in a healthy adult female baboon

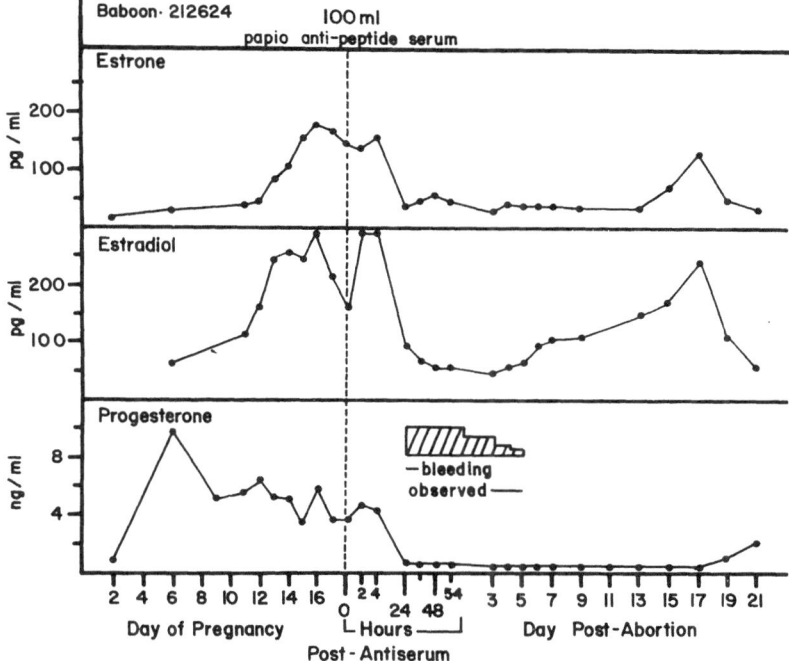

Figure 8.5 Disruption of pregnancy in a baboon by the intravenous administration of baboon anti-HCG peptide serum on day 18 of gestation. Hormone levels, within the normal range prior to the passive immunization, dropped markedly within 24 h and menstrual bleeding was initiated. The animal began a new menstrual cycle, with normal hormonal patterns and sex skin changes, a few days after the induced abortion.

100 ml of an antiserum from a baboon immunized with peptide β-HCG–111–145 to a non-immunized pregnant baboon promptly disrupted gestation, as evidenced by menstrual bleeding and a rapid decline in serum hormone levels (Figure 8.5). Despite the limited cross-reactivity of anti-β-HCG peptide antibodies with baboon CG, disruption of placental function at an early stage of pregnancy can be induced. These observations strongly suggest the feasibility of using a synthetic β-HCG peptide as an immunogen for an anti-fertility vaccine.

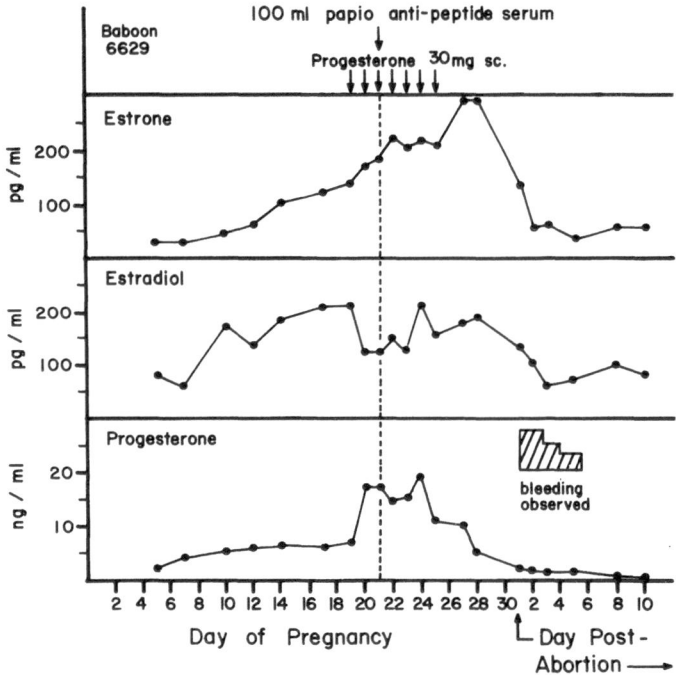

Figure 8.6 Delayed abortion in a pregnant baboon passively immunized with baboon anti-HCG peptide serum receiving injections of progesterone 2 days prior to, and 5 days following, the intravenous instillation of antiserum

Abortions induced with anti-peptide serum to date have been done during the early weeks of gestation when the maintenance of pregnancy is dependent upon ovarian production of progesterone. In order to study the mechanism of action of these pregnancy disruptions, an experiment was conducted to ascertain whether the administration of exogenous progesterone prior to the passive immunization could block the action of the antibodies. As seen in Figure 8.6, the subcutaneous administration of progesterone 2 days prior to, and 5 days following, the intravenous instillation of anti-peptide serum prevented immediate menstrual bleeding. Oestrogen levels remained in the normal range. When progesterone therapy was discontinued, menstrual bleeding occurred within 5 days and a new cycle was initiated, as evidenced by sex skin deturgescence. This experiment suggests, but does not prove, that the action of antisera disrupts placental function or damages its tissues directly, and the replacement of ovarian progesterone merely supports the maternal endometrium and prevents bleeding. Should further study confirm this suggestion, it would indicate that the anti-fertility effects of antibodies to HCG in women could not be reversed by the administration of progesterone following conception.

ANTI-FERTILITY EFFECTS OF ACTIVE IMMUNIZATION

Several adult fertile female baboons have been immunized with numerous conjugates of the β-HCG peptide 111–145. In recent years, most conjugates have been peptide coupled either to tetanus toxoid or to flagellin. A few animals have been immunized with carriers only prior to testing their fertility.

Table 8.1 Fertility rates in female baboons immunized with conjugates of β-HCG peptide 111–145

Immunogen*	Anti-HCG mating titre (ng/ml)	Number of baboons	Number of matings	Number of pregnancies	Percentage fertility
None (untreated controls)		44	96	78	81.3
Tetanus toxoid		6	8	6	75.0
Flagellin β-HCG (111–145)	< 50		13	3	23.1
	51–150		1	0	0.0
	151–400		1	1	100.0
	> 401		0	0	
TOTALS		7	15	4	26.7
Tetanus toxoid β-HCG (111–145)	< 50		22	4	18.2
	51–150		9	1	11.1
	151–400		5	0	0.0
	> 401		3	0	0.0
TOTALS		19	39	5	12.8
Total for all matings		26	54	9	16.7

* Injected with 'complete Freund's adjuvant'

Results of some breeding experiments of normal females, carrier-immunized females, and females immunized with tetanus toxoid and flagellin conjugates are shown in Table 8.1. In these studies females were introduced into a cage with a male of proven fertility for 5 days at their mid-cycle fertile period. This 5-day exposure to a male was considered one mating. Some immunized females were mated only once, and others as many as three times if no pregnancy resulted.

Also shown in Table 8.1 is the antibody level at the time of exposure to the male. Despite a few exceptions, the antifertility effects of immunizations appeared to be related to the antibody level at the time of mating. Pregnancies in females with relatively high levels to HCG showed lower affinities than antisera from animals not conceiving, and had a lower cross-reactivity with baboon CG. Which, if either of these factors, was related to the failure of these immunizations to prevent sustained pregnancy is not known from present data.

While the pregnancy rate in these baboons is not one that would be acceptable for human application, a clear reduction in fertility from control animals is apparent. It must be remembered that the immunogen used here was related to the human antigen and low cross-reactivity with the baboon hormone was present in all antisera. Should these antibody levels represent total reactivity to the homologous CG, a much lower fertility rate would probably have been observed.

PROBLEMS AND PROSPECTS FOR DEVELOPMENT OF A VACCINE

The probability of developing a vaccine to inhibit fertility in women using synthetic β-HCG peptides now appears high. Nonetheless, several serious problems still exist before confidence that a safe and effective method will be forthcoming. First of all, a higher efficacy rate must be demonstrated either by increasing the response to peptides in non-human primates or by immunizing with an immunogen with inherently higher cross-reactivity. This latter approach could be accomplished by using peptides derived from baboon CG for studying anti-fertility efficacy from baboon immunizations. Unfortunately, no peptides representing the COOH terminal portion of baboon β-CG are now available for study. An alternative to an homologous immunization for higher cross-reactivity is the use of chimpanzees for immunizing with the human βCG peptide. Antibodies raised in this species would likely react to chimpanzee CG much more than to baboon CG. However it is unlikely that adequate numbers of adult, fertile, female chimpanzees to conduct a statistically valid anti-fertility trial (including controls) could be acquired at a feasible cost. Therefore, if complete anti-fertility efficacy is to be demonstrated, efforts must be directed towards:

(1) producing a more immunogenic β-HCG peptide conjugate for baboon immunizations; and/or

(2) the isolation, sequence analysis and synthesis of COOH peptides from baboon beta subunit for evaluations in baboons.

Active immunization of female baboons, for assessment of anti-fertility effects, have to date been performed by incorporating the HCG-peptide immunogen in Freund's complete adjuvant. This adjuvant was used to provide maximum immunostimulation for antigen evaluation but certainly could not be used in any human experimentation. Therefore, other adjuvants suitable for human use must be identified before vaccine development can be completed. Several synthetic compounds without toxic or other undesirable properties have been shown to be effective adjuvants in laboratory animals, and some of these are currently being evaluated for their ability to enhance the immune response to HCG-peptide antigens. Preliminary results are encouraging that one or more synthetic adjuvant compounds can be used in a HCG vaccine, although much more testing will be required in animals before the safety and efficacy of such adjuvants is established. Thus, adjuvant development is a vital aspect of the overall vaccine development programme.

Another major problem with this approach to fertility regulation is the determination of vaccine safety. The observations that anti-peptide sera reacts slightly with extracts of normal tissues causes concern that immunization of women could result in autoimmune damage. Carefully designed, intensive studies in appropriate animal species must be conducted before a vaccine, even if shown to be effective, can be applied to human populations[14]. Homologous baboon or chimpanzee CG peptide immunizations in these species would be the best models for evaluating the safety of a vaccine.

The reversibility of this approach to fertility regulation has not been established. While baboons with low antibody levels, and those whose levels waned after several months, have conceived and maintained pregnancies until term, method reversibility has been too little studied at present. A statistically valid number of animals must be mated at varying periods after immunity has been lost in order to determine whether normal gestation, without abortions, can be expected after use of the method has ceased. Also, the effects on the fetus of inadvertent immunizations during an established pregnancy must be evaluated in animals. There are no theoretical reasons to expect teratological effects from this treatment, but adequate testing must precede human trials.

The data discussed here, representing several years of study, reflect only the early development phase of a safe and effective vaccine for human application. While there is every reason to be optimistic that this approach will result in a valuable tool for fertility regulation, the patience to persist on a strict, step-by-step, well-designed development plan is mandatory. Since the entire concept of purposeful immunological manipulation of the human reproductive system is without precedent in medicine, this caution is not believed to be unwarranted.

Acknowledgements

Studies reported here received financial support from the World Health Organization.

References

1. Stevens, V. C. (1974). Fertility control through active immunization using placental proteins. In Diczfalusy, E. (ed.) *Immunological Approaches to Fertility Control*, pp. 357–375. 7th Karolinska Symposium. Suppl. 194, *Acta Endocr. (Kbh)*, 1915. (Copenhagen: Bogtrykkeriet Forum)
2. Talwar, G. P., Dubey, S. K., Salahuddin, M., Das, C., Ramakrishman, S., Kumar, S. and Hingorani, V. (1976). Isoimmunization against HCG with conjugates of processed β subunit of the hormone and tetanus toxoid. *Proc. Natl. Acad. Sci. USA*, **73**, 218
3. Hearn, J. P. (1976). Immunization against pregnancy. *Proc. R. Soc. Lond.*, **195**, 149
4. Stevens, V. C. (1978). Immunological approaches to fertility regulation. *Bull. WHO*, **55**, 179
5. Stevens, V. C. and Crystle, C. D. (1973). Effects of immunization with hapten-coupled HCG on the human menstrual cycle. *Obstet. Gynecol.*, **42**, 485
6. Vaitukaitis, J. L., Braunstein, G. D. and Ross, G. T. (1972). A radioimmunoassay which specifically measures human chorionic gonadotropin in the presence of luteinizing hormone. *Am. J. Obstet. Gynecol.*, **113**, 751
7. Stevens, V. C. (1976). Actions of antisera to hCG-β: *in vitro* and *in vivo* assessment. In *Proceedings of the Fifth International Congress of Endocrinology*, Vol. I, p. 379. (Hamburg: Excerpta Medica International Congress Series No. 402)
8. Das, C., Talwar, G. P., Ramakrishman, S., Salahuddin, M., Kumar, S. and Hingorani, V. (1978). Discriminatory effect of anti-Pr-β-hCG-tt antibodies on the neutralization of the biological activity of placental and pituitary gonadotropins. *Contraception*, **18**, 35
9. Morgan, F. J., Birken, S. and Canfield, R. E. (1973). Human chorionic gonadotropin: a proposal for the amino acid sequence. *Mol. Cell. Biochem.*, **2**, 97
10. Louvet, J. P., Ross, G. T., Birken, S. and Canfield, R. E. (1974). Absence of neutralizing effects of antisera to the unique structural region of human chorionic gonadotropin. *J. Clin. Endocrinol. Metab.*, **39**, 1155
11. Matsura, S., Ohashi, M., Chen, J. and Hodgen, G. (1979). A human chorionic gonadotropin-specific antiserum against synthetic peptide analogues to the carboxyl-terminal peptide of its β-subunit. *Endocrinology*, **104**, 396
12. Chen, H., Hodgen, G. D., Matsura, S., Lin, L. J., Gross, E., Reichert, L. E., Birken, S., Canefield, R. E. and Ross, G. T. (1976). Evidence for a gonadotropin from nonpregnant subjects that has physical, immunological, and biological similarities to human chorionic gonadotropin. *Proc. Natl. Acad. Sci. USA*, **73**, 2885
13. Robertson, D. M., Suginami, H., Hernandez-Montes, H., Puri, C. P., Choi, S. K. and Diczfalusy, E. (1979). Studies on a chorionic gonadotropin-like material present in nonpregnant subjects. *Acta Endocrinol.*, **89**, 492
14. Anon (1978). Evaluating the safety and efficacy of placental antigen vaccines for fertility regulation. (Task Force on Immunological Methods for Fertility Regulation, WHO). *Clin. Exp. Immunol.*, **33**, 360

9
Vaccines Based on the Beta-subunit of HCG

G. P. TALWAR

CHEMISTRY AND CHARACTERISTICS OF THE SUBUNIT

The beta-subunit of HCG is a glycoprotein consisting of a polypeptide of 145 amino acid residues with six carbohydrate moieties[1,2]. Two of the sugar chains are linked to asparagine residues and the remaining four are attached to the serines located in the C-terminal end. The carbohydrate chains end with sialic acids, which contribute to the acidic charge of the molecule. The primary structure of the subunit is known. It bears large homologies with β-HLH. Figure 9.1 gives the comparative structure of the two hormonal subunits. It will be noted that β-HCG differs from β-HLH at 51 amino acid residues, 30 of which reside in the C-terminal part of the molecule. There are also some important amino acid substitutions in other parts of the molecule. A notable feature of the chemistry of this glycopeptide is the presence of 12 half-cytines. There is nevertheless, no titrable 'SH' groups in the native subunit, suggesting the existence of six intra-chain disulphide loops. These contribute to the conformation of the molecule in an important way, as reduction and alkylation results in the loss of the biological activity.

INDICATIONS OF IMMUNOLOGICAL INTEREST FROM BASIC CHEMISTRY

The primary structure of β-HCG is suggestive of the possibility of using the C-terminal portion of the molecule as antigen to obtain antibodies, which are completely non-reactive with HLH. The 30-amino acid unique portion at the

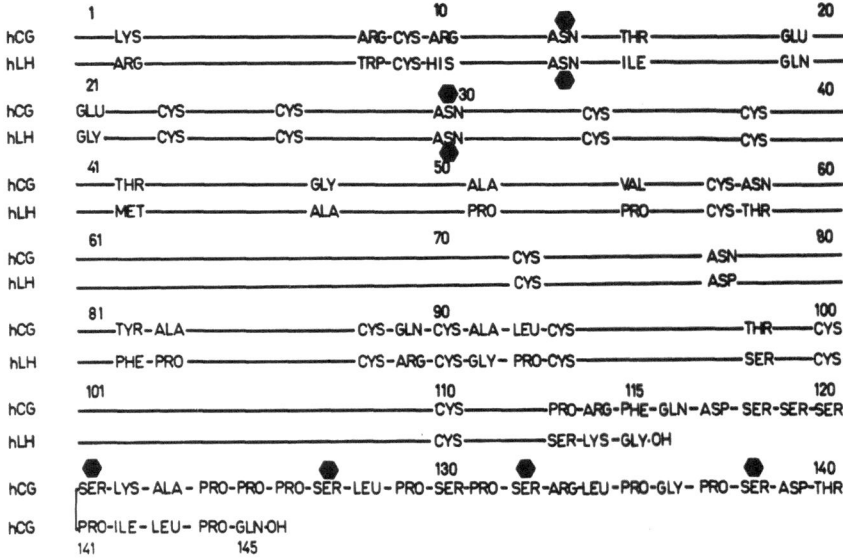

Figure 9.1 Amino acid sequence of the beta-subunit of HCG as proposed by Morgan *et al.*[2] and the beta-subunit of HLH according to Sairam and Li[3]. Solid lines indicate the positions at which identical amino acid residues are present. The location of cystine residues and the amino acid substitutions are individually represented. ● Symbol indicates the oligosaccharide chains linked to asparagine and serine residues. Note the presence of unique C-terminal sequence of 30 amino acid residues in β-HCG which has four serine linked sugar residues. The asparagine linked carbohydrates are present at identical places (13 and 30) in both the subunits

C-terminus has, however, no aromatic amino acids; it has nine prolines and eight serine residues. Circular dichroism studies show lack of any helical and beta-structures in this region (unpublished data).

The C-terminal peptides are poor immunogens as we have reported elsewhere[4]. Antibodies raised against the whole HCG and/or against the beta-subunit of HCG seldom bind to the C-terminal peptides; out of the 20 sera from monkeys and 13 sera from baboons checked by us, none contained antibodies reactive with epitopes located in the C-terminal end. However, if the tertiary structure is destroyed by breaking the S–S bonds, the anti-sera against the reduced alkylated β-HCG attain the ability to react with the C-terminal synthetic peptides.

Several factors suggest the presence of HCG unique conformations in β-HCG, as the sera raised with the subunit react preferentially with HCG and at times can be highly specific. The SB_6 serum of NIH raised by Vaitukaitis *et al.*[5] permitted the assay of HCG in presence of HLH. Similar sera have been obtained by many other investigators in a variety of animal species[6]. The immune system can thus recognize conformations in the β-HCG, which are distinct from those in β-HLH, besides the presence of overlapping regions, in the two hormonal subunits.

RELEVANT AREAS IN β-HCG FOR BIOLOGICAL ACTIVITY

The biologically active hormone is an associated molecule of two subunits, the alpha and the beta. This is the state in which relevant conformations are created for optimal biological activity. The alpha-subunit of HCG is, however, very nearly identical to that of LH, FSH and TSH[7,8] and as such the use of the total hormone as immunogen would provoke widespread cross-reaction with other pituitary hormones[9]. It is for this reason that beta-subunit of HCG is the first reductive possibility for an anti-HCG vaccine.

The beta-subunit by itself has very low biological activity. The dis-association of HCG, reduces the biological activity by 400-fold[10]. β-HCG has, however, some intrinsic biological activity. Figure 9.2 summarizes the pertinent experiments. Using Leydig cell bioassay system, it was noted that β-HCG could induce a dose-dependent increase in testosterone production. The C-terminal peptides were completely devoid of this capability. However, the synthetic peptide 39–71 as well as the enzyme cleaved fragment 1–40 . . . 50–114 had some capacity to stimulate steroidogenesis in the cells. These results suggest:

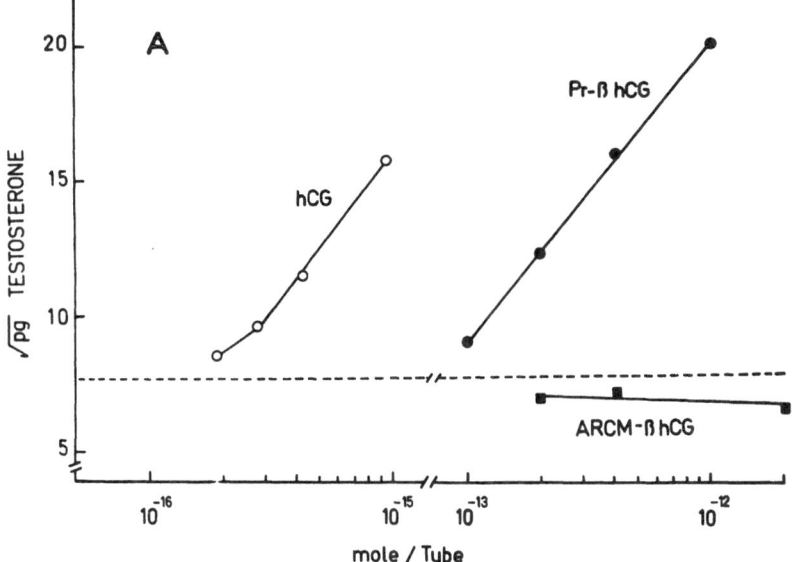

Figure 9.2a   Tissue receptor recognition of determinants in β-HCG. Effect of HCG (○) and immunochemically purified beta-subunit of HCG (●) on testosterone production by mouse Leydig cells *in vitro*. The assay was according to the method reported elsewhere[19]. The values shown are mean of quadruplicate determinations. Broken line denotes the basal production of testosterone by the Leydig cells in the absence of added gonadotropic stimulus. The reduced carboxymethylated derivative of asialo-β-HCG (ARCM-β-HCG) failed to stimulate steriodo-genesis up to a concentration of 2 pmol/assay tube.

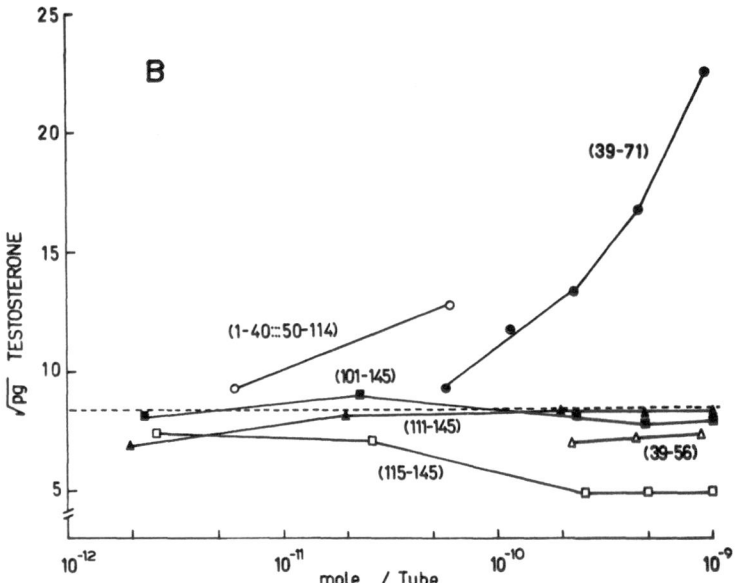

Figure 9.2b   Tissue receptor recognition of determinants in β-HCG. Effect of synthetic peptides and an enzyme-cleaved fragment of beta-subunit of HCG on testosterone production by mouse Leydig cells *in vitro*. □, C-terminal peptide 115–145; ▲, C-terminal peptide 111–145; ■, C-terminal peptide 101–145; △, Core 18 amino acid peptide 39–56; ●, Core 33 amino acid peptide 39–71; ○, thermolysin-cleaved fragment of asialo-β-HCG in which fragment 1–40 was linked to fragment 50–114 with disulfide bonds. (Data from Ramakrishnan *et al.*[10])

(1) The importance of the alpha- and beta-subunit association for obtaining the most appropriate conformations for biological activity.

(2) The residual presence of some conformations in β-HCG, recognized by the tissue receptors.

(3) The likely presence of some of these determinants in the core part of the molecule.

It is obvious that a vaccine to be effective must generate antibodies neutralizing the biological activity. This could best be done by intervention at sites binding to the receptors on the target tissue, though antibodies of high avidity reacting at other sites can theoretically scavenge the hormone and make it unavailable for sensitization of the target cells. All antibodies need not neutralize the hormonal activity as has been reported for β-TSH[11]. Some antibodies may even potentiate the activity by increasing its biological half-life in circulation, without masking the activity sites of the hormone. Louvet *et al.*[12] described the inability of the antibodies against the 23-amino acid C-terminal peptide obtained by enzyme cleavage of β-HCG to neutralize the biological activity of HCG. Similar observation has been made with antibodies generated against the last 30 amino acid residues (116–145) by Matsuura et al.[13].

THE β-HCG BASED VACCINE (Pr-β-HCG-TT)

Females are tolerant to HCG and will not normally evoke an immune response if HCG or a part thereof is administered. It can be rendered immunogenic by modification with haptenic groups or by linking it to immunogenic carriers. A vaccine was developed by conjugating immunochemically purified beta-subunit of HCG (Pr-β-HCG) to tetanus toxoid[14, 15]. A molar ratio of 10–12 β-HCG linked to each tetanus toxoid (TT) molecule was indicated to be appropriate by experiments in mice[16]. The conjugate Pr-β-HCG-TT was immunogenic in almost all species investigated. Antibodies were produced against both HCG and TT, conferring to the recipient an additional immunoprophylactic benefit of protection against tetanus. The antibodies reacted with HCG, were devoid of cross-reaction with TSH, FSH, GH and HPL and had only marginal cross-reaction with HLH. The association constants for binding with HCG ranged from 10^9–10^{11} L/M and for HLH 10^8–10^{10} L/M, showing that the antibodies had 5–10-fold higher affinity for HCG than for HLH[17]. The differential reactivity of the antibodies with HCG was also reflected in in vivo and in vitro experiments in which antibodies neutralized preferentially the biological activity of HCG, sparing by and large the LH bioactivity. An amount of antiserum inhibiting completely the HCG induced ovulation in primed mice, did not abolish oLH induced ovulation[18]. Injection of HCG (1500–6000 iu) to rhesus monkeys (actively immunized with Pr-β-HCG-TT) in the late luteal phase, did not result in a rise in plasma progesterone, whereas administration of HLH (75–180 iu) at similar periods of the cycle caused an increase in plasma progesterone values[19]. These experiments indicate that even though the antibodies had a certain degree of cross-reaction with HLH in the radioimmunoassays, the low cross-reaction did not suppress the biological action of LH. Monkeys, baboons and human subjects immunized with Pr-β-HCG-TT continued to ovulate normally with regular menstrual cycles in spite of circulating antibodies neutralizing HCG in vivo[20, 21] and in vitro[22].

The main advantages of using Pr-β-HCG-TT vis-à-vis the C-terminal peptides are:

(1) A much better immunogenicity than that observed with the C-terminal synthetic peptides.

(2) The properties of antibodies to neutralize the biological activity of HCG. An average of two to three antibody molecules are bound to one molecule of HCG, in contrast to essentially a monovalent binding obtained with antibodies produced against the C-terminal peptides[4].

SIDE-EFFECTS

Immunization with Pr-β-HCG-TT did not lead to any observable change in reproductive, endocrine, metabolic or organ function. There was no evidence of autoantibodies formation against DNA, rheumatoid factor, and the antisera did not react with other tissues.

The antibodies could effectively scavenge the exogenously administered HCG, forming biologically inactive complexes[19]. The complexes were not deposited in kidney and the choroid plexus. Autopsy of eight immunized animals repeatedly challenged with HCG did not reveal any gross or microscopic pathology[23].

EFFICACY

Immunization with β-HCG has been reported to prevent pregnancy in marmosets[24] and in baboons[25]. In a limited series of animals, we also found that baboons actively immunized with Pr-β-HCG-TT did not conceive on repeated matings[26]. There were however some who became pregnant. This may be due to the low and variable cross-reaction of the (baCG) antibodies with baboon chorionic gonadotropin. The baboon is an inappropriate model for the efficacy studies on the grounds of poor cross-reactivity of anti-β-HCG antibodies with baCG. There are differences in hormonal profiles in pregnancy and the dependence of chorionic gonadotropin support for luteal function is of short duration in this species as compared to the human. Chen and Hodgen[27] have further reported the relative lack of cross-reactivity of the antiserum raised against the C-terminal peptide of β-HCG with baCG when tested *in vitro*. If these results are valid *in vivo*, the baboon may not be an ideal model for studies with the vaccines based on the C-terminal peptides of β-HCG, and only marginally suitable for studies with β-HCG based vaccines.

Some recent experiments carried out by Atul Tandon in our laboratory, demonstrate the ability of the antibodies raised in·monkeys against Pr-β-HCG-TT to terminate pregnancy in baboons, although the quantity of immunoglobulins required to achieve this was substantial.

PHASE I CLINICAL TRIALS

Phase I clinical trials with this vaccine have been carried out in 63 women in six centres located in Delhi, Bombay, Helsinki, Uppsala, Santiago and Bahia. The women received three or four injections of Pr-β-HCG-TT given at fortnightly or monthly intervals. The amount of Pr-β-HCG injected ranged from 80 µg to 160 µg of β-HCG coupled to 10 Lf of TT. per injection. Antibodies reacting with HCG were detectable in circulation after a lag period of 6 weeks (Figure 9.3). The titres went up after the completion of the injection schedule. The antibodies persisted in circulation for a variable time period after which they declined to nearly zero levels. In each case the response was reversible. The duration of the antibody response in 'good' responders was between 300 and 500 days[15, 16, 28].

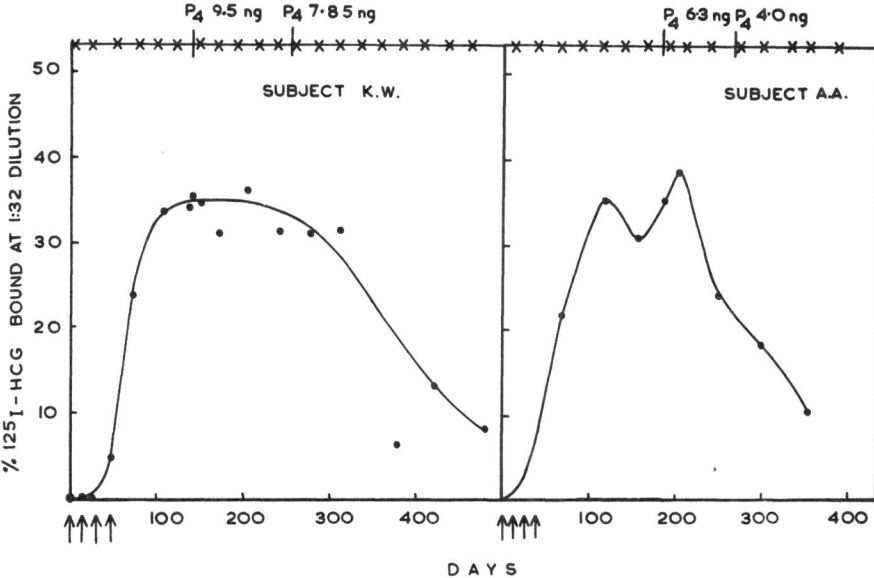

Figure 9.3 Representative picture of the kinetics of antibody response in two subjects immunized with the vaccine Pr-β-HCG-TT. The vaccine (80 μg Pr-β-HCG conjugated to 10 Lf of TT) was given intramuscularly at two contralateral sites adsorbed on alum. Arrows denote the time at which four injections of the vaccine were given. Ordinates represent the capacity of the sera for binding radioiodinated HCG. Crosses at the upper line denote the menstrual cycles. P_4 are the progesterone values in the luteal phase indicative of the ovulatory cycles.

The antibodies had the ability to recognize and neutralize HCG as is clearly shown by the clearance tests carried out in several immunized subjects[16, 20]. HCG alone did not act as a booster, and administration of the total conjugated material was required for the secondary immune response.

The immunized women had regular menstrual cycles with no significant change in the number of bleeding days and cycle length[29, 30]. Ovulation was evident by the level of plasma progesterone in the luteal phase and the endometrial biopsies carried out in some cases. All immunized subjects were examined clinically at periodic intervals, and extensive laboratory investigations carried out show the normalcy of metabolic, endocrine and other organ functions[30]. No evidence for autoantibodies such as rheumatoid factor, anti-DNA, anti-microsomal antibodies was observed[31]. Some of the women have now been under observation for a period of over 5 years, and no side-effects of any kind have been detected. In all immunized cases, the vaccine produced also anti-TT antibodies.

PROBLEMS

The main problem noticed in course of these studies, is the wide variability in immune response of individuals. Some women produce good antibody response (about 75 ng HCG binding per ml serum). Others produced modest and some had low titres. Some low responders became pregnant, the titres in them ranged from 1 to 6 ng/ml at the time when conception occurred. In many cases, pregnancy took place at a time when the immunization schedule of four injections was not completed. These observations indicate the absolute necessity of having high antibody titres to achieve efficacy. Research must continue to devise immunopotentiating agents, which are non-toxic and permissible for human use.

ECTOPIC SYNTHESIS OF HCG

Many reports have appeared recently on the synthesis and secretion of HCG by non-placental tissues[32-34]. Several trophoblastic and non-trophoblastic tumours make this fetoplacental protein[35-37]. It may be appropriate to investigate the possible utility of anti-HCG immunization in the suppression of metastasis of such tumours. Anti-β-HCG antibodies have been found to exercise cytotoxic effect on Bewo choriocarcinoma cell lines *in vitro*[38] in the presence of complement. Whether anti-HCG immunization can have similar suppressive effect *in vivo* remains to be seen.

Acknowledgement

This chapter was written during the tenure of Jawahar Lal Nehru Foundation Fellowship.

References

1. Morgan, F. J., Birken, S. and Canfield, R. E. (1973). Human chorionic gonadotropin: a proposal for the amino acid sequence. *Mol. Cell. Biochem.*, **2**, 97
2. Morgan, F. J., Birken, S. and Canfield, R. E. (1975). The amino acid sequence of human chorionic gonadotropin. The alpha-subunit and beta-subunit. *J. Biol. Chem.*, **250**, 5247
3. Sairam, M. R. and Li, C. H. (1975). Human pituitary lutropin. Isolation, properties and complete amino acid sequence of the beta-subunit. *Biochim. Biophys. Acta*, **412**, 70

4. Ramakrishnan, S., Das, C., Dubey, S. K., Salahuddin, M. and Talwar, G. P. (1979). Immunogenicity of three C-terminal synthetic peptides of the β-subunit of hCG and properties of the antibodies raised against 45-amino acid C-terminal peptide. *J. Reprod. Immunol.*, **1**, 249

5. Vaitukaitis, J. L., Braunstein, G. D. and Ross, G. T. (1972). A radioimmunoassay which specifically measures human chorionic gonadotropin in the presence of human luteinizing hormone. *Am. J. Obstet. Gynecol.*, **113**, 751

6. Salahuddin, M., Ramakrishnan, S., Dubey, S. K. and Talwar, G. P. (1976). Immunological reactivity of antibodies produced by Pr-β-hCG-TT with different hormones. *Contraception*, **13**, 163

7. Morgan, F. J., Birken, S. and Canfield, R. E. (1973). Comparison of human chorionic gonadotropin and luteinizing hormone: a note on a proposed significant structural difference in the β-subunit. *FEBS Lett.*, **31**, 101

8. Pierce, J. G., Faith, M., Giudice, L. C. and Reeve, J. R. (1976). Polypeptide hormones. Molecular and cellular aspects. *Structure and Structure–Function Relationships in Glycoprotein Hormones*. Ciba Foundation Symposium No. 41, pp. 225. (Amsterdam: Elsevier Excerpta Medica North-Holland)

9. Vaitukaitis, J. L., Ross, G. T., Reichert, L. E. Jr. and Ward, D. N. (1972). Immunologic basis for within and between species cross reactivity of luteinizing hormone. *Endocrinology*, **91**, 1337

10. Ramakrishnan, S., Das, C. and Talwar, G. P. (1978). Recognition of the beta-subunit of human chorionic gonadotropin and sub-determinants by target tissue receptors. *Biochem. J.*, **176**, 599

11. Beall, G. N., Chopra, I. J., Solomon, D. H., Pierce, J. G. and Cornell, J. S. (1973). Neutralizing and non-neutralizing antibodies to bovine TSH and its subunits. *J. Clin. Inves.*, **52**, 2979

12. Louvet, J. P., Ross, G. T., Birken, S. and Canfield, R. E. (1974). Absence of neutralizing effect of antisera to the unique structural region of human chorionic gonadotropin. *J. Clin. Endocrinol. Metab.*, **39**, 1155

13. Matsuura, S., Ohashi, M., Chen, H. C. and Hodgen, G. D. (1979). A hCG specific antiserum against synthetic peptide analogs to the C-terminal peptide of its beta-subunit. *Endocrinology*, **104**, 396

14. Talwar, G. P., Sharma, N. C., Dubey, S. K., Salahuddin, M., Shastri, N. and Ramakrishnan, S. (1976). Processing of the preparations of β-subunit of human chorionic gonadotropin for minimization of cross-reactivity with human luteinizing hormone. *Contraception*, **13**, 131

15. Talwar, G. P., Dubey, S. K., Salahuddin, M. and Shastri, N. (1976). Kinetics of antibody response in animals injected with processed beta-hCG conjugated to tetanus toxoid (Pr-β-hCG-TT). *Contraception*, **13**, 153

16. Talwar, G. P., Sharma, N. C., Dubey, S. K., Salahuddin, M., Das, C., Ramakrishnan, S., Kumar, S. and Hingorani, V. (1976). Isoimmunization against human chorionic gonadotropin with conjugates of processed β-subunit of the hormone and tetanus toxoid. *Proc. Natl. Acad. Sci. (USA)*, **73**, 218

17. Shastri, N., Dubey, S. K., Vijaya Raghavan, S., Salahuddin, M. and Talwar, G. P. (1978). Differential affinity of anti-Pr-β-hCG-TT antibodies for hCG and hLH. *Contraception*, **18**, 23

18. Das, C., Talwar, G. P., Ramakrishnan, S., Salahuddin, M., Kumar, S., Hingorani, V., Coutinho, E., Croxatto, H., Hemmingson, E., Johansson, E., Luukkainen, T., Shahani, S., Sundaram, K., Nash, H. and Segal, S. J. (1978). Discriminatory effect of anti-Pr-β-hCG-TT antibodies on the neutralization of the biological activity of placental and pituitary gonadotropins. *Contraception*, **18**, 35

19. Ramakrishnan, S., Das, C. and Talwar, G. P. (1978). Progesterone levels in monkeys immunized with Pr-β-hCG-TT after injection of hLH and hCG during luteal phase. *Contraception*, **18**, 51

20. Ramakrishnan, S., Dubey, S. K., Das, C., Salahuddin, M., Talwar, G. P., Kumar, S. and Hingorani, V. (1976). Influence of hCG and tetanus toxoid injections on the antibody titers in a subject immunized with Pr-β-hCG-TT. *Contraception*, **13**, 245

21. Ramakrishnan, S., Das, C. and Talwar, G. P. (1978). Nature of immune complexes formed in rhesus monkeys immunized with Pr-β-hCG-TT on challenge with hCG. *Contraception*, **18**, 71

22. Das, C., Salahuddin, M. and Talwar, G. P. (1976). Investigations on the ability of antisera produced by Pr-β-hCG-TT to neutralize the biological activity of hCG. *Contraception*, **13**, 171

23. Gupta, P. D., Nath, I. and Talwar, G. P. (1978). Immunofluorescence and electron microscopic studies on kidney, choroid plexus and pituitary in rhesus monkeys immunized with the anti-hCG vaccine Pr-β-hCG-TT. *Contraception*, **18**, 91

24. Hearn, J. P. (1979). Long term suppression of fertility by immunization with hCG-β subunit and its reversibility in female marmoset monkeys. In Talwar, G. P. (ed.) *Recent Advances in Reproduction and Regulation of Fertility*, pp. 427–438. (Amsterdam: Elsevier/North-Holland)

25. Stevens, V. C. (1976). Prospectives of development of a fertility control vaccine from hormonal antigens of the trophoblast. In *Development of Vaccines for Fertility Regulation*, pp. 93–110. (Copenhagen: Scriptor)

26. Talwar, G. P., Das, C., Tandon, A., Sharma, M. G., Salahuddin, M. and Dubey, S. K. (1979). Immunization against hCG: efficacy and tetarological studies on baboons. *Proceedings of the VIIth Congress of the International Primatological Society, Bangalore*, 8–12 January (In press)

27. Chen, H. C. and Hodgen, G. D. (1976). Primate chorionic gonadotropins: antigenic similarities to the unique carboxyl terminal peptide of hCG-β subunit. *J. Clin. Endocrinol. Metab.*, **43**, 1414

28. Hingorani, V. and Kumar, S. (1979). Anti-hCG immunization – Phase I clinical trials. In Talwar, G. P. (ed.) *Recent Advances in Reproduction and Regulation of Fertility*, pp. 467–472. (Amsterdam: Elsevier/North-Holland)

29. Shahani, S. M., Kulkarni, P. P. and Patel, K. L. (1979). Evaluation of immunological and safety data in women treated with Pr-β-hCG-TT vaccine. In Talwar, G. P. (ed.) *Recent Advances in Reproduction and Regulation of Fertility*, pp. 473–476 (Amsterdam: Elsevier/North-Holland)

30. Kumar, S., Sharma, N. C., Bajaj, J. S., Talwar, G. P. and Hingorani, V. (1976). Clinical profile and toxicology studies on four women immunized with Pr-β-hCG-TT. *Contraception*, **13**, 253

31. Nath, I., Whittingham, S., Lambert, P. H. and Talwar, G. P. (1976). Screening for antoantibodies in human subjects immunized with Pr-β-hCG-TT. *Contraception*, **13**, 225

32. Braunstein, G. D., Rasor, J. and Wade, M. E. (1975). Presence in normal testes of a chorionic gonadotropin like substance distinct from human luteinizing hormone. *N. Engl. J. Med.*, **293**, 1339

33. Chen, H. C., Hodgen, G. D., Matsuura, S., Lin, L. J., Gross, E., Reichert, L. E. Jr., Birken, S., Canfield, R. E. and Ross, G. T. (1976). Evidence for a gonadotropin from non-pregnant subjects that has physical, immunological and biological similarities to hCG. *Proc. Natl. Acad. Sci. (USA)*, **73**, 2885

34. Yoshimoto, Y., Nolfsen, A. A. and Odell, W. D. (1977). Human chorionic gonadotropin like substance in non-endocrine tissues of normal subjects. *Science*, **197**, 575

35. Braunstein, G. D., Vaitukaitis, J. L., Carbone, P. P. and Ross, G. T. (1973). Ectopic production of hCG by neoplasms. *Ann. Intern. Med.*, **78**, 39

36. Gilani, S., Chu, T. M., Mussbaum, A., Ostrander, M. and Christoff, N. (1976). HCG in non-trophoblastic neoplasms. *Cancer*, **38**, 1684

37. Braunstein, G. D. (1979). Human chorionic gonadotropin in non-trophoblastic tumours and tissues. In Talwar, G. P. (ed.) *Recent Advances in Reproduction and Regulation of Fertility*, pp. 389–397. (Amsterdam: Elsevier/North-Holland)

38. Gupta, S. K., Buckshee, K. and Talwar, G. P. (1979). Effect of anti-hCG antibodies on tumour cells secreting hCG. Presented at the *4th Asian Cancer Conference*, December 4–8, Bombay

10
The Immunobiology of Chorionic Gonadotrophin

J. P. HEARN

INTRODUCTION

The last 10 years have seen a revolution in our understanding of the structure and functions of chorionic gonadotrophin (CG). Until the early seventies it was thought to be a glycoprotein hormone restricted to pregnancy in primates. It was known to be secreted by the trophoblast and assumed to be a major component of the luteotrophic stimulus that supports the corpus luteum of primates until the luteoplacental shift is completed[1-3]. While this role in early pregnancy, backed by a great deal of circumstantial evidence, is still accepted, we are now fairly certain that the hormone is restricted neither to pregnancy nor to primates.

The prospect of using antibodies raised against the β-subunit of human chorionic gonadotrophin (HCG-β) or synthetic fragments of it as a vaccine for long-term fertility control, generated widespread studies on this hormone in recent years; providing a great deal of new information on the hormone itself as well as on its biological effects. This is perhaps a little surprising as CG is also one of the oldest known hormones. Its discovery in the urine of pregnant women by Ascheim and Zondek in 1927[4] led to a vast literature over the subsequent 30 years. Indeed its presence was suspected earlier by Halban[54], who in 1905 suggested that the placenta was the source of substances that exerted profound effects on the mother during pregnancy and by Aschner[5], who in 1913 experimented with human placental extracts on guinea-pigs.

The new era for CG started in 1971 when Canfield et al.[55] and Pierce et al.[56] discovered the subunit structure of the gonadotrophins and thyroid stimulating hormone, showing that they exist in the form of α- and β-subunits; the α-subunit being immunologically similar in LH, FSH, TSH and HCG while the β-subunit was immunologically distinct and contained these hormones' biological specificity. Their finding explained the lack of immunological specificity seen between antisera raised against the whole hormones and allowed a fresh start to be made in efforts to immunize against pregnancy using the specific β-subunit of HCG. Previous attempts had failed because antibodies to whole HCG cross-reacted with LH and FSH, preventing follicular development and ovulation both in baboons and in women[6,7]. The current status of the field, including the attempts to apply vaccines against HCG-β as a method of fertility control in women, is reviewed by Stevens and Talwar in Chapters 8 and 9 respectively. In this chapter I will review briefly the occurrence of CG outside pregnancy and summarize our own studies on the long-term effects of immunizing female marmoset monkeys against HCG-β, concentrating on their fertility and on the reversibility of the 'vaccine'; and discussing the roles of CG in addition to that as a luteotrophin in early pregnancy.

CHORIONIC GONADOTROPHIN DURING PREGNANCY

In primates, the secretion of CG by the trophoblast is thought to be responsible for the 'rescue' of the corpus luteum when it would normally decline at the end of the luteal phase of the cycle, transforming it into the corpus luteum of pregnancy[2,8,9]. The maternal endocrine system 'recognizes' pregnancy through this mechanism (Figure 10.1) and its result is the continued secretion of progesterone, essential for the support of early pregnancy until implantation has occurred and the luteoplacental shift in progesterone production is well advanced. We know that in the human[1], the marmoset[10] and the Rhesus monkey[11], ovariectomy or luteectomy does not interrupt pregnancy after the 6–7th week, by which time the placenta is sufficiently established to produce sufficient progesterone on its own.

With the assays that are available, the first measurement of CG in pregnancy in primates coincides with the timing of early implantation (Table 10.1). While an early claim[12] suggested the possible secretion of CG by the pre-

Table 10.1 The days of gestation when embryo attachment and the first detection of chorionic gonadotrophin are reported for five primate species

Species	Days of gestation		
	Embryo attachment	CG first detected	References
Human	5½–6	7–8	14, 15
Chimpanzee	9–10	11	16
Baboon	8–9	12	17
Rhesus	8–9	12	18
Marmoset	After 8	10	19

implantation blastocyst, the balance of current opinion is that CG secretion is initiated once embryo attachment and trophoblast penetration of the endometrium has commenced. However it is not yet possible for us to measure the secretion of CG at the implantation site and the above opinion may have to be revised in the next few years. In non-primates there have been intermittent claims for the secretion of steroids or gonadotrophins by the blastocyst (for a summary see reference 8) and in a recent paper Fischel and Surani[13] have demonstrated for the first time the synthesis and release of a major glycoprotein by the preimplantation mouse blastocyst. In the Rhesus monkey, Batta and Channing[31] have isolated a secretory product of the preimplantation blastocyst cultured *in vitro* that is capable of stimulating progesterone production by granulosa cell cultures.

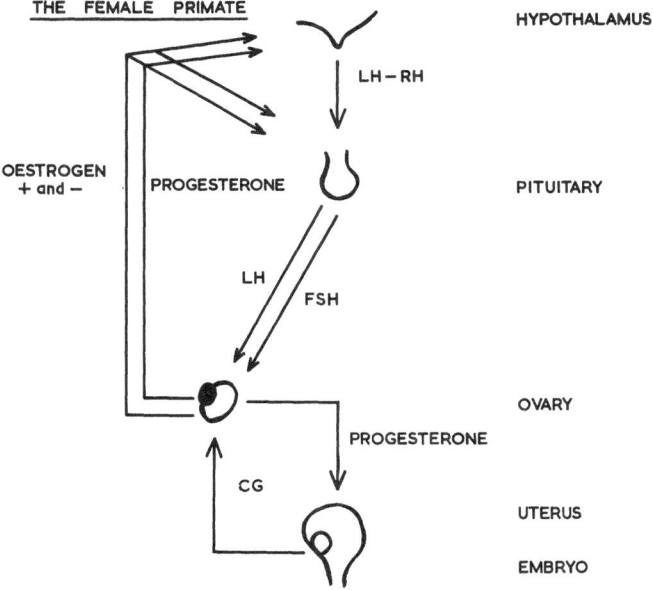

Figure 10.1   During early pregnancy in primates the corpus luteum depends on a luteotrophic stimulus, of which CG from the conceptus is thought to be a major part. Immunization against the specific β-subunit of CG should therefore cause premature luteal regression. Specific antisera raised against the β-subunit should not cross-react with the other gonadotrophins or TSH

The restriction of chorionic gonadotrophin to primates may need reconsideration as Wide and Hobson[20] have found biologically active gonadotrophins, with a similar chromatographic profile to HCG and its subunits, in the placentae of the rat, mouse and hamster. Moreover, Haour *et al.*[21] measured elevated 'gonadotrophin' levels from day 10–16 in the rat. We know that pituitary LH is necessary for pregnancy in the rat and mouse until day 10–11[22] and perhaps the placenta has a role in the gonadotrophic support of later pregnancy in these species. There are also reports of CG like proteins with biological activity during pregnancy in the rock hyrax and springhare[23].

Returning to the human, the profile of chorionic gonadotrophin shows a rapid rise to peak levels between weeks 8 and 14 of pregnancy, then declining to still considerable levels that are secreted throughout the remainder of pregnancy[24]. Noting that pregnancy can proceed after luteectomy in the 7th week of pregnancy[1], before CG levels have even reached their peak, one must ask whether the role of this hormone is restricted merely to the support of the corpus luteum? If so, there is an awful lot of redundant hormone being secreted through the remainder of pregnancy. Additional functions of CG in pregnancy for which evidence, although circumstantial, is accumulating, are in the stimulation and differentiation of the fetal gonads[25] and as an immunosuppressant, protecting the fetal allograft from maternal immune rejection[26-29].

The role of CG as an immunosuppressant in pregnancy or tumours has become something of a bandwagon and the data supporting this claim are critically reviewed by Des Cooper in Chapter 2. The recent demonstration by Muchmore and Blaese[30] that contaminants in the available preparations of CG have the immunosuppressant effects that have been attributed to the hormone calls the previous claims into question. Certainly if all of the 'immunosuppressant effects' claimed for a series of steroid and protein hormones during pregnancy were valid, the human species would be extinct as pregnant women would be extraordinarily vulnerable to infection. However, high local concentrations of CG or other substances at the maternal–fetal interface might exert an immunosuppressive or masking effect without jeopardizing the general maternal immune system where much lower concentrations would be circulating.

CHORIONIC GONADOTROPHIN APART FROM PREGNANCY

The production of CG by trophoblast tumours has been recognized for many years and the tumours have been monitored by measurement of CG production[32,33]. Over the last 5 years reports have proliferated on the secretion of CG from non-trophoblastic tumours, non-neoplastic lesions and, indeed, from normal tissues in men and women. The bulk of the evidence suggests that CG is not a pregnancy specific hormone and may have biological roles in normal tissues. While many of the reports can be questioned on the basis of inadequately validated assays, there is undoubtedly enough evidence from highly specific assays used with meticulous control material to support the widespread production of CG apart from that in pregnancy and from trophoblastic tumours.

With the advent of assays that could distinguish between HCG and HLH and thereby measure circulating levels of CG below those of circulating LH, it became possible to measure the low levels of CG that are secreted by non-trophoblastic tumours. The data from the retrospective and prospective studies of several investigators showed that CG was secreted in 19.3% of 3880 patients examined[34]. The highest proportions of positive CG secreting tumours were found in patients with gynaecological, breast, lung, gastro-intestinal tract tumours and in malignant melanomas. Braunstein suggests[34] that far higher proportions of tumours produce CG in low levels. A large series of investigations show that CG may also be measured in the serum of normal subjects or those with benign diseases, although the proportion of positive cases is small, for example 14.2% in gynaecological ($n = 120$), 8% in gastrointestinal ($n = 255$) and 4.6% in breast ($n = 152$) disorders, giving an overall incidence of CG production in 5.4% of patients with benign diseases ($n = 1085$) and of 0.6% in normal subjects ($n = 1577$)[33, 34].

It is therefore not surprising that since Ghosh and Cox reported the production of CG by HeLa cells *in vitro*[35], the reports of CG production by malignant cell lines *in vitro* have also multiplied. Recently Rosen *et al.*[36] found that 13 of 33 malignant cell lines examined produced HCG or its β-subunit.

Many of the reports of production of CG outside pregnancy and trophoblastic disease are stretching the available assays to the limit, using the uppermost end of the standard curve where both precision and specificity are poorest. Further improvements in the assays will be required before we are fully confident of the results. The very low levels measured by immunological reactions in test tubes may be genuine, but they may also be measurements of metabolic products of gonadotrophins that share enough amino acids and immunological determinants to be bound by specific antisera, while not necessarily retaining the biological effects of the whole hormone or its subunits. But if studies of the structure and biological effects of CG found in non-pregnant normal patients confirm its presence we will need to recognize that the genome responsible for CG production in the trophoblast is not fully suppressed in the adult.

IMMUNIZATION AGAINST HCG-β SUBUNIT IN MARMOSETS

The current status of attempts to produce vaccines against pregnancy based on HCG-β subunit or on synthetic fractions of it is summarized by Vernon Stevens in Chapter 8 and Pran Talwar in Chapter 9. The latter also gives details of preliminary clinical trials. In our studies since 1972 we have used the marmoset monkey as an animal model, first to demonstrate the efficacy of antibodies to HCG-β in interrupting early pregnancy and suppressing subsequent fertility; and secondly to examine the reversibility of the treatment.

We chose the common marmoset, *Callithrix jacchus* (Figure 10.2) for these studies for the simple reason that it is a primate that breeds well in captivity. With a mean cycle length of 16 days and a pregnancy of 144 days, normal production of twins and sexual maturity at 18 months[10, 37–40], the marmoset can be established in self-supporting colonies in a relatively short time providing high quality laboratory primates for research. Elevated levels of CG can be measured from day 10 of pregnancy in this primate and preliminary results show that implantation commences between days 8 and 10[10, 39]. With its rapid rate of reproduction, lack of seasonal breeding and early attainment

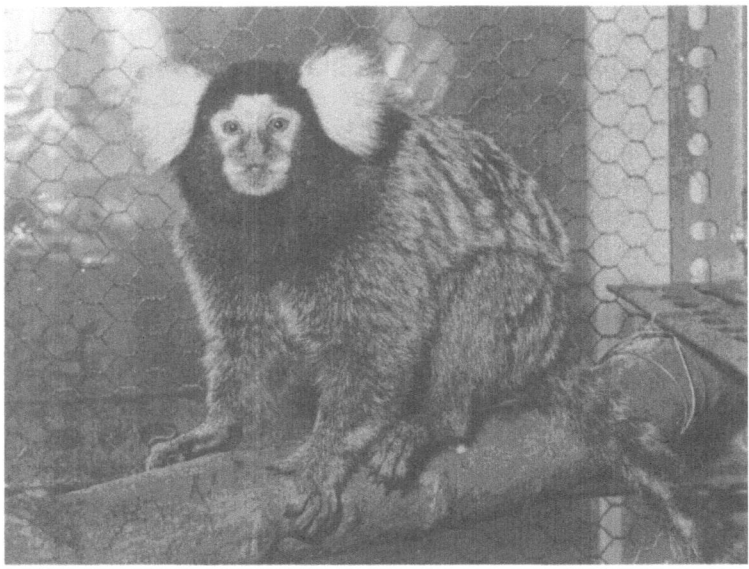

Figure 10.2   The marmoset, *Callithrix jacchus*, is a small New World primate (adult body weight about 400 g). Marmosets breed throughout the year and normally produce twins. They have an ovarian cycle with a mean of 16 days and a pregnancy of 144 days. They settle well to captive breeding and are easy to train for experimental procedures

of sexual maturity, when compared with any of the more conventional primate models, long-term studies on the reversibility of HCG immunization were possible. Marmosets were kept in stable male–female pairs throughout the studies outlined below, with any young produced living with the family group until they reached the onset of puberty at about 14 months of age.

Active immunization

After active immunization, using a dose of 100 μg HCG-β emulsified in Freund's adjuvant and injected in 6–10 subdermal sites, antibody titres rose in all animals immunized to plateau levels within 6–10 weeks. High levels of antibody could be measured within 10 days. Animals that were in early pregnancy (< 6 weeks) aborted within 25 days and remained infertile for 8–16 months until antibody titres declined[41, 42]. Control animals immunized against Freund's adjuvant alone showed no disruption of pregnancy.

Animals immunized between 6 and 10 weeks of pregnancy resorbed their fetuses, without any apparent risk to the mother, while those immunized after the 10th week of pregnancy showed no interruption and the pregnancies proceeded to term. Controls immunized against Freund's adjuvant alone showed no disruption of pregnancy.

Passive immunization

Plasma collected from actively immunized marmosets with high, plateau levels of circulating antibodies to HCG-β was pooled and used in experiments employing passive immunization. With a dose of 0.5–1.0 ml of this pooled antiserum, early pregnancy could be terminated within 2 days after the injection (intramuscular), but at this dose level no effects were produced if immunization was carried out after the 6th week of pregnancy. Controls, in all cases given the same doses of normal marmoset plasma, showed no interruption of pregnancy[41, 42].

Reversibility

As antibody titres declined, we noted that the cycle lengths of immunized marmosets were becoming extended. The animals experienced recurrent abortions that occurred later in pregnancy as antibody titres continued to wane. Some produced live young after apparently normal pregnancies but this was no guarantee of a return to normal fertility as additional abortions followed. A summary of the breeding history of one such monkey is shown in Figure 10.3.

Booster immunization with HCG-β, given 2½ years after primary immunization, led to a rapid return of high antibody titres and to 'normal' cycles. 3–4 months after booster immunizations, the uteri of experimental and control animals were flushed during the luteal phase 6–8 days after ovulation. Apparently normal blastocysts, still in their zonae, were recovered indicating that circulating antibodies to CG do not interfere with preimplantation embryo development.

As antibody titres declined once more, the same phenomenon of recurrent abortions experienced earlier became apparent. The fetoplacental unit was recovered through hysterotomy from three immunized and three control animals at an estimated 1 week before predicted abortion in the immunized monkeys. Analysis of peripheral and uteroovarian vein progesterone levels showed no significant differences from the normal controls and light microscopy showed no lesions in the placenta or fetus that might explain the recurrent abortions[43, 44]. There was no evidence that recurrent pregnancies, with their production of endogenous CG, boosted the circulating levels of antibodies to HCG; similar findings have been reported by Talwar in tests where he has administered injections of HCG to women with declining titres of anti-HCG-β[45].

Table 10.2 summarizes our findings using active or passive immunization against HCG-β to suppress the fertility of marmoset monkeys.

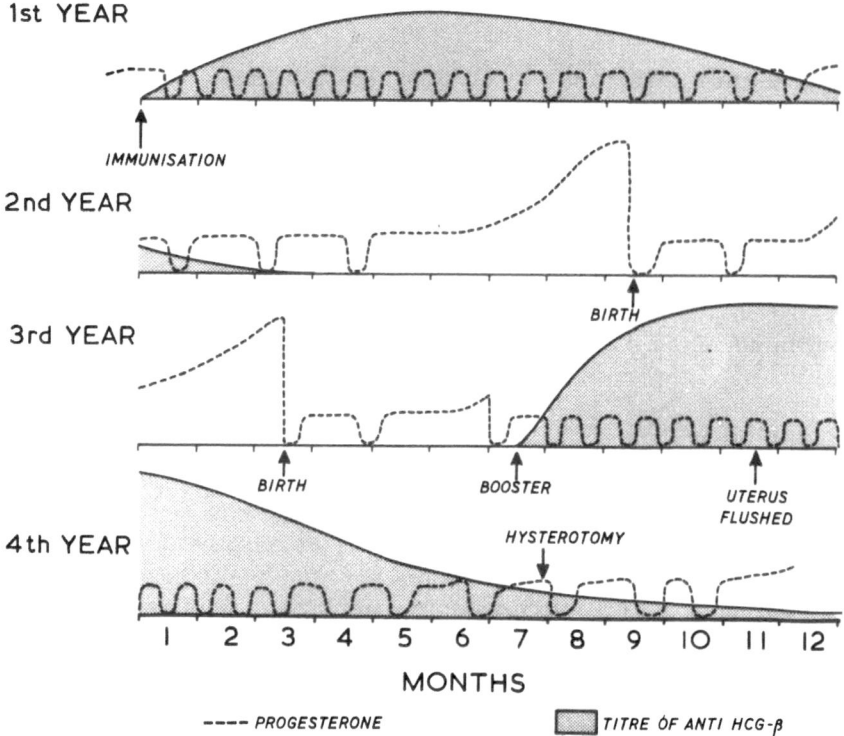

Figure 10.3 A summary of the breeding history, over 4 years, of a female marmoset immunized against HCG-β subunit. When antibody titres were high pregnancy did not extend beyond the length of the normal cycle, but with decline of antibody titres cycles became extended and recurrent abortions were noted. Pregnancies were diagnosed by RIA and by uterine palpation. When pregnancies went beyond the 12th week of gestation they proceeded to term and apparently normal young were born. This did not mean a resumption of normal fertility as such births were usually followed by a return to recurrent abortions.

A booster injection 2½ years after immunization caused a repetition of events seen after the primary immunization. Blastocysts were recovered at uterine flushing 5 days after ovulation in animals with high titres, indicating that the process of ovulation, fertilization and blastocyst formation continued in presence of antibodies. There was no evidence that successive pregnancies boosted antibody titres during the period of decline. In animals hysterotomized 1 week before predicted abortion, there were no histopathological or endocrine changes that might explain the causes of the abortions

Table 10.2 Summary of effects of active and passive immunization against HCG-β on pregnancy and on resumption of fertility in 10 (active) and 15 (passive) immunized female marmosets when compared with controls (4 per group). The normal gestation period in the marmoset is 144 ± 2 days

	Active immunization	Passive immunization
Ovarian cycles	Continue as normal when titres high, become extended as titres begin to decline	Not examined
Early pregnancy (<42 days)	Abortion 17–25 days after immunization. Dose: 100 μg HCG-β in Freund's adjuvant	Abortion 2 days later. Dose: 0.5–1.0 ml marmoset anti-HCG antiserum of high titre
Mid pregnancy (42–84 days)	Resorption of fetuses with no risk to mother. Dose: as above	Pregnancy proceeds. Dose: 0.5–1.0 ml
Late pregnancy (84–144 days)	Pregnancy proceeds. Dose: as above	Pregnancy proceeds. Dose: as above
Resumption of fertility	8–16 months after immunization depending on titre and affinity of antibodies	2–4 weeks after immunization
Complications	Recurrent abortions over 2–3 years as titres decline	None apparent

Antibodies to HCG-β in fetal fluids

Figure 10.4 shows the levels of antibodies to HCG-β measured in maternal plasma and in fetal fluids in three marmoset monkeys 24 h after passive immunization with 0.5 ml anti-HCG-β. Similar results were obtained after active immunization. Clearly the antibodies can pass easily through the placenta into the fetal fluids.

Antibodies to HCG-β in milk

Figure 10.5 shows the levels of antibodies to HCG-β measured in the peripheral plasma and milk of a lactating marmoset over a 40-day period after passive immunization with 0.5 ml anti-HCG-β. Clearly the antibodies can pass easily into the milk.

Affinity of antibodies to HCG-β

The measure of titre allows us to monitor the presence and amounts of circulating antibody in the plasma or other fluids of marmoset monkeys after active or passive immunization against HCG-β, but the affinity of the antibodies is more important in interpreting their effects. In a recent study[46] we

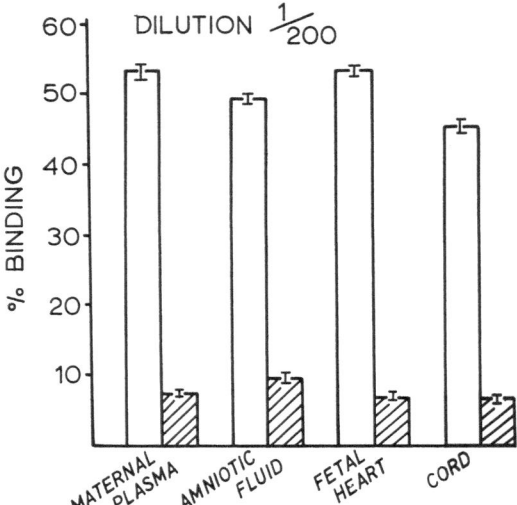

Figure 10.4 The levels of antibodies to HCG-β subunit, 24 h after intramuscular injection with 0.5 ml marmoset anti-HCG-β, in maternal plasma, amniotic fluid, fetal heart and cord plasma of three monkeys and six fetuses. Maximal binding was found in all cases indicating that antibodies easily cross the placenta. The hatched bars are the levels in control animals injected with 0.5 ml normal marmoset plasma, indicating the non-specific binding inherent in the assay

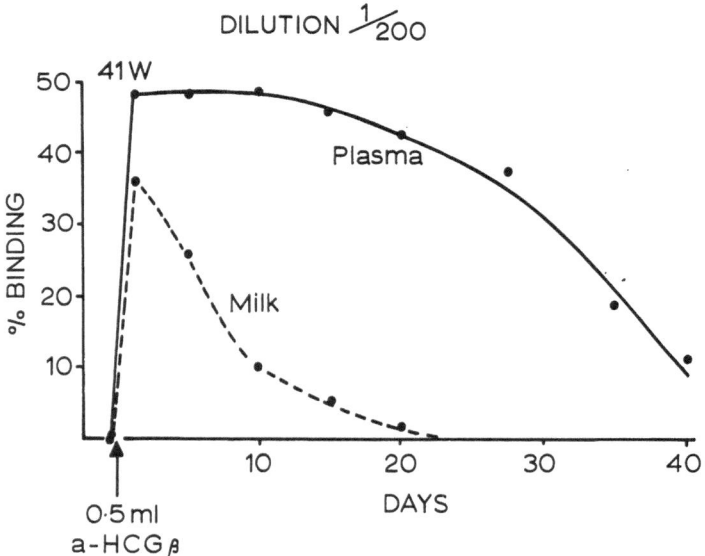

Figure 10.5 The levels of antibodies to HCG-β in the peripheral plasma and milk of marmoset 41W for 40 days after intramuscular injection of 0.5 ml marmoset anti-HCG-β. The results show that antibodies pass into the milk. Values shown are corrected for 8–10% non-specific binding found in control plasma

showed that affinity is not correlated to titre and, when marmosets with declining antibody titres become pregnant, there is a transient drop in antibody affinity. It may be that this is simply a preferential removal of high affinity antibodies by the endogenous CG produced by the pregnancy, but low affinity antibodies would be less able to bind CG in competition against high affinity sites in the corpus luteum, allowing pregnancy to proceed in the presence of antibodies to CG.

Effects on the fetus

When antibody titres and affinities are high, pregnancy does not proceed beyond the normal length of the cycle, implying that implantation is blocked. The recovery of blastocysts from marmosets with high antibody titres shows that immunization of the mother against HCG-β subunit does not suppress ovulation by cross-reacting with endogenous LH, nor does it prevent conception and development of the blastocyst. However, with falling antibody titres the recurrent abortions described show that antibodies terminate early pregnancy, though it is not clear whether they do so by neutralizing luteotrophic support or by direct effects on the trophoblast. Morisada[29] has shown that antibodies to CG can have cytotoxic effects on trophoblastic tissues.

Whatever the mechanisms of suppression of fertility by antibodies to HCG-β subunit, they terminate pregnancy at or after implantation, so that the method is an abortifacient and not a contraceptive.

Once the antibody affinity has declined to the degree that a proportion of pregnancies can proceed in marmosets, there are no evident effects on the young born. Five female and two male marmosets born to females with low levels of circulating antibodies, studied up to 4 years of age, showed normal growth and endocrine development to sexual maturity. Both males have successfully sired young and four of the females have produced young; the last female is approaching sexual maturity. Consequently there do not appear to be any adverse effects of exposure to low levels of anti-HCG-β during fetal or neonatal life on these animals' subsequent reproductive performance. It may well be that once antibody affinities are low, receptor sites in the fetal gonads can compete successfully for CG from weakly bound antibody–antigen complexes that would be circulating. In any event suggestions that CG is required for fetal gonadal differentiation are still based almost entirely on circumstantial evidence[25].

FUTURE PROSPECTS

It is one thing to demonstrate a mechanism on which a potential new approach to fertility control may be based. It is quite another to develop the approach for widespread application to human fertility. The demonstration, in the mid-1970s, that HCG could be made immunogenic and that antibodies would prevent pregnancy in primates[41, 45, 47] led to optimistic forecasts of rapid development for use in women. The strong investigative tool that immunization against HCG-β gave us to study the production and function of CG is showing that the secretion and biological functions of this hormone may be more widespread and complex than our simplistic views supposed of its restriction to the support of the corpus luteum. There is still inadequate knowledge of the mechanisms of action and of possible toxicological or teratological effects, as well as of the reversibility of the method.

The poor immunogenecity of HCB-β in women, reported in Chapter 9 and elsewhere[48, 49], suggests that advances are required in the development of acceptable adjuvants. There is as yet no demonstration that adequate antibody titres of sufficiently high affinity can be produced in women to protect against pregnancy. Those women that have been immunized have experienced short-duration, low-level antibody levels that tell us nothing of the potential immune complex problems that could be attached to high-affinity antibodies circulating for long periods necessary to provide effective fertility regulation. The dilemma is that such data in primates, unless immunized against homologous hormone, are questionable and provision of the data would take several more years to accumulate.

The criticism that HCG used in primate models is of limited value because of its heterologous nature may also be levelled at the effects we have seen in marmosets that show recurrent abortions. We know that marmoset CG does not cross-react avidly with HCG-β *in vitro*, i.e. in radioimmunoassay[50]. On the other hand it can be argued that cross-reaction in a test tube is quite irrelevant, as the biological cross-reaction *in vivo* is a great deal wider, both between hormones and between species. We know that marmoset chorionic gonadotrophin and HCG will cross-react strongly *in vivo*[51]. We also know from the vast literature on CG stimulation that receptors in the testis and ovary will bind CG. A further problem is that antibodies raised to the whole HCG-β subunit, even in the most purified form currently available, will bind to the pituitary and cross-react to a limited extent with HLH[53].

The recent findings[52] that normal men, women and children may have naturally occurring low-affinity antibodies to HCG circulating in their blood adds another dimension to the uncertainty over the occurrence and functions of CG in the body. The next few years may show that claims for the presence of CG or antibodies to it in normal tissues are artefacts of rapidly developing assay technology but until it does we should proceed with caution in any attempts to immunize humans with HCG.

With the availability of purer preparations of CG from humans as well as from primates, and perhaps the development of monoclonal antibodies, we should have excellent tools with which to study the functions of CG during and outside pregnancy. Apart from the scientific knowledge this will provide in our understanding of cellular mechanisms, implantation and fetal development, there may be opportunities to assist with problems of embryonic loss due to hormonal insufficiency or with the improved diagnosis and control of CG secreting tumours.

Whatever the future holds, CG is no longer a hormone that is restricted to early pregnancy in primates.

Acknowledgements

I am grateful to Mr Stephen Lunn and Mrs Pamela Chambers for their help in aspects of this work, to Mr Frank Burden for the care and maintenance of the animals and to the Medical Research Council for their financial support. I thank Professor Bob Canfield and the National Institutes of Health, USA, for supplies of HCG-β subunit.

References

1. Csapo, A. I., Pulkkinen, M. O., Ruttner, B., Sauvage, J. P. and Wiest, W. G. (1972). The significance of the human corpus luteum in pregnancy maintenance. *Am. J. Obstet. Gynecol.*, **112**, 1061
2. Short, R. V. (1969). Implantation and the maternal recognition of pregnancy. In *Ciba Foundation Symposium on Fetal Autonomy*, pp. 2–26. (London: Churchill)
3. Heap, R. B. and Perry, J. S. (1974). The maternal recognition of pregnancy. *Br. J. Hosp. Med.*, July, 8
4. Aschheim, S. and Zondek, B. (1927). Hypophysenvorderlappenhormon und Ovarialhormon im Harn von Schwangeren. *Klin. Wochenschr.*, **6**, 1322
5. Aschner, B. (1913). Ueber brunstartige Erscheinungen (Hyperämie und Hämorrhagie am weiblichen Genitale) nach subkutaner Injektion von Ovarial oder Placentarextrakt. *Arch. Gynaekol.*, **99**, 534
6. Stevens, V. C. and Crystle, C. D. (1973). Effect of immunisation with hapten-coupled hCG on the human menstrual cycle. *Am. J. Obstet.*, **42**, 485
7. Stevens, V. C. (1975). Antifertility effects from immunisation with intact, subunits and fragments of hCG. In Edwards, R. G. and Johnson, M. H. (eds.) *Physiological Effects of Immunity Against Reproductive Hormones*, pp. 249–274. (Cambridge: Cambridge University Press)
8. Heap, R. B., Flint, A. P. and Gadsby, J. E. (1979). Role of embryonic signals in the establishment of pregnancy. *Br. Med. Bull.*, **35**, 129
9. Knobil, E. (1973). On the regulation of the primate corpus luteum. *Biol. Reprod.*, **8**, 246
10. Hearn, J. P. (1978). The endocrinology of reproduction in the common marmoset, *Callithrix jacchus*. In Kleiman, D. G. (ed.) *Biology and Conservation of Marmosets*, pp 163–171. (Washington: Smithsonian Institution)
11. Meyer, R. K., Wolfe, R. and Arslan, M. (1968). Implantation and maintenance of pregnancy iin progesterone treated ovariectomised monkeys (*Macaca mulatta*). *Proc. 2nd Int. Cong. Primatology*, Vol. **2**, 30
12. Saxena, B. B., Hasan, S. H., Haour, F. and Schmidt-Gollwitzer, M. (1974). Radioreceptor assay of human chorionic gonadotropin: detection of early pregnancy. *Science, N.Y.*, **184**, 793

13. Fishel, S. B. and Surani, M. A. H. (1980). Evidence for the synthesis and release of a glycoprotein from mouse blastocysts. *J. Reprod. Fertil.*, **59**, 181

14. Landesman, R. and Saxena, B. B. (1976). Results of the first radioreceptor assays for the determination of human chorionic gonadotrophin. *Fertil. Steril.*, **27**, 357

15. Ortiz, M. E. and Croxatto, H. B. (1979). Observations on the transport, ageing and development of ova in the human genital tract. In Talwar, G. P. (ed.) *Recent Advances in Reproduction and Fertility Control*, pp. 307–318. (Amsterdam: Elsevier/North Holland)

16. Reyes, F. I., Winter, J. S. D., Faiman, C. and Hobson, W. C. (1975). Serial serum levels of gonadotrophins, prolactin and sex steroids in the non-pregnant and pregnant chimpanzee. *Endocrinology*, **96**, 1447

17. Hendrickx, A. G. and Enders, A. C. (1980). Implantation in non-human primates: 2. Endocrinology. In Anand Kumar, T. C. (ed.) *Non-human Primate Models for Study of Human Reproduction*, pp. 109–115. (Basle: Karger)

18. Atkinson, L. E., Hotchkiss, J., Fritz, G. R., Surve, A. H., Neill, H. D. and Knobil, E. (1975). Circulating levels of steroids and chorionic gonadotropin during pregnancy in the rhesus monkey, with special attention to the rescue of the corpus luteum in early pregnancy. *Biol. Reprod.*, **12**, 335

19. Hearn, J. P. (1980). The endocrinology and timing of implantation in the marmoset monkey, *Callithrix jacchus*. In Leroy, F. (ed.) *Ovum Implantation*. (Basle: Karger)

20. Wide, L. and Hobson, B. (1977). Chromatographic studies on a chorionic gonadotropic activity in the placenta of the rat, mouse and hamster. *Uppsala J. Med. Sci.*

21. Haour, F., Tell, G. and Sanchez, P. (1976). Mise en évidence et dosage d'une gonadotrophine chorionique chez le rat (rCG). *C. R. Acad. Sci. (D) Paris*, **282 (12)**, 1183

22. Madhwa Raj, H. G. (1976). Antigonadotrophins and the endocrine function of the ovary. In Edwards, R. G. and Johnson, M. H. (eds.) *Physiological Effects of Immunity against Reproductive Hormones*, pp. 187–204. (Cambridge: Cambridge University Press)

23. Gombe, S. and Else, J. (1980). New models for studies in human fertility from African mammals. In Serio, M. (ed.) *Animal Models in Human Reproduction*. (New York: Pergamon Press)

24. Braunstein, G. D., Rasor, J., Adler, D., Danzer, H. and Wade, M. E. (1976). Serum human chorionic gonadotropin levels throughout normal pregnancy. *Am. J. Obstet. Gynecol.*, **126**, 678

25. Jaffe, R. (1980). Fetal differentiation. In Serio, M. (ed.) *Animal Models in Human Reproduction*. (New York: Pergamon Press)

26. Borland, R., Loke, Y. and Wilson, D. (1975). Immunological privilege resulting from endocrine activity of the trophoblast *in vivo*. In Edwards, R. G., Howe, C. and Johnson, M. H. (eds.) *Immunology of the Trophoblast*, pp. 157–170. (Cambridge: Cambridge University Press)

27. Loke, Y. W., Brook, S. S. and Allen, G. E. (1977). Surface IgM on lymphocytes from pregnant women. *Am. J. Obstet. Gynecol.*, **127**, 847

28. Amoroso, E. C. and Perry, J. S. (1975). The existence during gestation of an immunological buffer zone at the interface between maternal and foetal tissues. *Phil. Trans. R. Soc. Lond. B.*, **271**, 343

29. Morisada, M., Yamaguchi, H. and Iizuka, R. (1976). Immunobiological function of the syncytiotrophoblast: a new theory. *Am. J. Obstet. Gynecol.*, **125**, 3

30. Muchmore, A. V. and Blaese, R. M. (1977). Immunoregulatory properties of fractions from human pregnancy urine: evidence that hCG is not responsible. *J. Immunol.*, **118**, 881

31. Batta, S. K. and Channing, C. P. (1979). Preimplantation of rhesus monkey blastocyst: secretion of substance capable of stimulating progesterone secretion by granulosa cell cultures. *Life Sci.*, **25**, 2057

32. Braunstein, G. D., Vaitukaitis, J. L., Carbone, P. P. and Ross, G. T. (1973). Ectopic production of hCG by neoplasms. *Ann. Intern. Med.*, **78**, 39

33. Vaitukaitis, J. L. (1977). Human chorionic gonadotropin. In Fuchs, F. and Hopper, A. (eds.) *Endocrinology of Pregnancy*, 2nd edn, pp. 63–75 (New York: Harper and Row)
34. Braunstein, G. D. (1979). hCG in non-trophoblastic tumours and tissues. In Talwar, G. P. (ed.) *Advances in Reproduction and Regulation of Fertility*, pp. 389–398. (Amsterdam: Elsevier/North Holland)
35. Ghosh, M. K. and Cox, R. P. (1976). Production of hCG in HeLa cell cultures. *Nature (London)*, **259**, 415
36. Rosen, S. W., Waintraub, B. D. and Aronson, S. (1978). Ectopic hCG production by malignant cell lines. *Clin. Res.*, **26**, 537A
37. Hearn, J. P. and Lunn, S. F. (1975). The reproductive biology of the marmoset monkey, *Callithrix jacchus*. In Perkins, F. J. and O'Donoghue, P. N. (eds.) *Breeding Primates for Developmental Biology. Laboratory Animal Handbooks*, **6**, 191
38. Hearn, J. P., Abbott, D. H., Chambers, P. C., Hodges, J. K. and Lunn, S. F. (1978). Use of the common marmoset, *Callithrix jacchus*, in reproductive research. *Primates Med.*, **10**, 40
39. Chambers, P. L. and Hearn, J. P. (1979). Peripheral plasma levels of progesterone, oestradiol-17β, oestrone, testosterone, androstenedione and chorionic gonadotrophin during pregnancy in the marmoset monkey, *Callithrix jacchus*. *J. Reprod. Fertil.*, **56**, 23
40. Abbott, D. H. and Hearn, J. P. (1978). Physical, hormonal and behavioural aspects of sexual development in the marmoset monkey, *Callithrix jacchus*. *J. Reprod. Fertil.*, **53**, 155
41. Hearn, J. P., Short, R. V. and Lunn, S. F. (1976). The effects of immunising marmoset monkeys against the β-subunit of hCG. In Edwards, R. G. and Johnson, M. F. (eds.) *Physiological Consequences of Immunity against Hormones*, pp. 229–247. (Cambridge: Cambridge University Press)
42. Hearn, J. P. (1976). Immunisation against pregnancy. *Proc. R. Soc. Lond. B.*, **195**, 149
43. Hearn, J. P. (1978). Immunological interference with the maternal recognition of pregnancy in primates. In *Maternal Recognition of Pregnancy*. (Ciba Foundation Symposium 64), pp. 353–376. (Amsterdam: Elsevier/North Holland)
44. Hearn, J. P. (1979). Long term suppression of fertility by immunisation with hCG-β subunit and its reversibility in female marmoset monkeys. In Talwar, G. P. (ed.) *Advances in Reproduction and Regulation of Fertility*, pp. 427–438. (Amsterdam: Elsevier/North Holland)
45. Talwar, G. P., Sharma, N. C., Dubey, S. K., Salahuddin, M., Das, S., Ramakrishnan, S., Kumar, S. and Hingorani, V. (1976). Isoimmunization against human chorionic gonadotropin with conjugates of processed β-subunit of the hormone and tetanus toxoid. *Proc. Natl. Acad. Sci. USA*, **73**, 218
46. Thanavala, Y. M., Hearn, J. P., Hay, F. C. and Hulme, M. (1979). Characterisation of the immunological response in marmoset monkeys immunised against hCGβ-subunit and its relationship with their subsequent fertility. *J. Reprod. Immunol.*, **1**, 263
47. Stevens, V. C. (1976). Perspectives of development of a fertility control vaccine from hormonal antigen of the trophoblast. In *Development of Vaccines for Fertility Regulation*, pp. 93–110. (Copenhagen: Scriptor)
48. Talwar, G. P., Ramakrishnan, S., Das, C., Dubey, S. K., Salahuddin, M., Shastri, N., Tandon, A. and Om Singh (1979). Anti-hCG immunisation. In Talwar, G. P. (ed.) *Recent Advances in Reproduction and Regulation of Fertility*, pp. 453–466. (Amsterdam: Elsevier/North Holland)
49. Hingorani, V. and Kumar, S. (1979). Anti-hCG immunisation – phase 1 clinical trials. In Talwar, G. P. (ed.) *Recent Advances in Reproduction and Regulation of Fertility*, pp. 467–471. (Amsterdam: Elsevier/North Holland)
50. Chen, H. C. and Hodgen, G. D. (1977). Primate chorionic gonadotrophins. Antigenic similarities to the unique carboxyl terminal peptide of hCG-β subunit. *J. Clin. Endocrinol. Metab.*, **43**, 1414
51. Hobson, B. and Wide, L. (1972). A comparison between chorionic gonadotrophins extracted from human, rhesus monkey and marmoset placentae. *J. Endocrinol.*, **55**, 363

52. Wass, M., McCann, K. and Bagshaw, K. D. (1978). Isolation of antibodies to hCG/LH from human sera. *Nature (London)*, **274**, 368

53. Pala, A., Donini, P. and Carenza, L. (1979). Characterisation of antibodies against hCG-β raised in rabbits and in humans. In Talwar, G. P. (ed.) *Advances in Reproduction and Regulation of Fertility*, pp. 439–452. (Amsterdam: Elsevier/North Holland)

54. Halban, J. (1905). Die innere secretion von Ovarium und Placenta und ihre Bedeutung fur die Function der milchdruse. *Arch. Gynaekol.*, **75**, 353

55. Canfield, R. E., Morgan, F. J., Kammerman, S., Bell, J. J. and Agosto, G. M. (1971). Studies of human gonadotrophin. *Rec. Prog. Horm. Res.*, **27**, 121

56. Pierce, J. G., Liao, T. H., Howard, S. M., Shome, B. and Cornell, J. S. (1971). Studies on the structure of thyrotrophin: its relationship to luteinising hormone. *Rec. Prog. Horm. Res.*, **27**, 165

Index

abortifacient, 239
abortion, 66, 235, 236
  delayed and HCG immunization, 212
acrosin, 110, 181
  antibodies, 113
acrosome
  antigens, 106, 110, 112
  enzymes, 110
  gamete recognition, 11
  staining, 125, 131
  zona binding, 175
ACTH; see adrenocorticotrophic hormone
actinomycin D, 127
Addinsonian adrenal disease, 134
adjuvants, 166, 167; see also Freund's
adrenocorticotrophic hormone (ACTH), 133
allantois, 7
allograft
  conceptus analogy, 33–40
  definition, 34
alloincompatibility, intracellular in
      invertebrates, 5
alopecia, 134
amenorrhoea, 134, 165
AMP, cyclic, 153, 154
anaemia
  autoimmune haemolytic, 51
  pernicious, 134
angiotensin II, 85
antibody; see also immunoglobulins
  anti-neutrophil, 54
  anti-sperm, 112, 113, 117, 120
    clinical significance and sex, 128–31
    detection, 122–7
    fertility correlation, 124
    and genital pathology, 131
    head, 125–31
    immunofluorescence, 124, 125
    WHO collaborative programme, 122
  blocking, 51, 52
  enhancing, 17
  haemagglutinating, 17
  HCG, 174–85, 217–24
    kinetics of response, 223, 224
    peptide, reaction, 207
  LHRH and reproductive function, 143–67

local, reproductive tract, 118, 119
  ovarian, 179
  production and steroids, 45
  smooth muscle, 113
antigenic disparity, mother–fetus, 21
antigens; see also HLA
  aspermatogenic, 106
  blood group, 36, 38, 89, 114
  conceptus, pre-implantation, 13, 14
  detection technique, 37
  fetal, 84
    expression of, 15
  histocompatibility; see HLA
  ova, 188–92
  ovarian, 188–94
  paternal, fetal expression, 53
  platelet, 54
  polymorphism in invertebrates, 5, 6
  pregnancy-associated, 69–72
  rhesus, 54
  semen, 111–15
  sperm, 105–11, 114
    – brain shared, 115
    differentiation, 114, 115
    t-locus, 114, 115
    TA1 and 2, 40
    teratoma F–9, 115
    transplantation, 115
    trophoblastic, 37
    zona, 173–97
antiluteolysin, 72
antilymphocyte serum, 44
antisera; see also antibodies
  conformational, 145
  sequential, 145
alpha_1-antitrypsin, 93
aortic hyperplasia, 85
arcuate nucleus lesions, 160, 162
aspermatogenesis, 108
ataxia telangiectasia, 134
atherosis in pre-eclampsia, 85, 95
auto-immunity, 50, 121–35
  reproductive tract, pathogenesis, 106,
    ˙119–21

baboons, 204–14, 222

bacteria, antigen modification, 113
blastocyst
    recovery of, 239
    surface immunogens, 13, 14
blood group system, 122
    incompatibilities, 49, 53
    and infertility, 113
blood transfusion, 47, 84
Bordetella pertussis, 146
bursa of Fabricius, 8

Callithrix jacchus, 65, 234
    HCG *beta*-subunit immunization, 233
Candida albicans, 45
    pregnancy infections, 46
candidiasis, mucocutaneous, 134
carbodi-imide, 144
carcinoma; *see also* tumours
    prostrate, 107
Cebus albifrons, 65
cell fusion, 12
cell-mediated immunity
    assessment to male antigens, 126
cerebral haemorrhage, 83
ceruloplasmin, 93
cervix, immunological activity, 117
chemotaxis, 11
alpha-chlorohydrin, 107
chorionic gonadotrophin (HCG), 153, 165
    alpha-subunit, 64, 219, 229, 230
    antibody-peptide specificity, 207–11
    antiserum, 208
    beta-subunit 64, 204, 205, 217–24, 229
        amino-acid sequence, 205, 217, 218
        antiserum, 204–13
        clinical trials, 222–4
        conjugation, 221, 229
        C-terminal antigen, 205, 217
        cross-reactivity, 204, 205, 208, 221, 229, 231
        detection in monkeys, 65
        in equidae, 67, 68
        immunization
            and breeding history, 236
            effects in marmosets, 233–9
            and fertility, 213, 214, 234, 235
            fetal fluid antibodies, 237, 238
            milk antibodies, 237, 238
            reversibility, 235
        clearance of IgG, 211
        ectopic synthesis, 224, 232, 233
        female tolerance, 203, 221
        hapten coupling, 203
        and immune response, 19, 41, 43
        immunization and gestation disruption, 204, 211, 212, 214
        immunobiology, 229–41
        in non-human primates, 64–7

peptide length and vaccine, 205, 206, 209
    specificity, 208, 209
    and uterine weights, 210
pregnancy diagnosis, 63
preimplantation detection, 66, 67
species range, 68
synthetic anti-pregnancy vaccines, 203–15, 220
chorionic membranes, 85
clotting system activation in pre-eclampsia, 83, 95
CMI; *see* immunity, cell-mediated
coitus, immune response after, 9
complement, 35, 53, 117, 128
    levels and menstrual cycle, 118
    in pre-eclampsia, 91–3
    in pre-eclamptic sera, 93
concanavalin A, 44
    zona receptors, 175
conceptus; *see also* fetus
    allograft analogy, 33–40
    antigenic immaturity, 13, 14
    immunization by, 47
    immunocompetence, development of, 20, 21
contraception
    HCG *beta*-subunit vaccination, 222
    HCG synthetic, 203, 214
    immunological, 108, 135, 173
    LHRH antagonists, 157
    LHRH inhibitors, 165
    zona antigens, 196, 197
corals, graft rejection, 6
corpus luteum, 4, 231
    maintenance of, 66, 72
    progesterone secretion, 72
    in reptiles, 7
corticosteroids, 19, 44, 132, 133
cortisone, 41, 44, 45
    levels in pregnancy, 44
Cowper's gland, 120
cumulus oophorus, 12, 174, 176
cytotoxicity, cell-mediated in annelids, 6
cytotrophoblast
    HLA antigens on, 39
    proliferation, 85

diabetes mellitus, 134
diagnosis of early pregnancy, 63–75
    accuracy, 73, 74
    false positives, 74
    sheep, 71
    substances used, 63
diazsulphanilic acid, 108
dithiothiestol, 112
DNA
    egg-induced synthesis, 12
    sperm, 125

early pregnancy factor, 41, 44, 75
   and E-rosettes, 44
   preimplantation diagnosis, 63, 64
   time of appearance, 69
ectoplacental cone, 15
embryonic mortality, 109
endocrine disorders and autoimmune disease,
   134
endometrium giant cells, 68
epididymis, 120, 121
Epiperipatus trinidadensis
   oviduct development, 4, 5
equine endometrial cups, 19

Fallopian tubes, 117
   fluid antibodies, 118
fertility
   after anti-sperm antibody test, 128, 129
   in rat and immunization type, 190
   regulation; *see* contraception
fertilization
   gamete recognition, 10–12
   sea urchin, 11
   vaccine inhibiting, 173
   zona immunization, 182
fertilizin, 11
alpha-fetoprotein
   effects on lymphocytes, 19
   levels in pregnancy, 42, 43
   pregnancy immunosuppression, 41–3
   in primates, 70
   and T-cell reactivity, 42, 43
fetuin, 19
fetus
   immune competence, 20
   and maternal HLA antibodies, 52, 53
   – mother relationship, 3–22
      antigenic disparity, 21
      barriers, 13, 18
      post-implantation separation, 14, 15
   tissue rejection, 14
fibrinoid barrier, 14, 15
flagellin, 206, 213
follicle stimulating hormone (FSH), 143, 221,
   230
   effect of LHRH antibody, 148–51, 157
   and ovariectomy, 158
follicular fluid and local immunity, 119
Freund's adjuvant, 106, 119, 144, 146, 166,
   203, 213
FSH; *see* follicle stimulating hormone

gelatin, 123
genes, Ir, 50
genital tract
   male autoimmunization, 119–21, 131
   occult lesions, 131, 132
   pathology, 131

gill placentation, 7
giraffe, 68
beta-globulin, 122
alpha$_1$-acid glycoprotein, 93
alpha$_2$-glycoprotein
   pregnancy-associated and
      immunosuppression, 41, 43, 44
   SPT, 70
beta$_1$-glycoprotein, 19
   pregnancy-specific, 41
glyoxylase, 35
gonadal dysgenesis, 45
Gorilla gorilla gorilla, 65, 67
grafts
   reaction in invertebrates, 6
   rejection and phylogeny, 9
   survival and hormones, 19
growth hormone, 221

haemagglutination inhibition assays, 64
   HCG, 65, 66
   PMSG, 67
   pregnancy-associated antigen in sheep, 70,
      71
haemolytic disease, 47
Hashimoto's thyroiditis, 134
HCG; *see* chorionic gonadotrophin
HeLa cells, 233
Hemimerus talpoides
   pseudoplacenta, 4
histocompatability loci
   fetal expression, 15
   and graft rejection, 36
   major, 35, 36; *see also* HLA
   minor, 36; *see also* blood group
   polymorphism in invertebrates, 5, 6
HLA antibodies and pre-eclampsia, 88
HLA antigens, 122; *see also* microglobulin
   A and B, proposed structure, 34
   antibody development, maternal, 52
   antigen sharing in pre-eclampsia, 87
   –A on sperm, 114, 115
   DR$_w$, 36, 88
      proposed structure, 35
   extracellular, 34
   homozygosity and pre-eclampsia, 88
   and infertility, 113
   linkage map, chromosome, 6, 35
   papain effects, 34, 35
   placental antibodies, 36
   pregnancy response in pre-eclampsia, 50
   sperm, 114, 115
   Y and sex determination, 115
HLH; *see* luteinizing hormone
hormones
   inhibition by immunization, 150
   protein in pregnancy, 19
   sex and meat production, 166

hormones (*continued*)
　steroid in pregnancy, 18, 19, 45, 72–4
　　and immune system, 45
　trophoblast produced, 18
hyaluronidase, 110, 176
　antibodies, 113
hydatidiform mole, 66, 85, 86
hydrops fetalis, 85, 86
hyperplacentosis, 86
hypertension
　chronic immune disorder, 94
　familial, 94
　lymphocyte transference of experimental, 94
　placental damage, 85
　pregnancy-induced; *see* pre-eclampsia
hypoparathyroidism, 134
hypothalamus, 143
hysterotomy, 235, 236

immune complex, 51, 86, 107
　complement fixing and pre-eclampsia, 92, 93
　and pre-eclampsia, 91, 95
　in pregnancy, 91
immune responses
　and hormones, 18, 19, 90
　invertebrate, 5, 6
　phylogeny of, 9
　post-coital, 9
　vertebrate, 8, 9
immunity, cell-mediated
　cytotoxicity, 46–8
　maternal, 46
immunization; *see also* HCG, Zona
　sperm antigens, response to 108, 109
　　and fertility, 108, 109
immunocompetence
　fetal, 20, 21
　in pregnancy of thymectomized mice, 21
immunofluorescence, 111–13, 124, 125, 180, 184, 185
immunogens, 13, 15, 16
　paternal, 17
immunoglobulins
　in agnatha, 6, 8, 9
　F_{ab} preparation, 125
　IgA, 9, 45, 118
　　cervical, 117, 125
　　F_c fragment stickiness, 127
　　follicular fluid concentration, 118, 119
　　secretory, composition, 117, 118
　　seminal plasma, 121
　IgD, 9
　IgE, 9
　IgG, 9, 123, 125, 127
　　antigen receptors, 9
　　cervical, 117

　　clearance in baboon, 211
　　complexes, 92, 93
　　depressed in pre-eclampsia, 91
　　follicular fluid concentration, 118, 119
　　G_1 and G_2, 20
　　HCG, peptide antibody, 209
　　immunosupressive, maternal, 90
　　at implantation, 20
　　placental transfer, 49
　　seminal plasma, 121
　　sperm immobilization, 131
　IgM, 9, 91, 123, 125, 209
　　cytotoxic in blastocyst, 20
　　sperm immobilization, 131
　　phylogeny, 8, 9
　placental transfer, 53
　pregnancy response to G_m, 46, 47
　transfer after gestation, 20
immunological privilege, 16
immunological relationships, mother–fetus, 33–55
immunosuppression, 36, 39, 117
　agents, 40–2
　antigen-specific, 48
　HCG, 232
　lymphocytes, 41, 69
　non-specific in pregnancy, 17–19, 40–9, 69
　therapy, 132, 133
implantation, 12, 13
　and anti-ovary antiserum, 183
　cell fusion, 12
　delayed, 14
　LHRH inhibition, 164
infertility
　immunological factors in, 105–35
　immunological investigations, 121–7
　immunological tests
　　cell-mediated immunity, 126
　　cervical mucus, 125, 126
　　complement dependent sperm immobilization, 123, 124, 129–31
　　gelatin agglutination, 123, 130
　　immunofluorescence, 124, 125, 129
　　post-coital test, 127
　　results and fertility, 129, 130
　　seminal plasma antibody, 126
　　sperm microagglutination, 122, 123, 129, 130
　　sperm-mucus contact test, 127
　　sperm-mucus penetration test, 127
　immunological, treatment of, 132, 133
　male, 130–2
　and sperm immunization, 108, 109
insemination, intra-uterine, 132, 133
invertebrates immune system, 5, 6
isolating mechanisms, 10

kidney

kidney (*continued*)
  function in pre-eclampsia, 83
  immune complex deposition, 91
  lesion in pre-eclampsia, 50, 51
  placental common antigens, 50, 86

lactic dehydrogenase-X
  isoantibodies in infertility, 113
  non-specific, 110
  sperm, 109, 110
lactoferrin, 113
lamina propria, 8, 9, 118
leukocytes in annelids, 6
Leydig cells, 155
  effect of LHRH immunization, 153, 154
  HCG bioassay, 219
  HCG stimulation, 154
LH; *see* luteinizing hormone
LHRH; *see* luteinizing hormone-releasing
    hormone
lupus erythematosus, disseminated, 92, 93
luteinizing hormone (LH)
  alpha-subunit, 230
  amino acid sequence, 205, 217, 218
  beta-subunit, 153, 205, 230
  effect of anti-LHRH antibody, 148–51
    and LHRH agonist, 163, 164
    and ovariectomy, 158, 159, 163
  /HCG bioassay, 66
  HCG cross-reaction, 173, 204, 205, 208,
    221
  oestrogen variable effects, 156, 157
  and pregnancy, 231
  and prostaglandins, 160
  surge, 157–60
    causes, 160
    and oestradiol benzoate, 159
luteinizing hormone-releasing hormone
    (LHRH)
  antibodies
    generation, 144–6
    and reproductive function, 143–67
    site of action, 147, 148
  antibody titre
    and hormone levels, 151
    progesterone in monkeys, 161
    and testicular biopsy, 152
  conjugation to carrier, 144, 145
  effects on
    FSH, 148, 149, 151, 157, 158, 160
    LH, 148–51, 158–60, 163, 164
    oestradiol, 162
    testosterone, 148–51, 153–5
  immunization
    and hormone levels, 148–64
    and LHRH agonist effects, 163, 164
    and ovulation induction, 161
  inhibition

implantation, 164
in vivo, 146–8
  in female, 156–65
  in male, 148–56
  and meat production, 166
  practical applications, 165–7
long-term inhibition, 160–4
octapeptide precursor, 167
and ovulatory cycle, 157, 158
receptors, 164
structure, 143, 144
lymph nodes, peripheral, 9
lymphocytes
  antigen recognition, 9
  B, 8, 9, 206
  breast milk, 20
  fetal cord blood, antigens, 53
  inhibitory factors, 41–5
  maternal, response in pregnancy, 17, 90
  peptide sensitization, 206
  placental transfer, 20
  suppressor in uterus, 17
  T, 9, 206
    and *alpha*-fetoprotein, 42, 43
    and rejection, 34
    suppressor, 41, 51

Macaca arctoides, 161
  M.mulatta, 65
  M.speciosa, 65
alpha$_2$-macroglobulin, 19
  pregnancy-associated, 70, 90
macrophage, 116, 119, 120
mare, pregnancy-associated antigen, 72
marmoset; *see Callithrix*
median eminence, 148
membrane
  egg and embryo protection, 7
menopause, premature, 134
menstrual cycle and mucus
    immunoglobulins, 118
MHC; *see* histocompatability, major
beta$_2$-microglobulin (HLA light chain), 34,
    37, 38
  antigens on sperm, 114
MIH; *see* histocompatability, minor
  milk
    progesterone in cows, 73
    transfer in, 20
miscarriage and pre-eclampsia, 84
mitogens, 42, 44
mixed lymphocyte reaction (MLR), 41–3, 90
monkeys
  gestation length, 65
  ovarian cycle, 65
morula, cell function, 12
mother
  –fetus relationships, 3–22, 33–55

antigenic, 87–9
specific suppression of responses, 16–19
mucus
antibodies in, 125, 126
cervical, 112, 117, 123
preparation of, 125, 126
sperm contact test, 127
sperm penetration, 127
mumps, 135
Mycobacterium butyricum, 167

neonatal purpura, 54
neuraminidase, 15, 19
neutropenia, 54

occlusion therapy, 133
oestradiol, 45
–17 *beta*, 157
levels and HCG antiserum, 211, 212
plasma levels and LHRH immunization, 162
oestradiol benzoate
effect on LH levels and ovariectomy, 159
oestriol, 90
oestrogens, 45, 90, 231
effects on LH, 156, 157
and graft survival, 18
oestrone levels and HCG antiserum, 211, 212
oestrone sulphate, 63
pregnancy test, 74, 75
Opsanus tau
embryo invasion, 16
oral contraceptives, 43, 45
orchidectomy, 107
orchitis
epididymo–, 131
experimental allergic, 106, 119
mumps, 120
ova
antibodies to cumulus-free, 189–91, 193
ovarian failure, autoimmune, 134, 135
ovariectomy, 18, 157, 159, 163
ovary
antibodies to, 179, 182, 188, 190, 192
antigen preparation, 188
gonadotrophin receptors, 134
oviduct, fluid antibodies, 118
oviparity, 3
ovomucoid, 19
ovulation and LHRH immunization, 161, 162

Pan troglodytes, 65, 67
Papio anubis, 65
Papio cynocephalus, 65
parathyroid allograft rejection, 16
peptides
HCG antisera action *in vivo*, 209–13

immunogenicity of synthetic HCG, 206, 207
specificity of HCG, 207–9
pergonal, 208
Peyer's patches, 8
phagocytosis, sperm, 116, 119, 120, 131
pheromones, 4
phospholipid, bovine sperm, 109
phytohaemagglutinin, 19, 42, 90
pituitary gland, 133
effects of LHRH immunization, 153
gonadotrophic histochemistry, 153
HCG activity, 66, 208
primitive in tunicates, 3, 4
placenta
allograft success, factors affecting, 22, 54
antigenic, 38, 85, 86
chorioallantoic types, 8
connective tissue, 86
eluate, immunosuppressive, 41
HLA antibody production, 38
hormones, 18
immunoadsorbant, 52, 53
immunosuppression, 17, 18
infarction, 85
ischaemia, 83, 85
mass and immunity, 21
and pre-eclampsia, 86
polysaccharide, 86
in pre-eclampsia, 50, 84–9
renal antigen cross-reaction, 86
uterine invasion, 8
vascular pathology in pre-eclampsia, 84, 85
yolk sac, first description, 6
placental lactogen; *see*
somatomammotrophin
placental transcortin, 41
placentation
invertebrate, 4, 5
marsupial, 8
phylogeny, 3–8
pseudo–, 4
teleost, 7
vertebrate, 6–8
platelet, 54
PMSG; *see* pregnant mares serum
gonadotrophin
poliomyelitis, 46
polyspermy, barriers to, 177, 178
Pongo pygmaeus, 65, 67
porifera graft reaction, 6
pre-eclampsia, 49–52, 83–95
and complement system, 91–3
fetal survival and HLA homozygosity, 88
and immune complexes, 91
immune function, maternal, 89
incidence, 83
and pregnancy number, 50, 84

Pre-eclampsia (*continued*)
  inheritance, 49, 50, 89
  placenta, 84–7
    bed-vessels in, 50
  proteinuric, 83
  and suppressor T-cell function, 51, 52
  symptoms, 49, 83
pregnancy
  –associated antigens
    domestic animals, 70–2
    non-human primates, 70
  corpus luteum in, 231
  diagnosis, immunological, 63–75
  disruption by anti-HCG serum, 181
  mother–fetus relationship and, 3–22
  non-specific immunosuppression, 17–19,
    40–9, 69
  rates and infertility, 128, 129
  stage and diagnosis, 63
  test, non-human primates, 65
    progesterone, 72–4
    accuracy, 73
pregnant mares' serum gonadotrophin
  (PMSG), 63, 67, 68, 75
  serum levels, 67
  subunits, 67
progesterone, 63, 64, 90, 122, 221, 231
  and anti-HCG serum, 211, 212
  immunosuppressant, 19, 41, 45
  levels in pregnancy, 45
  LHRH immunization, 161, 162
  in marsupials, 18
  and pregnancy diagnosis, 72–4
    accuracy, 73, 74
  in reptiles, 7
prolactin, 165, 221
prostaglandin E, 117
  and LH release, 160
prostrate, 120, 121, 165
  involution, 153
protamine, 125
proteins, pregnancy-associated, 19
Pygathrix nemaeus, 65, 67

radioimmunoassay, 64, 66
  HCG, 66, 207, 208
  LHRH, 145, 147
    sensitivity, 157
  oestrone sulphate, 75
  PMSG, 67
  progesterone, 72–4
radioreceptor assays, 67
Raji cell assay, 91
renin, uterine, 85
reverse transcripticase, 13
rhesus incompatability, 16
  pregnancy, response to, 46, 47
  severity, reasons for, 49

Ricinus communis, 175
RNA, maternal messenger, 13
rosette inhibition test. 41. 44. 69
Saimiri sciureus, 65
Salamandra atron
  cannibalism, 7
scaferrin, 113
semen
  antigenic spectrum, 111–15
  hypersensitivity, 110, 113
  isoimmunization in female, 115–19
  plasma
    antibodies, 126
    antigens, 110
    glycoprotein, 117
seromucoid, 93
Sertoli cells, 119
serum
  goat anti-human, 44
  pregnancy immunosuppressive, 41
sheep
  conceptus antisera raising, 71
  pregnancy-associated antigen, 70, 71
    purification, 71
  progesterone pregnancy test, 74
sialomucin, 38
Soay ram sex hormones
  effect of anti LHRH serum, 148, 149
somatomammotrophin (placental lactogen),
  41, 64, 90
  origin, 68
  time of detection, 68
species evolution, 10
spermatogenesis suppression, 133
spermatozoa; *see also* acrosome
  agglutination, 11, 111–13
    gelatin, 123
    head to head, 122, 123, 126
    micro–, 122, 123, 129
    tail to tail, 123, 126
  alloantigens, 114, 115
  autoantibody, head, 125, 131
  autoimmunization, 106–8
  behaviour and eggs, 10, 11
  capacitation, 119
    and zona binding, 174–6
  cell-mediated immunity, 107
  complement-dependent immobilization,
    111–13
  cytotoxicity to, 109, 119, 127
  entry in sea urchin, 11
  enzymes, 109, 110
  guinea-pig antigen spectrum, 106, 107
  histocompatability antigens, 9, 114, 115
  immobilization test, 123, 124
    and fertility, 129
  isoimmunization, 108–11
    contraceptive effects, 108, 109

spermatozoa (*continued*)
  midpiece and neck, 112
  non-motile in rabbit, 10
  post-nuclear cap, 112
  selection by female tract, 10
  smooth muscle antibodies, 113
  storage in bats, 10
  tail, 112, 125
  tail end-piece, 112, 125
  transplantation antigen sensitization, 115
  washing and insemination, 133
  zona binding, 179, 186–95
    assay, 186–93
spleen phylogeny, 9
staphylococcal protein A, 127
surinam toad, 7
syncitiotrophoblast, 38, 39
  coated vesicles, 53

testicular atrophy, 131
testicular infusion, hot water, 107
testicular trauma and orchitis, 119, 120
testis
  biopsy, 152
  HCG binding and LHRH immunization,
    156
  involution, 150, 153, 165
  LH/HCG receptors, 155
  weight and LHRH antibodies, 151
testosterone, 45, 66, 122, 133
  effect of anti-LHRH antibody, 148–51, 153
  HCG *beta*-subunit stimulated, 219
  HCG response, 153–5
tetanus toxoid, 206, 207, 213
  HCG linked, 173, 221
tetraploidy, human, 66
thrombocytopenia purpura, 134
thymus
  ontogeny, 21
  phylogeny, 8, 9
  replacement, 134
thyroid stimulating hormone (TSH), 221
  alpha-subunit, 230
  beta-subunit, 220
thyrotoxicosis, 134
transplantation reactions
  kidney, 36
    immune injury, 85
  recognition molecules, 12
triploidy, 85
trophoblast, 8, 47, 54, 74, 230
  differentiation, 12
  disease, 232, 233
  HLA antigens, 36, 37, 86
  immunogenicity, 13, 15
  microvilli, 39
  protection by blocking antibody, 51, 52
  villus, antigens on, 38, 39

xenoantigens, 39
trophoblastin, 72
trypsin, 204
tumours, 165
  HCG-secreting, 224, 233, 234
  placental, 66
  trophoblastic, 36, 38, 47, 232
Turner's syndrome, 134

urine
  post-menopausal, 208
  pregnancy test, 66
uterus, 85
  immunological privilege, 16
  response to spermatozoa, 9, 10
  weight and HCG antiserum, 210

vaccine, 184
  anti-pregnancy and synthetic HCG,
    203–15
  HCG *beta*-subunit, 217–24
    clinical trials, 222–4
  HCG peptide selection, 205, 206
  LHRH, 167
  spermatozoal, 109
vagina, immunological inactivity, 117
vaginal infections, 116
vasculitis, 93
vasectomy, 107
  immunological concomitants, 120, 121, 125
  patchy orchitis, 120
  reversal, persistent antibodies, 121
virus disease
  oncornavirus, 90
  in pregnancy, 46
  response, 90
vitelline membranes, 7
vitiligo, 134
viviparity, 3
  and altitude, 7
  in invertebrates, 4

Wampole UCG test, 71

yolk test, 7, 8

zebra, 68
zona pellucida, 7, 11, 14
  active immunization, 183–96
  antibodies to, 135, 179
    and conception in rat, 194–6
    and fertilization, 179
    titre and sperm binding, 187–96
  blastocyst protection, 14
  -free eggs, hamster, 11
  function, 175–9
    post-fertilization, 178

zona pellucida, function (*continued*)
    and trypsin, 178
  immunization against, 173–97
  immunoprecipitation and sperm binding,
    180, 181, 184, 185
    cross-reactivity, 183, 184
    in vitro activity, 179–82

    in vivo activity, 182–96
    passive immunization, 182–183
  spermatozoa binding, 174–81, 186–96
    assay, 186–93
  spermatozoa receptors, 11, 179, 184
  structure, 174, 175
zona reaction, 177

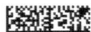